Nutrition, Weight Control, and Exercise

Nutrition, Weight Control, and Exercise

FRANK I. KATCH
Professor and Chairman
Department of Exercise Science
University of Massachusetts
Amherst, Massachusetts

WILLIAM D. McARDLE
Professor
Department of Health and Physical Education
Queens College
City University of New York
Flushing, New York

THIRD EDITION

LEA & FEBIGER • PHILADELPHIA
1988

Lea & Febiger
600 South Washington Square
Philadelphia, Pa. 19106 U.S.A.
(215)922-1330

About the Authors

Drs. Katch and McArdle are actively engaged in experimental research in the exercise sciences. Having published over 150 articles in national and international scientific journals, and presented their research at over 225 scientific meetings and conferences, they are also the authors or co-authors of 7 books. The recipients of numerous research grants from government and private industry, both doctors serve as reviewers and associate editors of various professional journals. Professors Katch and McArdle are elected Fellows of the Research Council of the American Association of Heath, Physical Education, Recreation, and Dance, and the American College of Sports Medicine. They serve on the Scientific Advisory Boards for numerous companies in the health and fitness field. They also contribute articles to and are consultants for popular magazines such as Vogue, Harper's Bazaar, Mademoiselle, Self, Shape, Muscle and Fitness, and Weight Watchers.

Library of Congress Cataloging-in-Publication Data

Katch, Frank I.
Nutrition, weight control, and exercise.

Bibliography: p.
Includes index.
1. Nutrition. 2. Reducing. 3. Exercise—Physiological aspects. 4. Food—Caloric content.
I. McArdle, William D. II. Title. [DNLM:
1. Exertion. 2. Nutrition. 3. Obesity—prevention & control. QT 255 K186n]
RA784.K32 1988 613.7 87-2785
ISBN 0-8121-1114-1

Printed in the United States of America

Print Number: 5 4 3 2 1

We dedicate this book to our parents, Roma Katch, and Claire and Harry McArdle, our wives Kerry and Kathy, and our children David, Kevin, and Ellen, and Kevin, Amy, Theresa, and Jennifer.

Preface

SINCE THE publication, in 1983, of the second edition of *Nutrition, Weight Control, and Exercise,* the importance of total fitness to human well-being has become firmly established. Courses such as aerobic conditioning, circuit training, jazzercize, figure control, and aerobic dancing are flourishing in the universities, public schools, health clubs, and Y's in this country and abroad. Private industry has also instituted many of the aspects of complete fitness programs, and more small and large corporations now provide full-fledged facilities for their employees (including families). Furthermore, programs that focus on weight loss for both children and adults are recognizing the unique interrelationships between food restriction, psychologic and behavioral support, and regular exercise for long term success.

Although opportunities for participation in vigorous physical activities had long been available to men, the involvement of women in such fitness-oriented programs was relatively new. In the past, activity for women was generally relegated to the figure salon and health spa where a woman could be passively exercised by machines and patronized by gadgetry. But this is clearly no longer the case. Opportunities to engage in vigorous exercise for women and men are now commonplace—and research shows that the training process and physiologic adaptation for both sexes are essentially the same. We have indeed come a long way, and we are very much encouraged by the public's response, enthusiasm, and desire for knowledge regarding the importance of regular, vigorous exercise in one's daily life. What is still amazing, however, is the proliferation of misinformation by self-serving zealots and charlatans who make unwarranted and false claims about nutrition and diet, weight control, and physical conditioning. We believe that providing sound, scientifically based information as to both the "why" and "how" of the multi-dimensional aspects of fitness can help stem the tide of "hucksterism" that exploits the admirable goal of good health and fitness. It is our hope that with the appropriate information more people will become intelligent and sophisticated consumers in the fitness marketplace, and not simply believe everything put forth about yet another "miracle plan" sure to solve their problem.

In the third edition of *Nutrition, Weight Control, and Exercise,* we have attempted to incorporate up-to-date and relevant information in each of the chapters. The book has been somewhat reorganized to provide for easier reading. The appendices of the caloric cost of physical activities and the energy value of foods have been updated, including an expansion of the nutritive value of foods at 14 "fast-food" restaurants. Considerable new information has been added about carbohydrate feeding and exercise performance, osteoporosis, cholesterol, dietary fiber, iron requirement and exercise, fluid replacement, exercising during pregnancy, spot reduction, muscular strength, body composition, aerobic and anaerobic training, and cardiovascular health. As with the second edition, no attempt was made to be all inclusive or to cover the numerous related topic areas as done in exercise physiology textbooks. We feel the content is appropriate for nutrition, weight control, exercise, and physical fitness courses at the university level, for the various exercise programs for men and women offered at health spas and clubs, as well as the professional preparation of exercise specialists in physical education, exercise science, and the health-related disciplines.

The book is divided into three main parts with chapter sub-divisions. Part One discusses nutrients in food, optimum nutrition for exercise and sport, energy and oxygen delivery systems for exercise, and energy value of food and physical activity. Part Two deals with the evaluation of body composition, obesity, weight control through exercise and diet, and the modification of eating and exercise behaviors. Part Three considers training for muscular strength and conditioning for anaerobic and aerobic power, as well as aging, exercise, and cardiovascular health. The appendices contain the energy expenditure for a wide variety of physical activities, the evaluation of body composition, the nutritive value of commonly used foods, and basic free weight resistance exercises for the trunk, and upper and lower extremities.

As with the second edition, we have based our factual information on the research findings of many of our colleagues in physical education and exercise science, applied physiology, medicine, and nutrition. We have also included data from recent experiments in our laboratories in Massachusetts and New York. We are particularly grateful to Dr. Albert Behnke for his helpful suggestions with Chapter 5, and to the numerous people throughout the country who provided constructive suggestions and helpful hints about the overall presentation of material. A special thanks goes to Debbie Southworth who toiled skillfully with her computer and hard disc in typing the manuscript, to J. Hirsch, E. A. Simms, and George and Revea Orsten for providing original photographs, and Fitness Technologies, Inc., Ann Arbor, for making arrangements to process the questionnaires for the computer dietary and exercise plan in Appendix A.

Amherst, Massachusetts FRANK I. KATCH

Flushing, New York WILLIAM D. MCARDLE

Contents

PART I. *Nutrition and Energy For Exercise* 1

1. Nutrients in Food 3
2. Optimal Nutrition for Exercise and Sport 39
3. Energy Systems for Exercise 53
4. Energy Value of Food and Physical Activity 93

PART II. *Body Composition and Weight Control* 113

5. Evaluation of Body Composition 115
6. Obesity 137
7. Weight Control 155
8. Modification of Eating and Exercise Behaviors 179

PART III. *Physiologic Conditioning for Total Fitness* 193

9. Conditioning for Muscular Strength 197
10. Conditioning for Anaerobic and Aerobic Power 217
11. Aging, Exercise, and Cardiovascular Health 239

General Readings (All Chapters) 259

Appendix A Computerized Meal and Exercise Plan 261

Appendix B Energy Expenditure in Household, Recreational, and Sport Activities (in kcal per min) 268

Appendix C Evaluation of Body Composition 278

Appendix D Nutritive Value of Commonly Used Foods 290

Appendix E Basic Free Weight Resistance Exercises for the Neck, Arms, Shoulders, Chest, Abdomen, Back, Buttocks, and Legs 328

INDEX 333

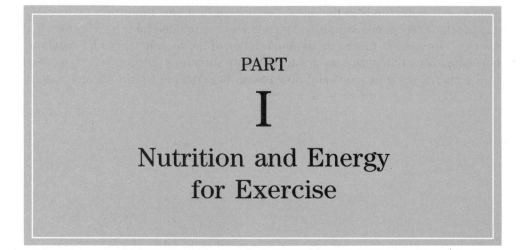

PART I
Nutrition and Energy for Exercise

THE NUTRIENTS CONSUMED in the daily diet provide the energy necessary to maintain bodily functions both at rest and during various forms of physical activity. Although the raw fuel for biologic work takes the form of carbohydrates, fats, and proteins, the efficient extraction and utilization of energy from these foods requires a delicate blending of other nutrients in the finely regulated watery medium of the cell. The different vitamins and minerals play important and highly specific roles in activating and facilitating energy transfer throughout the body. Fortunately, minute yet crucial quantities of these substances are readily obtained in the foods consumed in well-balanced meals. With proper nutrition, the need to consume vitamin or mineral supplements is both physiologically and economically wasteful.

In the transition from rest to more vigorous physical activity, the energy for muscular contraction is provided in several ways. Certain biochemical reactions can generate considerable energy quite rapidly for short periods of time without consuming oxygen. In sprint activities or all-out bursts of exercise, the body's capacity for this form of rapid energy production is critical in maintaining a high standard of performance. On the other hand, in performing exercise lasting longer than 2 minutes, energy must be extracted from food through reactions that do require oxygen. To be effective, the physiologic conditioning process necessitates a basic understanding of how energy is supplied as well as the energy requirements of a particular activity. This understanding is fundamental in formulating an effective yet prudent program of weight control.

This section presents a broad overview of nutrition and energy transfer. Each group of nutrients is discussed in terms of its general structure, function, and source in specific foods in the diet. The concept of optimal nutrition is explored, and practical recommendations and guidelines are provided for the active man and woman. Emphasis is placed on the importance of the food nutrients in sustaining physiologic function during moderate and more strenuous physical activity, as well as the energy value of foods and how energy is extracted from food and used to power various forms of physical activity.

1
Nutrients in Food

SIX CATEGORIES of nutrients compose the foods we eat: carbohydrates, fats, proteins, vitamins, minerals, and water. The nutrients are the basic substances the body uses for a variety of vital processes. These can be broadly classified as follows: (1) maintenance and repair of body tissues, (2) regulation of the thousands of complex chemical reactions that occur in cells, (3) provision of energy for muscle contraction, (4) conduction of nerve impulses, (5) secretion by glands, (6) synthesis of the various compounds that become part of the body's structures, (7) growth, and (8) reproduction. The sum of these processes in which the energy and nutrients from foods are made available to and utilized by the body is referred to as *metabolism.* A general understanding of the role of the nutrients in metabolism is important because proper nutrition not only affects the normal functioning of the body at rest, but also contributes to its efficient operation during the stress of physical activity.

Chemical Differences Between the Nutrients All the nutrients except water and minerals contain the element carbon. In fact, compounds containing carbon compose almost all the biologic substances within the body. Some of these compounds have relatively few carbon atoms while others contain hundreds or even thousands of carbon atoms joined together. A unique characteristic of a carbon atom is that it has four places to which other elements can be attached. These other elements are held in place by forces of attraction called *chemical bonds.* These bonds can be thought of as the chemical cement that helps to keep the atoms and molecules in a substance from coming apart readily.

Atoms of hydrogen and oxygen, in addition to carbon, also form the basic structural units for most of the biologically active substances within the body. Carbon, hydrogen, and oxygen atoms, organized in a specific way, form carbohydrates. Other combinations of the same elements make fats, while carbon, hydrogen, and oxygen, with the addition of nitrogen and other mineral substances, bind together to form proteins. These four elements—carbon, hydrogen, oxygen, and nitrogen—are the *organic* building blocks from which the nutrients are made.

Each nutrient can be distinguished by the type of bonding within the nutrient substance, and the size and complexity of the basic molecule.

In the sections that follow we will take a closer look at the six nutrients and attempt to answer the following questions: What are they? Where do they come from? What are their functions? In what foods are they found?

Carbohydrates

WHAT ARE CARBOHYDRATES?

Carbohydrates are compounds made up of atoms or carbon, hydrogen, and oxygen. A carbohydrate always contains, in addition to carbon, two atoms of hydrogen for each oxygen atom. The arrangement of the atoms of the simple carbohydrate molecule glucose is illustrated in Figure 1-1.

Glucose, also called dextrose or blood sugar, is composed of a chain of 6 carbon atoms to which 6 oxygen and 12 hydrogen atoms are attached. The chemical formula that describes this molecule in terms of its different atoms is $C_6 H_{12} O_6$. Glucose can be used in one of three ways: (1) directly by the cell for energy, (2) stored as glycogen in the muscles and liver, or (3) converted to fats for energy storage. Two other commonly known carbohydrates have the same chemical formula as glucose. One is fructose, or fruit sugar, the sweetest of the simple sugars, and is present in large amounts in fruits and honey; the other is galactose, produced in the mammary glands of lactating animals. Collectively these three sugars are known as *monosaccharides* because each molecule contains only one 6-carbon sugar group. The basic differences among the monosaccharides are the specific arrangements of the atoms within the molecules. The body easily converts both fructose and galactose to glucose for energy metabolism.

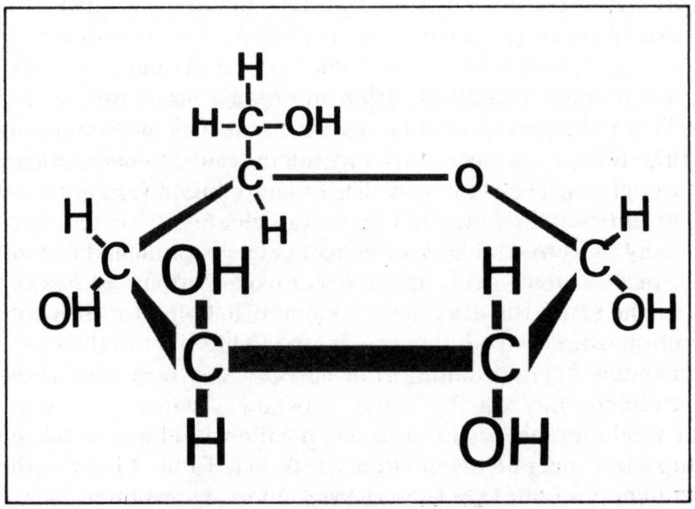
H
H-C-OH
C
O
H
H
H
C
OH
H
C
OH
OH
C
C
H
OH

Figure 1-1. *Three dimensional structure of the simple sugar molecule glucose. The molecule resembles a hexagonal plate to which the H and O atoms are attached.*

The joining of two simple sugar molecules forms a double sugar or *disaccharide;* sucrose, maltose, and lactose are examples. Sucrose (common table sugar) is formed from glucose and fructose, and is found mainly in sugar cane or sugar beet. In 1890, Americans consumed about 4 pounds of sugar a year, while they now average more than 130 pounds. This amounts to 30 teaspoons per day or about 50% of the total carbohydrate consumed in the United States! The mono- and disaccharides collectively make up what is commonly referred to as the simple sugars. These sugars are packaged under a variety of guises—brown sugar, corn syrup, invert sugar, corn sugar, fructose, dextrose, honey, and "natural sweeteners." Interestingly, honey contains the same two monosaccharides that make up table sugar. While sweeter, it is no more superior nutritionally or as an energy source. Excessive amounts of any simple sugar will draw fluid from the body into the intestinal tract and reduce fluid uptake, and may bring about a hormonal response that can actually cause a drop in blood sugar. Maltose is composed of two glucose molecules, while the disaccharide lactose is found in milk and breaks down during digestion into glucose and galactose.

The term *polysaccharide* is used when three or more sugar molecules combine. The most common polysaccharides are starch, cellulose, and glycogen. Three hundred to thousands of individual sugar molecules may join together in a starch molecule. Starch is found in corn and in various grains from which bread, cereal, spaghetti, and pastries are made. Large amounts are also present in beans, peas, and potatoes.

Cellulose and most other fibrous materials that are resistant to human digestive enzymes are another form of plant polysaccharide. They make up the fibrous or structural part of plants and are present in leaves, stems, roots, seeds, and fruit coverings; they are also found as mucilage and gums within the plant cell.

Although technically not a nutrient, dietary fiber has received considerable attention by researchers and the lay press. Because the Western diet is high in fiber-free animal foods and loses much of its natural fiber through processing, it is speculated that this accounts for the prevalence of intestinal disorders in this country, compared to countries that consume a more primitive-type diet high in unrefined, complex carbohydrates. For example, the typical American diet contains a daily fiber intake of 20 grams (g), whereas diets from Africa and India range between 40 and 150 g per day. Fibers hold considerable water and thus give "bulk" to the food residues in the small intestines, often increasing stool weight and volume by 40 to 100%. This bulking action aids in gastrointestinal functioning by shortening the transit time for the passage of food residues (and possibly cancer-producing materials) through the digestive tract. This may reduce the chances of contracting various gastrointestinal diseases later in life.

Fiber intake, especially the water soluble fibers such as pectin and guar gum present in oats, beans, peas, carrots and fruits, also lowers blood cholesterol. These fibers may depress the synthesis of cholesterol in the gut, while at the same time, facilitate the excretion of existing cholesterol bound to the fiber in the feces. In contrast, the water-insoluble fibers, such as cellulose found in wheat bran, show no cholesterol-lowering effect.

Present nutritional wisdom maintains that a dietary fiber intake of about 30 grams per day is an important part of a well-structured diet. Table 1-1 gives the fiber content of some common foods. As is the case with most nutrients, an excessive fiber intake may be counterproductive because increased dietary fiber can decrease the absorption of the minerals calcium, iron, magnesium, and phosphorus.

Table 1-1. *Fiber content of some common foods listed in order of overall fiber content*

FOODS	SERVING SIZE	TOTAL FIBER G	SOLUBLE FIBER G	INSOLUBLE FIBER G
100% Bran cereal	½ cup	10.0	0.3	9.7
Peas	½ cup	5.2	2.0	3.2
Kidney beans	½ cup	4.5	0.5	4.0
Apple	1 small	3.9	2.3	1.6
Potato	1 small	3.8	2.2	1.6
Broccoli	½ cup	2.5	1.1	1.4
Strawberries	¾ cup	2.4	0.9	1.5
Oats, whole	½ cup	1.6	0.5	1.1
Banana	1 small	1.3	0.6	0.7
Spaghetti	½ cup	1.0	0.2	0.8
Lettuce	½ cup	0.5	0.2	0.3
White rice	½ cup	0.5	0	0.5

Glycogen, or animal starch, is also a very large molecule. It can range in size from a few hundred to ten thousand or more glucose molecules linked together. Glycogen is not present to any large extent in the foods we eat. Instead, when glucose enters the muscles and liver, it is trapped and stored for later use as glycogen. Approximately 375 to 475 g of glycogen (about three-fourths to one pound) are stored mainly in the muscles and liver. The process of transforming glucose to glycogen in the liver is known as *glycogenesis.* When glucose is needed as an energy source, the glycogen in the liver is reconverted to glucose and transported in the blood for use by the working muscles. The term *glycogenolysis* is used to describe this reconversion process.

When glycogen is depleted via dietary restriction or exercise, glucose synthesis from the structural components of the other nutrients, especially proteins, tends to increase. This process is termed *gluconeogenesis.* For this reason, adequate carbohydrate intake should be maintained, especially for active people or those on a low calorie,* weight-loss diet. Starvation diets and diets with reduced carbohydrate intake result not only in depletion of glycogen reserves, but also in a possible protein deficiency and an accompanying loss of lean (muscle) tissue. The hormone *insulin* plays an important part in the regulation of liver and muscle glycogen stores by controlling the level of circulating blood sugar.

WHERE DO CARBOHYDRATES COME FROM?

The diagram in Figure 1-2 illustrates the general process of *photosynthesis,* by which carbohydrates are manufactured in green plants. The roots of plants and trees take up water in the soil. Carbon dioxide in the air comes into contact with

*A calorie is a unit of heat to express the energy value of food.

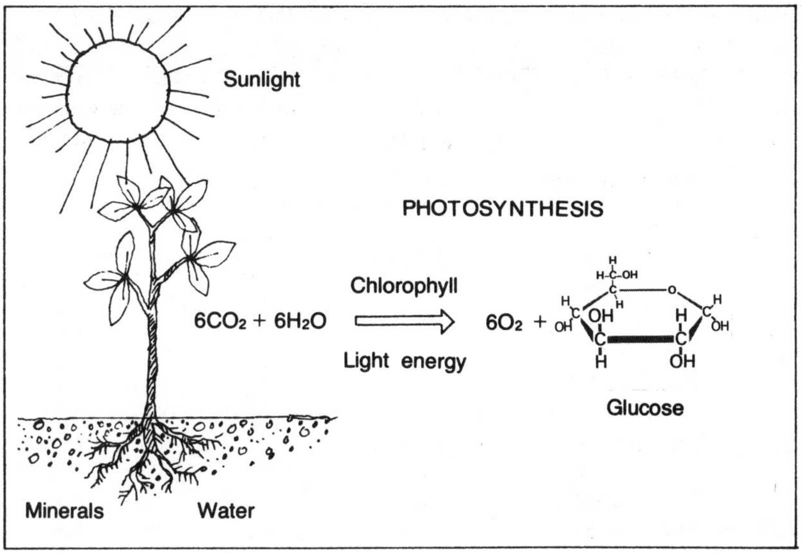
Sunlight
PHOTOSYNTHESIS
Chlorophyll
6CO2 + 6H2O
6O2 +
Light energy
Glucose
Minerals
Water

Figure 1-2. *The process of photosynthesis to make sugars from CO_2, H_2O, sunlight and chlorophyll.*

the leaves, while the solar energy from visible sunlight is absorbed by the leaves' green pigment, *chlorophyll.* The interaction of carbon dioxide in the atmosphere, water, sunlight, and chlorophyll provides the necessary ingredients for the synthesis of the carbohydrate molecule. When a carbohydrate molecule is formed, oxygen is released into the atmosphere to be used by animals in the life-sustaining process of energy metabolism.

FUNCTIONS OF CARBOHYDRATES

The major function of carbohydrates is to provide a continuous energy supply to the trillions of cells within the body. The carbohydrates in food, whether in the form of a disaccharide like table sugar or a more complex polysaccharide like starch in potatoes or rice, must eventually break down in digestion into simple 6-carbon sugar molecules before the bloodstream can absorb them from the intestines. Sugar is then transported in the blood to individual cells throughout the body. In the cell the bonds of the glucose molecule are broken through specific chemical reactions. As a result energy is provided to power the cell's vital functions. If the amount of glucose is inadequate to meet the cell's energy needs, the reserve glucose stored as glycogen is recruited as an energy source. The level of sugar in the blood is elevated immediately following a meal, however, and increases the transport of glucose into the cell. This excess sugar is then converted to glycogen and stored for later use. Once the capacity of the cell for glycogen storage is reached, the excess sugars are readily converted into fat and stored in the adipose (fat) tissue beneath the skin. This helps to explain how the body's fat content can increase when a person consumes excess calories, even though the diet is high in carbohydrates.

Adequate carbohydrate intake also serves to limit the use of body protein as an energy source: this spares this important nutrient for its vital role in maintenance, repair, and tissue synthesis. Aside from this role as a "protein sparer," carbohydrate serves two other functions; first, it facilitates the complete breakdown of fat in the body's energy releasing processes; second, it provides a continuous fuel supply for the proper functioning of the central nervous system. The symptoms of lowered blood glucose (called hypoglycemia) include feelings of weakness, hunger, and dizziness. This condition impairs exercise performance and may partially explain the fatigue associated with prolonged exercise.

Because comparatively little glycogen is stored in the body, it is important that adequate amounts of carbohydrate be consumed routinely. The quantity of liver and muscle glycogen can be modified considerably through the diet. For example, a 24-hour fast results in a large reduction in liver and muscle glycogen reserves. On the other hand, maintaining a carbohydrate-rich diet for several days enhances the body's carbohydrate stores to a level almost twice that obtained with a normal, well-balanced diet. The effect of enhanced carbohydrate storage on exercise performance is discussed in the next chapter.

CARBOHYDRATES IN FOODS

Approximately 50% of the calories consumed in the typical American diet consists of carbohydrates. Interestingly, the percentage of starch consumed has decreased by about 30% since the turn of the century, while the consumption of sugars has correspondingly increased from 31% to over 50% during the same pe-

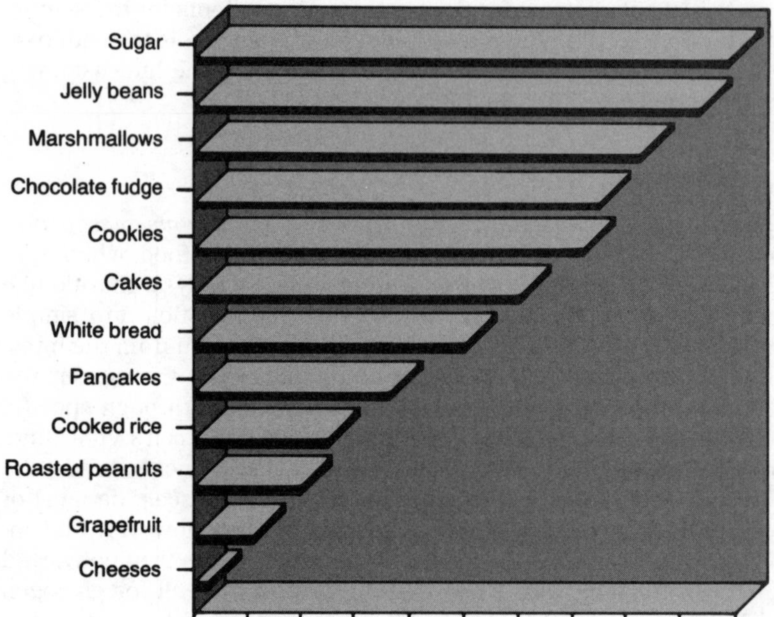
Sugar
Jelly beans
Marshmallows
Chocolate fudge
Cookies
Cakes
White bread
Pancakes
Cooked rice
Roasted peanuts
Grapefruit
Cheeses
0
10
20
30
40
50
60
70
80
90
100
Percent

Figure 1-3. *Percentage of carbohydrates in common foods as served. (Adapted from Handbook No. 8: Composition of Foods, United States Department of Agriculture, D.C., 1963.)*

riod. Some clinical nutritionists have suggested that this change in carbohydrate sources is associated with the increasing prevalence of dental caries, adult diabetes, and coronary heart disease.

Figure 1-3 graphically displays the percentage of carbohydrates in some common foods. As can be seen, cookies, candies, cakes, and white bread consist predominantly of carbohydrates. Because the values in Figure 1-3 are based on carbohydrate percentage in relation to total food weight, including water content, fruits and vegetables appear to be less valuable carbohydrate sources. However, the dried portion of these foods is almost pure carbohydrates.

WHAT IS A FAT?

A molecule of fat, like a carbohydrate molecule, is composed of carbon, oxygen, and hydrogen atoms linked together in a specific and unique way. Essentially, a fat consists of two different clusters of atoms. One cluster, *glycerol*, is the basic building block, and is composed of 3 atoms of carbon combined with 3 hydroxyl (OH) groups. The second cluster, known as a *fatty acid*, is attached to glycerol. The most common fatty acids contain between 16 and 18 atoms of carbon in each molecule. When glycerol and fatty acid molecules are joined chemically, they produce a molecule of "neutral fat" or *triglyceride*. The triglyceride represents the most plentiful fat in the body as more than 95% of body fat is of this form.

There are two types of fatty acids, saturated and unsaturated. Figure 1-4 illustrates the general differences in bonding and arrangement of hydrogens in saturated and unsaturated fatty acids. For simplification, the symbol R represents the rest of the molecule. For saturated fatty acids, only single bonds link the carbon atoms; therefore, at least two hydrogen atoms can attach to each of the carbon atoms of the main chain. The interconnected chain of carbon atoms holds as many hydrogens as is chemically possible. The molecule is said to be *saturated* with hydrogen atoms and is called a saturated fatty acid such as the predominant fatty

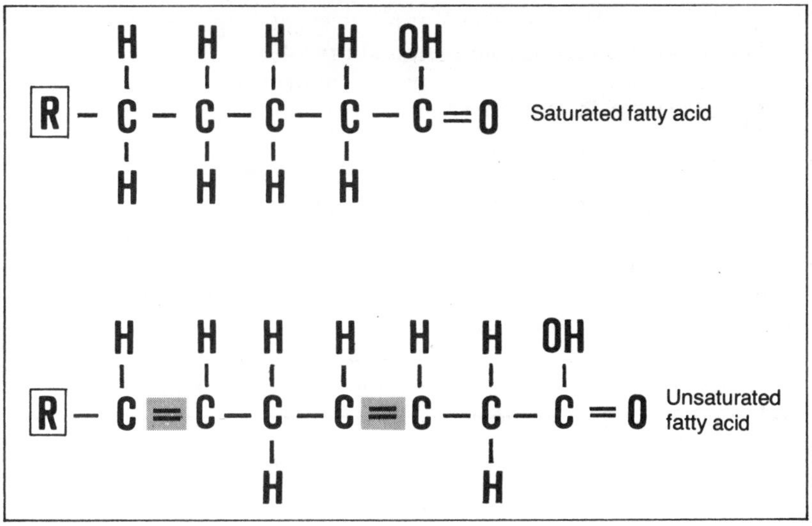
Saturated fatty acid
Unsaturated fatty acid

Figure 1-4. *The major structural difference between saturated and unsaturated fatty acids is the presence or absence of double bonds between the carbon atoms.*

acids in butter. In contrast, a fatty acid is *unsaturated* if it contains one or more double bonds along the main carbon chain. Each double bond in the chain takes the place of two hydrogen atoms. If the fatty acid has only one such double bond, it is *monounsaturated* as in olive or peanut oil. If it has two or more double bonds, the molecule is *polyunsaturated* as in corn or safflower oil. Fats from the plant kingdom are generally unsaturated. Regardless of the degree of saturation, all fats have essentially the same number of calories.

Saturated fat intake has steadily increased in the American diet to the point where the average person now consumes about 15% of total calories or over 50 pounds of saturated fat per year, most of which is animal in origin. This is in contrast to groups like the Tarahumara Indians of Mexico whose high complex unrefined carbohydrate diet contains only 2% of the total calories as saturated fat. Coincident with an increased consumption of saturated fats has been an increase in coronary heart disease. This relationship has led many nutritionists and medical personnel to suggest replacing at least a portion of the saturated fat in one's diet with fats that are mono- and polyunsaturated such as fats derived from vegetable sources (e.g., olive oil and corn oil) or the polyunsaturated oils of fish. Concern has been also expressed concerning the association of high-fat diets (both saturated and unsaturated) with breast and colon cancer, as well as the possibility that such high fat diets promote the growth of other cancers.

Aside from the triglycerides, several other fats are present in the body. One such group, the *phospholipids*, combines fat, phosphorous, and nitrogen compounds. These fats form in all cells. In addition to helping maintain the structural integrity of the cell, phospholipids are important in blood clotting. Other compound fats are the *glucolipids*, fatty acids bound with carbohydrate and nitrogen, and the *lipoproteins*, formed primarily in the liver from the union of either triglycerides, phospholipids, or cholesterol with protein.

Another perhaps more widely known fatty-like substance is *cholesterol*, present in all cells, and is either consumed in foods *(exogenous cholesterol)* or synthesized within the body *(endogenous cholesterol)*. Cholesterol is not contained in vegetable food sources and is negligible in egg whites and skimmed milk. Cholesterol is an important nutrient that is normally required in many of the complex functions of the body. It is utilized in the manufacture of bile (for digestion and absorption of fats) as well as the hormones estrogen, androgen, and progesterone, that are responsible for the development of male and female secondary sex characteristics.

Because cholesterol and triglycerides have been implicated as a possible associative factor in the development of heart disease, many people have attempted to reduce or eliminate these fats from their diets. Although the diet-heart disease controversy still rages, recent research indicates that lowering blood cholesterol has a direct and significant effect on reducing the incidence of heart attacks, and if an attack occurs, the chances for survival are improved. In fact, studies show that the improvement in one's heart disease risk is closely related to the decrease in cholesterol by the factor of 1:2—i.e., a 1% reduction in cholesterol caused a 2% reduction in risk! Such findings are encouraging because they provide an important "missing link" in the diet-heart theory and strongly support the efforts of health professionals who try to encourage people to attain and maintain reduced serum lipids through a concerted effort of good nutrition, exercise, and weight control. With this in mind, it is prudent to replace a portion of saturated fats and cholesterol (less than 300 milligrams (mg) daily) in the diet with unsaturated fats.

This is almost the amount of cholesterol contained in the yolk of one large egg and just about one half the cholesterol ingested by the average American male. It should be pointed out, however, that even on a cholesterol-free diet the body produces about 1.0 to 2.0 g of endogenous cholesterol each day.

The cholesterol and saturated fat content of some common foods is presented in Table 1-2. The intake of saturated fat also has a distinct serum cholesterol-raising effect regardless of the cholesterol content of the diet.

The lipoproteins are important because they constitute the main form of transport for fat in the blood. If blood lipids (Greek: lipos meaning fat) were not bound to protein or some other substance, they would float to the top like cream in milk that was not homogenized. Specifically, the *high density lipoproteins (HDL)* contain the largest amount of protein and correspondingly, the smallest amount of cholesterol. *Low and very low density lipoproteins (LDL and VLDL,* respectively) contain the greatest fat and least protein components. The LDL have the greatest affinity for the arterial wall as they help carry cholesterol into the cell. They are intimately involved in the process of arterial narrowing in coronary heart disease. The HDL may operate to protect against heart disease in two ways: (1) to carry cholesterol away from the arterial wall to the liver to be broken down to bile and excreted via the intestines, and (2) to compete with the LDL fragment for receptor sites on the arterial wall, thus blocking the entrance of LDL cholesterol into the cell.

The quantity of LDL and HDL as well as the specific ratio of these blood lipoproteins may provide a more meaningful signal than cholesterol per se in predicting the probability of contracting coronary heart disease. This ratio is improved with a low calorie-low saturated fat diet. It also appears that regular aerobic exer-

Table 1-2. *Cholesterol and saturated fat content of some common foods.*

FOODS	SERVING SIZE	CHOLESTEROL MG	SATURATED FAT G
Beef kidney	3 oz	680	3.8
Beef liver	3 oz	370	2.5
Egg	medium	275	1.7
Shrimp	3 oz	128	0.2
Beef hot dog	3 oz	75	9.9
Lean beef	3 oz	73	3.7
Ice cream	1 cup	59	8.9
Lean fish	3 oz	43	0.8
Whole milk	1 cup	33	5.1
Butter	1 tbsp	31	7.1
Chocolate bar	3 oz	18	16.3
Yogurt	1 cup	14	2.3
Skim milk	1 cup	4	0.3
Peanut butter	1 tbsp	0	1.5
Margarine	1 tbsp	0	2.1

cise and abstinence from cigarette smoking increase the HDL level and favorably affect the *LDL/HDL* ratio. This will be discussed more fully in Chapter 11.

WHERE DO FATS COME FROM?

Both plants and animals provide ready sources of fat. Plants manufacture fat by the same process of photosynthesis they use to make carbohydrates. Animals will use or store the fat they ingest, or synthesize fat from the carbon, hydrogen, and oxygen atoms present in the excess quantities of ingested carbohydrates and proteins.

One of the distinguishing properties of an unsaturated fat is its relatively low melting point. These fats tend to liquefy easily and generally take liquid form at room temperature. Unsaturated fats present as liquids are called oils. The more common vegetable oils are corn oil, cottonseed oil, and soybean oil. Unsaturated oils can be changed to semisolid compounds by a chemical process called *hydrogenation.* This process reduces a double bond in the unsaturated fat to a single bond, thereby allowing more hydrogen atoms to attach to the carbon atoms in the chain *thus causing the fat to behave as a saturated fat.* The most common hydrogenated fats include lard substitutes and margarine.

Saturated fats are derived mainly from animal sources and include the fat in meats such as beef, lamb, pork, and chicken, and in dairy products like egg yolk, cream, milk, butter, and cheese. Shellfish such as lobster, shrimp, and crab also contain a large amount of saturated fat and cholesterol. Coconut and palm oil, vegetable shortening, and margarine are sources of saturated fat from the plant kingdom and are present to a relatively high degree in commercially prepared cakes, pies, and cookies. In the United States, the fat consumed in the diet represents approximately 40 to 50% of the total calorie intake. This amounts to about 115 pounds of fat consumed per person each year, of which over 50 pounds or 16% of the total calories are saturated fat.

FUNCTIONS OF FAT

Energy Source

During light or moderate muscular exercise, such as jogging, energy is derived in approximately equal amounts from the body's stores of carbohydrates and fats. In prolonged exercise of an hour or more there is a significant increase in the amount of fat utilized to supply energy, and, if exercise is continued, the body's fat stores may supply nearly 90% of the total energy required for exercise. On the other hand, in intense but short-term exercise such as all-out running or swimming, essentially all the energy is generated from the glycogen stored in the specific muscles used in the activity.

The potential energy stored in the fat molecules of an average young adult male is about 100,000 calories. Because most of this fat is available for energy, this would be sufficient fuel to power a run from New York City to Madison, Wisconsin. Contrast this to the limited 2,000-calorie energy reserve of stored carbohydrate that becomes severely depleted during a 26-mile marathon run! In terms of its capability for energy storage, fat is remarkably efficient in that more than twice the energy is stored in a pound of body fat as in an equal weight of carbohydrate. This high energy density is due mainly to the amount of hydrogen in the fat molecule, which is larger than the amount of hydrogen in the carbohydrate molecule. Humans would be considerably larger if their energy reserves depended predominantly on carbohydrate storage. In addition, when the union of glycerol and fatty acid makes a fat molecule, it produces three molecules of water. In contrast, when glucose is stored as glycogen, 2.7 g of water are retained for each gram of dried glycogen. Thus, fat exists in a relatively concentrated form, whereas the addition of water to glycogen makes this a heavy fuel.

The preceding discussion is in no way intended to minimize the role of carbohydrate in energy metabolism for prolonged work. Although significantly less carbohydrate is used in long-term exercise than fat, a minimum amount must be available for energy if exercise is to continue. We will discuss the function of carbohydrates in both short- and long-term exercise more fully in Chapter 3.

Protection of Vital Organs

Approximately 4% of the total amount of fat in the body serves as a shock absorber and protective shield against internal and external trauma to vital organs such as the heart, liver, kidneys, spleen, brain, and spinal cord. Even during semistarvation for as long as a year or more, the protective layer of fat around these organs is reduced only slightly compared to the reduction in fat stored in the subcutaneous tissue just below the skin.

Insulation

Fat stored in the subcutaneous tissues acts as an insulator to protect the body against the thermal stress of a cold environment. Although this benefit may provide a comfortable rationalization for many of us who are exquisite insulators, it probably is of value to relatively few people, such as ocean or channel swimmers or occupational deep sea divers, who must work while submerged in water for prolonged periods. In fact, the insulation provided by excess body fat generally serves as a liability in temperature regulation. This is especially true in warm environments, where fat people are at a disadvantage in terms of dissipating body heat to the environment. It is common to observe that fat people sweat easily on warm days, while those who are relatively lean and possess less insulation can maintain body temperature for some time before relying on the cooling benefits of the sweat mechanism. This problem of heat regulation for fat people is magnified during sustained physical activity, where the body's heat production can increase 10 to 20 times above the resting level.

Other Functions

The fat consumed in the diet serves several functions besides protection, insulation, and energy storage. Dietary fat acts as the carrier of four vitamins, A, D, E, and K. These vitamins are fat soluble and are transported to the cells in conjunction with fat. As the amount of fat consumed in the diet is reduced, the availability and utilization of these important vitamins is also reduced. Thus, diets consistently low in fat content may ultimately lead to a deficiency of one or more of the fat-soluble vitamins.

Another function of fat is that its presence in the small intestines stimulates the release of a substance that has the effect of depressing "hunger pangs." These sensations frequently occur when there is a long interval between meals. Because fats are not completely absorbed from the small intestines for up to 4 hours after a meal, dietary fats may retard the feeling of hunger. This is one of the reasons why a limited amount of fat is often recommended in some reducing diets.

FATS IN FOOD

About 30 to 40% of the total dietary fat in the American diet is present in the "visible fats" in butter, lard, mayonnaise, cooking oils, and the visible fat in meat, while the remainder is derived from "invisible fats" in eggs, milk, cheese, nuts, vegetable, and cereals. For every 10 pounds of fat consumed, about 3.4 pounds come from vegetable fat, while the remaining 6.6 pounds are supplied from animal sources. The common vegetable oils are 100% fat, whereas margarine and mayonnaise possess about 80% fat. Most foods from animal sources range between 4 to 80% in fat content. As a frame of comparison, we have computed the fat content of popular fast food items from Appendix D. Expressed as a percentage of total calories, note that a McDonald's Big Mac is 52.8% fat, a Burger King Whopper is 51.0% fat, and a Wendy's double burger on a white bun is 54.6% fat! Other items are as follows: Roy Rogers bacon cheeseburger (60.4%), Jack in the Box Super Taco (54.6%), Burger King Chicken sandwich (54.8%), and McDonald's McNuggets (6 pieces without sauce—54.5%), onion rings from various sources (+50%), while a chocolate, vanilla, or strawberry shake has *only* 20 to 30% fat.

Protein

WHAT IS PROTEIN?

The structure of proteins is similar in one respect to that of carbohydrates and fats. Each molecule contains atoms of carbon, oxygen, and hydrogen. The major difference is that proteins also contain nitrogen, which makes up approximately 16% of the molecule. The basic units or "building blocks" of protein are *amino acids.* Amino acids are small organic compounds that contain at least one amino group and one group called an organic acid. The amino group, that forms the backbone of the amino acid, consists of two hydrogen atoms attached to a nitrogen atom (NH), while the *organic acid (COOH)* is made up of one carbon atom, two oxygen atoms, and one hydrogen atom. The chemical structure of the simple amino acid alanine is illustrated in Figure 1-5.

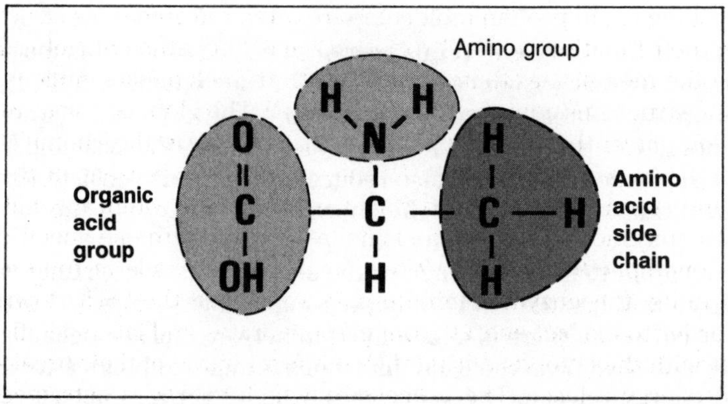
Amino group
Organic acid group
Amino acid side chain

Figure 1-5. *Structural arrangement of the amino acid alanine.*

There are 20 different amino acids present in proteins, although tens of thousands of the same amino acids may be present in a single protein. In the formation of protein, the number of possible combinations of amino acids and associated structures becomes almost infinite. Of the different amino acids, 8 (9 in children and stressed older adults) cannot be synthesized in the body at a sufficient rate to prevent an impairment in normal cellular function. These amino acids are called *essential* because they must be obtained through foods. The 12 amino acids that are manufactured within the body are termed *nonessential.* This does not mean they are unimportant, but simply that the body can synthesize nonessential amino acids from ingested nutrients in the diet.

WHERE DO PROTEINS COME FROM?

Proteins are found in the cells of all animals and plants. Plants make their own special kinds of proteins by incorporating nitrogen contained in the soil. Of the remaining elements, carbon, is obtained from the air, while oxygen and hydrogen are available from water absorbed directly by the roots. Animals, on the other hand, do not have the broad capability for amino-acid synthesis possessed by plants. In many instances, animals must rely on ingested protein sources such as the fruits and vegetables that grow from plants, or the animal protein in meat and in animal by-products such as eggs and milk.

FUNCTIONS OF PROTEINS

The protein content of an average living cell is approximately 15% of its total weight. However, the amount of protein contained in different cells varies considerably. For example, a brain cell is only about 10% protein, whereas protein constitutes 20% of the weight of the muscles, heart, liver, and glands. Furthermore, the protein contained in muscles strengthened through frequent resistance exercise is significantly greater than the protein in unexercised muscles. An increase in protein content contributes to an increase in muscle size that is readily apparent following a strength training program, especially in men. *However, simply ingesting large amounts of dietary protein does not cause a muscle to become larger.* The procedure for increasing the strength and size of muscles is discussed in Chapter 9.

Protein usually takes the shape of either a long, threadlike molecule or a more globular molecule. The long chain protein molecules are often referred to as structural proteins because their function is literally to hold the cell together. Structural proteins are present in the membranes that surround both the cell and its nucleus, as well as in the specific structures contained within the cell. The globular forms of protein make up the *enzymes;* these are substances that speed up the chemical reactions within the cell. As many as 1000 different enzymes are present in the fluids of a single cell and are in contact with surfaces of structures within the cell. One of the unique characteristics of an enzyme is its interaction with one specific substance to perform one specific function. When a protein molecule in food is split into amino acid units, the enzymes initiate and accelerate the breakdown process. Similarly, in order to extract energy from carbohydrates and fats, specific enzymes must interact with these foods during the complex course of their breakdown and subsequent energy release. The process by which energy is extracted from food for use by the body is discussed in Chapter 3.

The importance of protein is further illustrated in a variety of other tissues. Hair, fingernails, and the protective outer layer of skin are composed of the protein *keratin.* The specialized cells that form bone, the *osteoblasts,* secrete a protein substance that ultimately forms the major portion of new bone. Specialized proteins, *thrombin, fibrin,* and *fibrinogen* are intimately involved in the clotting of blood. In muscles, the structural proteins *actin* and *myosin* "slide" past each other during muscular contraction. *Hemoglobin,* that carries oxygen and carbon dioxide in the red blood cells, consists of an iron-containing compound *heme,* and a large protein molecule *globin.* The *hormones* are protein substances secreted into the body from the endocrine glands that control and regulate the function of various processes. For example, the front portion of the small pituitary gland located under the brain secretes six different hormones. Underproduction of pituitary hormones can retard growth, slow the metabolic rate, and influence electrolyte balance, fertility, and the metabolism of carbohydrates, fats, and proteins.

PROTEIN IN FOOD

The proteins contained in food are classified as complete or incomplete, depending on their content of amino acids. A *complete* or *high quality* protein contains all the essential amino acids in both quantity and correct proportion required to promote normal growth. An *incomplete* or *lower quality* protein lacks one or more of the essential amino acids. Consequently, diets that contain predominantly incomplete protein may eventually hamper the ability of various cells to carry out their normal functions.

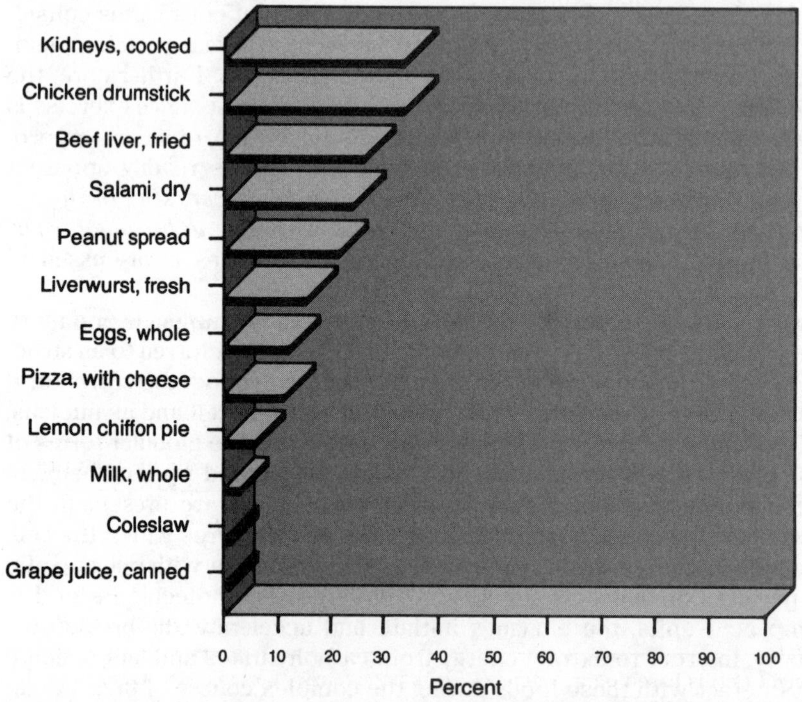
Kidneys, cooked
Chicken drumstick
Beef liver, fried
Salami, dry
Peanut spread
Liverwurst, fresh
Eggs, whole
Pizza, with cheese
Lemon chiffon pie
Milk, whole
Coleslaw
Grape juice, canned
0
10
20
30
40
50
60
70
80
90
100
Percent

Figure 1-6. *Percentage of protein in common foods as served. (Adapted from Handbook No. 8: Composition of Foods, United States Department of Agriculture, Washington, D.C., 1963.)*

The major sources of protein in the American diet are meat, fish, and poultry, whereas only 5% of the daily protein intake of Americans is in the form of peas, beans, or nuts. Generally, more than two-thirds of the protein in the American diet comes from animal sources compared to about one-half 70 years ago. Figure 1-6 illustrates the percentage of protein contained per 100 grams of some common foods.

THE RDA: A LIBERAL STANDARD

The Recommended Dietary Allowance or *RDA* for protein, as well as for the various vitamins and minerals required by the body, are standards for nutrient intake expressed as a daily average developed by the Food and Nutrition Board of the National Research Council/National Academy of Science and revised nine times since 1943. RDA levels are believed to represent a liberal yet safe level of excess to meet the nutritional needs of practically all healthy people. It is important to understand that the RDA reflects nutritional needs of a population over a long period of time. Malnutrition is the cumulative result of weeks, months, and years of a reduced nutrient intake. The RDA should be viewed as a probability statement for adequate nutrition; as nutrient intake falls below the RDA, the probability for malnourishment for that person is increased, and this probability becomes progressively greater as the nutrient intake becomes lower.

Table 1-3 shows the protein intake recommendations for adolescent and adult men and women. *On the average, the daily recommended intake is about 0.8 g of protein per kilogram (g/kg) of body weight.* Thus, a woman of 50 kg (110 lbs) would require about 40 g of protein per day. Heavier people require a greater intake. For an average-sized man who weighs 70 kg (154 lbs), the daily protein intake should be approximately 57 g; for a woman of 56 kg (123 lb), protein intake should be 45 g each day. For infants, a higher intake of protein is recommended, amounting to 2 to 4 g/kg of weight. Also, pregnant women and nursing mothers should increase their daily protein intake by 10 and 20 g, respectively. The protein requirement tends to decrease somewhat with increasing age, while more protein is required when a person is under stress, infection, and excessive heat. The body has no protein reserve; once the protein requirement is consumed, the excess is either used for energy or stored as fat.

Table 1-3. *Recommended dietary allowances of protein for adolescent and adult men and women living in the United States.*

	MEN		WOMEN	
RECOMMENDED AMOUNT	ADOLESCENT	ADULT	ADOLESCENT	ADULT
Grams per day per kg body weight	0.9	0.8	0.9	0.8
Grams per day based on average weight[a]	60.0	65.0	49.0	44.0

[a]Average weight (kg) is based on a "reference" man and woman. For adolescents (ages 14–18), average weight is approximately 145 pounds (65.8 kg) for boys and 123 (55.8 kg) pounds for girls. For adult men, average weight is 154 pounds (70 kg). For adult women, average weight is 125 pounds (56.7 kg).

The Vegetarian Approach to Sound Nutrition

Proteins that contain the essential amino acids are found in *both* animal and vegetable food sources. There is nothing "better" about a specific amino acid from an animal compared to one of vegetable origin. It is simply that sources of high quality protein are animal in nature such as eggs, milk, meat, fish, and poultry. The mixture of essential amino acids present in eggs has ben judged to be the best among food sources.

It should be emphasized that *all* of the essential amino acids can be obtained by consuming a *variety* of vegetable foods, each with a different quality and quantity of amino acids. *Plant sources meet nutritional needs for protein provided a sufficient variety of foods such as grains, fruits, and vegetable are incorporated in the diet.* There are champion athletes whose diet consists predominantly of nutrients from varied vegetable sources as well as some dairy products. In fact, two-thirds of the people in the world are adequately nourished on essentially vegetarian diets using only small amounts of animal protein. For these highly active individuals a basic problem is taking in sufficient calories on a high residue vegetarian diet to match their extremely high energy outputs. With few exceptions (calcium, phosphorus, and vitamin B) a strict vegetarian's nutritional problem is one of getting ample complete proteins. This is easily resolved with a lactovegetarian diet that allows the addition of milk and related products such as ice cream, cheese, and yogurt. The *lactovegetarian* approach minimizes the problem of getting sufficient protein and increases the intake of calcium and phosphorus. By adding an egg to the diet *(lacto-ovovegatarian diet)*, an intake of high-quality protein is assured. The vegetarian approach has additional "spin-off" because foods from the plant kingdom are rich sources of vitamins and minerals, are high in fiber, and generally low in calories and fat, especially saturated fatty acids with cholesterol.

Vitamins

WHAT IS A VITAMIN?

A vitamin is an organic substance needed by the body in very small amounts to perform specific metabolic functions within cells. For example, just 1 ounce of vitamin B would supply the daily needs of nearly 5 million people! Because the body cannot synthesize these substances, it must obtain them in food or through vitamin supplements.

Vitamins were discovered at the turn of the century by scientists who were experimenting with the effects of different foods in the diet. Rats fed a diet consisting of pure carbohydrates, fats, proteins, and adequate water and minerals soon became sick and died. However, if a small amount of milk was added to the diet the rats recovered and thrived. The scientists concluded that the milk must have contained small amounts of a substance that was essential for normal growth and good health. Before these experiments, the importance of vitamins was recognized in an indirect way by sailors who stayed at sea for long periods without being able to replenish their food supplies. In the absence of fresh fruit many sailors died from scurvy, a disease that causes muscle cramps, dizziness, loss of appetite, excessive bleeding of the gums, skin deterioration, infection, and finally death. Around 1750, a British physician conducted an experiment to determine the effect of different food supplements on this disease. Sailors who were fed citrus fruits as a supplement thrived, while those fed supplements without citrus fruits became ill. Based on these results, all ships of the British Navy were required to carry adequate supplies of lime juice. Consequently, British sailors were called "Limeys," a term still used today.

Before World War I, scientists in Europe and the United States had made considerable progress in their quest to determine exactly what those "special substances" were that were so essential for the normal functioning of the body. It was discovered that they could be classified into two different groups depending on their particular chemical properties. One group of chemicals was *fat soluble.* They were dissolved and stored in fat and the fatlike compounds within the body. Daily ingestion of these substances was *not* absolutely necessary because they tended to be retained within the body. Four fat-soluble vitamins are composed entirely of the elements carbon, hydrogen, and oxygen. They are vitamins A, D, E, and K. Vitamin A was discovered in 1913 as the cure for night blindness (poor vision in dim light). The ancient Greeks were aware that eating certain vitamin A-rich fatty foods, such as chicken livers and oils, cured this disease. Note, however, that consuming large doses of vitamin A for long periods can have a toxic effect on both infants and adults. In young children 1 to 3 years of age, an excessive intake of vitamin A (called *hypervitaminosis A*) has been shown to cause irritability, swelling bones, weight loss, and dry, itching skin. In adults, symptoms can include nausea, headaches, drowsiness, loss of hair, diarrhea, and loss of calcium from bones, causing brittleness. Discontinuing such high intakes of vitamin A reverses these symptoms. Large dosages of two other fat-soluble vitamins, D and K, can also produce undesirable toxic side effects, and they should not be consumed in excess without proper medical supervision.

The other group of vitamins is classified as *water soluble* because they are transported in the watery medium of tissues and cells. Because of their solubility in water, these vitamins are not stored in the body to any appreciable extent and are normally voided in the urine. Thus, the water-soluble vitamins must be consumed in the daily diet, or at least within a several day period. The 9 water-soluble vitamins include vitamin C (ascorbic acid) and what are commonly referred to as the B-complex vitamins. Included in this group are thiamine (B_1), riboflavin (B_2), niacin, pyridoxine (B_6), folacin, pantothenic acid, biotin, and cobalamin (B_{12}). These vitamins act as part of *coenzymes*—small protein molecules that can combine with another protein to make it an active enzyme.

Any excess of the water-soluble vitamins is usually excreted in the urine on a daily basis. An excess intake of the fat-soluble vitamins is maintained within the body tissues and in some instances produces a toxic "vitamin overdose." Thus, ingesting more vitamins than recommended will be of little or no benefit.

WHERE DO VITAMINS COME FROM?

With the exception of vitamin B_{12} that is synthesized *only* in animals, vitamins are manufactured in the green leaves and roots of plants by the process of photosynthesis that we have already discussed. The synthesis of vitamins involves the

Table 1-4. *Vitamins—their functions and symptoms of their deficiency.*

VITAMINS	FUNCTIONS	SYMPTOMS OF DEFICIENCY
A (Retinol)	Vision, growth	Poor vision (night blindness), failure of bones to grow in length, skin and respiratory infections, failure of tooth enamel
D	Bone calcification	Bone diseases
E (Tocopherol)	Not clear in humans	Unclear, possibly anemia
K	Blood coagulation and energy metabolism of the cell	Prolonged blood-clotting time
B_1 (Thiamine)	Metabolism of nutrients in cells	Beriberi—the degeneration of nerves and muscles, loss of appetite, mental depression, and neurological dysfunction
B_2 (Riboflavin)	Reactions that release energy in the cells	Lesions of the skin, eye, mouth, and retardation of growth
Niacin	Release of energy from the breakdown and synthesis of carbohydrate, fat, and protein	Diseases of the skin, gastro-intestinal tract, and nervous system, resulting in dermatitis, diarrhea and depression
B_6 (Pyridoxine)	Synthesis and breakdown of amino acids	Usually no deficiency because this vitamin is so readily available in foods
Pantothenic acid	Metabolism of carbohydrates, fats, and proteins, important in the formation of cholesterol	Subclinical symptoms such as irritability, restlessness, easy fatigue, muscle cramps
Folacin	Formation of normal red blood cells and of DNA and RNA	Toxemia of pregnancy and anemia and retarded production of white blood cells
B_{12}	Normal growth, maintenance of neural tissue, and formation of blood	Pernicious anemia (sore tongue, weight loss, mental and nervous disorders, degeneration of the spinal cord)
Biotin	Removal or addition of carbon dioxide in chemical reactions and metabolism of carbohydrate and protein	Dermatitis, such as scaling or hardening of skin, loss of appetite, nausea, muscle pains, high blood cholesterol levels

Table 1-4. *(continued)*

VITAMINS	FUNCTION	SYMPTOMS OF DEFICIENCY
C (Ascorbic acid)	Important for collagen formation that acts as "cement" to bind connective tissue cells together, tooth formation	Scurvy, sore joints, poor healing of wounds

integration of the energy from sunlight with carbon dioxide, water, and minerals in the soil. Animals obtain their vitamins from the plants, seeds, grains, and fruits they eat, or from the meat of other animals that have previously consumed these foods. There is essentially no difference between a vitamin synthesized in the laboratory and a so-called "natural" vitamin pre-formed from a plant or animal source.

Most animals are able to manufacture some of the vitamins within their own cells. Vitamin C, for example, can be synthesized by all animals with the exception of humans, monkeys, guinea pigs, and several species of birds. Several of the vitamins, notably vitamins A, niacin, and folacin, are converted to an activated form in the body from precursor substances known as *provitamins.* The most well known of the provitamins are the *carotenes,* the yellow and yellow-orange pigments that give color to vegetables and fruits such as carrots, squash, corn, pumpkins, sweet potatoes, apricots, peaches, and melons. *Carotenes,* the precursors of vitamin A, are also present in all green plants, but the green pigment chlorophyll masks their color. They are converted to vitamin A in the walls of the intestines and in the liver. Besides playing an important role in the prevention of night blindness and other eye diseases, this vitamin prevents some digestive and urogenital tract diseases and, in carotene form, may provide protection against several forms of cancer. Another provitamin substance in the skin is converted to vitamin D when the skin is exposed to the ultraviolet rays of the sun or to artificial ultraviolet light. Niacin, the B-complex vitamin that prevents pellagra (a skin disease), is converted to an active form by its precursor, the essential amino acid *tryptophan.*

FUNCTIONS OF VITAMINS

Vitamins perform many different functions. They generally serve as essential links and regulators in the chain of metabolic reactions within cells. If there is a dietary deficiency in either the vitamin or its precursor, the resulting defect in cellular function manifests itself in a variety of symptoms. The more important functions of the vitamins and the symptoms resulting from vitamin deficiencies are summarized in a general way in Table 1-4.

VITAMINS AND EXERCISE PERFORMANCE

Contrary to popular belief, vitamins themselves contain no usable energy. However, it is well established that 5 or 6 vitamins of the B-complex group interact with various enzymes that are important in the energy-yielding reactions during the metabolism of fats and carbohydrates. This has led many coaches, athletes, and fitness enthusiasts to believe that supplements of these vitamins will enhance or "supercharge" energy production, and consequently lead to improved physical performance. However, there is little experimental evidence to support this practice.

This is also the case for vitamins other than the B-complex group such as vitamins C and E. While there is some indication that the vitamin C requirement is increased in humans in times of stress, *it has yet to be demonstrated that an excess of this vitamin is needed during physical training.* Studies have shown that supplements of vitamin C had negligible effects on endurance and on the rate, severity, and duration of injuries compared to treatment with a placebo. In addition, the combined findings from several studies showed only a slight reduction in frequency, duration, and severity of colds in individuals on vitamin C supplementation compared to counterparts taking a placebo. Its major effect may be to act as an antihistamine to reduce cold symptoms. It has never been firmly established with careful research that a deficiency state for vitamin E exists, let alone that vitamin E supplements are beneficial to stamina, circulatory function, energy metabolism, aging, the effects of air pollution, or sexual potency.

VITAMIN SUPPLEMENTATION

Only in rare instances do healthy people who eat well-balanced meals require vitamin supplements. It has been estimated that the American consumer spends between $400 million and $800 million annually on unnecessary vitamin supplements! While most nutritionists feel that taking a daily multivitamin capsule of the recommended dosage will do little harm (the psychologic effects may even be beneficial), it is of great concern that some men and women resort to taking *megavitamins,* or doses of at least *tenfold* and up to 1,000 times the RDA in the hope of improving health or exercise performance. Except in cases of specific serious medical illness, this practice can be harmful. Once the enzyme systems that are catalyzed by specific vitamins are saturated, the excess vitamins in the megadose function as chemicals in the body.

Generally, an excess of the water soluble vitamins will be excreted in the urine on a daily basis. However, there may be specific and serious exceptions to this general rule. For example, a megadose of the water soluble vitamin C can raise serum uric acid levels and precipitate gout in people predisposed to this disease. Also, some American blacks, Asians, and Sephardic Jews have a genetic metabolic deficiency that can be activated to hemolytic anemia by excesses of vitamin C. In individuals who are iron-deficient, megadoses of vitamin C destroy significant amounts of vitamin B_{12} in the diet. In healthy people, vitamin C supplements frequently irritate the bowel and cause diarrhea. It is now believed that an excessive intake of vitamin B_6 may produce liver disease and nerve damage, whereas a megadose of nicotinic acid inhibits the uptake of fatty acids by cardiac muscle during exercise.

An excess intake of the fat soluble vitamins is maintained within the body tissues and, in some instances, produces a toxic "vitamin overdose." Possible side effects of vitamin E megadose include headache, fatigue, blurred vision, gastrointestinal disturbances, muscular weakness, and low blood sugar. This is ironic because it is difficult to even "construct" a vitamin E-deficient diet among individuals in a natural setting. The toxicity to the nervous system of megadoses of vitamin A and the damaging effects to the kidneys of excess vitamin D have been well demonstrated.

Perhaps the misuse and abuse of vitamins by individuals hoping to improve athletic performance can be put in proper perspective by the following quotation:

"The sale of vitamins is probably the biggest rip-off in our society today. Their only effect would appear to be a highly enriched sewage around athletic training or competition sites."

Minerals

WHAT IS A MINERAL?

The body is composed of at least 31 known chemical elements, of which 24 are considered to be essential for sustaining life. These essential elements are combined in thousands of different ways to form the various structures within the body. The most abundant nonmetal, chemical element is oxygen that amounts to 65% of a person's body weight. Three other nonmetal elements constitute 31% of the body mass; these are carbon (18%), hydrogen (10%), and nitrogen (3%). In addition to the organic elements oxygen, carbon, hydrogen, and nitrogen, the remaining 4% that would amount to about 5 pounds for a 125-pound woman, is composed of a group of 22 mostly metallic elements called *minerals.* Although the total quantity of minerals present in the body is relatively small, each of them is vital for proper cell functioning. For example, minerals play a *regulatory* role as part of enzymes, hormones, and vitamins. They also provide *structure* in the formation of bones and teeth. Calcium and phosphorus in teeth and bones account for 58 to 85% of the total percentage of minerals in the body. Minerals such as sodium, potassium, and chlorine are important in a *functional* sense for maintaining normal heart rhythm, muscular contractility, nerve conductivity, and the acid-base balance of the body. The remaining minerals include trace amounts of iron, zinc, selenium, manganese, iodine, copper, fluorine, and chromium. The body even contains small quantities of aluminum, silver, tin, lead, barium, and gold. If purchased in a store, the total worth of the body's minerals would be only about 12 cents!

WHERE DO MINERALS COME FROM?

Minerals occur freely in nature and are found mainly in the waters of rivers, lakes, and oceans, in topsoil, and beneath the earth's surface. Small amounts of minerals are absorbed into the natural foods, the carbohydrates, fats, and proteins. Minerals then become part of the body structure of animals who must consume food and water in order to survive. Similarly, the human supply of minerals is obtained almost exclusively from water and food.

FUNCTIONS OF MINERALS

Minerals are present in all living cells. They are part of the cell membranes, cell nucleus, and various cellular structures such as the "powerhouse" of the cell, the *mitochondrion,* that converts food nutrients to energy. They are intimately involved in *catabolism*—the breakdown of the nutrient substances glucose, fatty acids, and amino acids to their end products, carbon dioxide and water. In this process considerable energy is extracted from the food and used to maintain the body's energy supply. Minerals are also required for the reverse process, *anabo-*

lism, that refers to the synthesis of glycogen from glucose, fat from fatty acids and glycerol, and protein from amino acids.

Minerals also serve as important parts of the structure of various hormones, enzymes, and other substances that help to regulate the chemical reactions within cells. For example, in the previous section we mentioned that the mineral iodine was necessary for the synthesis of thyroxin, the hormone that accelerates the rate of energy metabolism in cells. Underproduction of thyroxin causes a decreased metabolic rate that could result in the development of obesity. As will be seen, the mineral iron is an important component of compounds involved in oxygen transport and utilization.

Calcium, the body's most abundant mineral, combines with the mineral phosphorus to form the bones and teeth. Calcium is also essential in maintaining the normal function of muscles, as well as for blood clotting, and the transport of fluid across cell membranes. Phosphorus is an essential component of the high energy compounds *adenosine triphosphate (ATP)* and *creatine phosphate (CP)*. As we will show in Chapter 3, these compounds are crucial in supplying the energy for all forms of biologic work. Phosphorus also combines with substances in the blood and acts to buffer the acid end products of energy metabolism. Because it can regulate the acid content of the blood, some coaches and trainers recommend that their athletes consume special "phosphate drinks" three to four hours prior to competition to improve their subsequent performance. Although some people have attributed enhanced performance to these drinks, scientific evidence in support of this practice is lacking. It is also possible that an excess intake of phosphorus, plentiful in red meats and diet soft drinks, can accelerate the rate of bone loss (osteoporosis) in athletic women who are relatively thin with a low percentage of body fat.

Magnesium plays a vital role in glucose metabolism by facilitating the reactions that synthesize glucose to glycogen in the liver and muscles. Magnesium is also involved in the breakdown of glucose, fatty acids, and amino acids to provide cellular energy. Futhermore, magnesium is important in bone formation, in maintaining normal muscle function, in the conduction of nerve impulses, and in the synthesis of fats and proteins from fatty acids and amino acids.

The minerals sodium, potassium, and chlorine have quite similar functions. Sodium and chlorine are present mainly in the fluids outside the cells, while potassium is found predominantly in the intracellular fluids. Collectively these three elements are called *electrolytes*, because they are present in the body as electrically charged particles called ions. A major function of electrolytes is to control and maintain the correct rate of fluid exchange within various fluid compartments of the body. In this way the constant flow of dissolved nutrients into the cell and waste products from the cell is properly regulated.

MINERALS IN FOOD

As with vitamins, healthy people who eat well-balanced meals consume enough of the essential mineral elements to maintain normal physiologic functioning and health. Mineral supplements may be necessary, however, in some geographic regions where mineral elements in the soil or water supply are relatively scarce. The mineral iodine, for example, is stored mainly in the thyroid gland and becomes part of thyroxin, a hormone that influences the rate of energy metabolism in cells. A diet deficient in iodine results in the over-enlargement of the thyroid gland as the gland attempts to produce an adequate supply of thyroxin. This disease, *goiter*, is one of the most prevalent nutrient deficiency diseases in the world. Iodine added to most common table salts (iodized salt) is an inexpensive, easily obtained iodine supplement. We will now take a closer look at the minerals iron, calcium, and sodium in terms of their requirements and relationship to exercise and good health.

Iron. A common mineral deficiency results from lack of iron in the diet. About 5 g or one-sixth of an ounce of iron is normally contained within the body. Two-thirds of this amount is combined with *hemoglobin*, the iron-protein compound manufactured in the marrow of long bones. This compound is found in red blood cells and increases the oxygen carrying capacity of the blood about 65 times. Iron is also part of *myoglobin*, a compound similar to hemoglobin, that aids in the storage and transport of oxygen within the cell. Small amounts of iron are also present in specialized substances called *cytochromes* that facilitate the transfer of energy within the cell. People who do not consume enough iron or have limited rates of iron absorption or high rates or iron loss can develop *anemia*, a condition that reduces the concentration of hemoglobin as well as the size of red blood cells. This condition, commonly referred to as *iron-deficiency anemia*, is characterized by general sluggishness, fatigue, and loss of appetite. Nutritionists estimate that between 30 to 50% of American women of childbearing age suffer some form of iron insufficiency. This is because women usually lose between 5 and 45 mg of iron during the menstrual cycle. This increases the iron requirement of females to almost twice that of males (18 versus 10 mg). Because the typical Western diet contains about 6 mg or iron per 1000 calories of food ingested, it is difficult for the average woman who consumes 2100 calories a day to obtain the required iron. A moderate iron deficiency is common during pregnancy when there is a greater demand for iron for both the mother and fetus.

Iron deficiency is corrected in most cases with a diet rich in iron-containing foods such as liver, nuts, legumes, dried uncooked fruits, oysters, shellfish, leafy green vegetables, egg yolk, and meats, especially kidney and heart. Iron supplements can be obtained in tablet or liquid form or in foods specifically fortified with iron. The Food and Nutrition Board's recommendations for daily intakes of iron for men and women of different ages are listed in Table 1-5.

Plant Versus Animal Sources of Iron. While the absorption of iron from the gut varies with iron need, a considerable difference in absorption occurs in relation to the composition of the diet. For example, only between 2 to 10% of the iron obtained from plants (non-heme iron) is absorbed, whereas 10 to 35% of the iron from animal sources (heme iron) is absorbed. This places women on vegetarian-type diets at greater risk of developing iron insufficiency than a female consuming a diet rich in foods from animal sources. This problem can be alleviated somewhat by including vitamin C-rich foods in the diet because ascorbic acid increases the absorption of non-heme iron in the intestines. The ascorbic acid in one glass of orange juice, for example, stimulates a three-fold increase in non-heme iron absorption from a breakfast meal.

Experiments have shown that individuals who suffer from iron deficiency anemia have a reduced capacity for sustaining even mild exercise. This occurs because lowered iron content in the red blood cells results in an inadequate supply of oxygen to the exercising muscles. This was illustrated in one experiment in which 29 iron-deficient, anemic men and women with low hemoglobin levels were placed into one of two groups: one group received intramuscular injections of iron

Table 1-5. *Recommended dietary allowances for iron.*

GROUP	AGE	IRON (MG)
Children	1–3	15
	4–10	10
Males	11–18	18
	19+	10
Females	11–50	18
	51+	10
	Pregnant	18+[a]
	Lactating	18

Source: Food and Nutrition Board, *Recommended Dietary Allowances*, 8th ed., National Academy of Sciences, Washington, D.C., Revised, 1980.

[a]Ordinary diets cannot meet this increased requirement; therefore the use of 30 to 60 mg of supplemental iron is recommended.

over an 80-day period, while the other group received intramuscular injections of colored saline solution. Both groups were tested for exercise capacity before receiving iron or placebo 4 to 6 days after receiving the first iron supplement or placebo, and after 80 days of treatment. The results of Table 1-6 clearly showed that the group given the iron supplement improved significantly in exercise response. Peak heart rate measured during a 5-minute stepping performance decreased from 155 to 113 beats per minute for men and from 152 to 123 beats per minute for the women. This translates into an average of 15% more oxygen delivered per heart beat. The heart rate and hemoglobin levels did not change for the group receiving the placebo treatment.

Added Iron Requirement with Exercise? Some researchers maintain that exercise training creates an added demand for iron that often outstrips its intake. To support the possibility of an "exercise induced anemia", data have been presented that marginal levels of hemoglobin concentration exist among endurance athletes, especially females, who have the greatest requirement and lowest intake of this important mineral. It is postulated that heavy training creates an augmented iron demand due to a loss of iron in sweat, or the loss of hemoglobin in the urine due to an actual destruction of red blood cells with increased temperature and circulation, or from actual mechanical trauma caused by pounding of the feet on the running surface.

Although there is undoubtedly some destruction of red blood cells with vigorous exercise and some loss of iron in sweat, it is yet to be adequately verified whether these factors are of sufficient magnitude to strain an athlete's iron reserves if iron intake is normal. Because adolescents and premenopausal women have a relatively high iron requirement, any increase in iron loss with training could strain an already limited iron reserve. This does not mean, however, that all individuals who undertake an exercise program should take supplementary iron! On the contrary, iron supplementation for those whose diet is sufficient in this mineral does not lead to an increase in hemoglobin or hematocrit (concentration

Table 1-6. *Hemoglobin (Hb) and exercise heart rate responses of anemic subjects to iron treatment.*

SUBJECTS	Hb (G PER 100 ML BLOOD) (AVERAGE)	PEAK EXERCISE HEART RATE (AVERAGE)
Normal		
Men	14.3	119
Women	13.9	142
Iron-Deficient Men		
Pre-treatment	7.1	155
Post-treatment	14.0	113
Iron-Deficient Women		
Pre-treatment	7.7	155
Post-treatment	12.4	123
Iron-Deficient Men		
Pre-placebo	7.7	146
Post-placebo	7.4	137
Iron-Deficient Women		
Pre-placebo	8.1	154
Post-placebo	8.4	144

From Gardner, G.W., et al.: Cardiorespiratory, hematological, and physical performance responses of anemic subjects to iron treatment. *American Journal of Clinical Nutrition, 28*:982, 1975.

of red blood cells). Furthermore, the indiscriminate use of iron supplements can cause iron to accumulate to toxic levels in the body and cause serious side effects. The prudent approach for athletes in training is to monitor iron status by periodic evaluation of blood characteristics as well as iron reserves.

Calcium. While growing children need more calcium on a daily basis than adults, many adults are deficient in their intake of this mineral. As a general guideline, adults need 800 mg of calcium daily or about the amount contained in three 8-oz glasses of milk. In reality, however, calcium is one of the most frequently lacking nutrients. For example, about 25% of all females in the United States consume less than 300 mg of calcium on any given day. Thus, the body must draw on its calcium reserve in bone to restore the deficit. If the imbalance is prolonged, the condition of *osteoporosis* (literally meaning porous bone) eventually sets in as the bone loses its mineral mass and progressively becomes porous and brittle; it eventually breaks under the stress of normal living. Osteoporosis affects nearly 20 million people in the United States. It accounts for nearly 1.2 million fractures annually, and more than 80% of the nearly 200,000 hip fractures among elderly females. The sites of the fractures are in the vertebrae (538,000 cases), the distal forearm (Colle's fracture—172,000 cases), and other limb sites (238,000 cases).

Twelve to 20% of hip fractures in the elderly are fatal, and it causes half of those who survive to go to nursing homes. The indirect and direct medical costs of osteoporosis in the United States exceeds 6.1 billion dollars annually!

Calcium, Exercise, and Osteoporosis. Osteoporosis begins early in life—perhaps because the average American teenager consumes suboptimal levels of calcium. An imbalance of calcium intake worsens into adulthood and by middle age, adult women consume only about one-third of the calcium they require for optimal bone maintenance. Starting at about age 50, the average man loses about 0.4% of bone each year, whereas women lose twice this amount starting at age 35. For men, the normal rate of bone mineral loss does not usually pose a problem until the seventh decade of life. Women, on the other hand, become susceptible to the ravages of osteoporosis at the menopause when bone loss accelerates to 1.0 to 3.0% per year. The increased susceptibility to osteoporosis among older women is closely associated with the decrease in *estrogen* production (estrogen facilitates calcium absorption and improves kidney conservation of calcium) that accompanies the menopause. The Food and Drug Administration has approved calcium, estrogen, and calcitonin that can be used to decrease bone resorption. Estrogen therapy, however, is not without risk because of the increased risk for cancers of the uterus, breast, and other organs. Combining estrogen with other hormones (progestins) may alleviate the higher risk of developing such cancers. The newer treatments will include transdermal patches (worn on the skin), as well as nasal sprays for administration of calcitonin, and fluoride therapy for osteoporosis.

A prime defense against bone loss with age seems to be adequate calcium intake throughout life, but the evidence is not fully complete. Many experts believe that the 800 mg RDA of calcium for adults is too low, and recommend an increase to 1000 mg with further increase to between 1200 to 1500 mg for women after menopause to assure positive calcium balance in later life. Good sources of calcium are milk and milk products, sardines and canned salmon, kidney beans, and dark green leafy vegetables. Calcium supplements (examples are calcium carbonate and calcium gluconate) portioned throughout the day can also help to correct dietary deficiencies. Adequate availability of vitamin D facilitates calcium metabolism, while excessive consumption of red meat, salt, coffee, and alcohol can inhibit calcium absorption. While upgrading the calcium content of the American diet is of utmost importance in the battle against the bone-wasting process of osteoporosis, emerging research suggests that this approach may be overly simplistic and that factors other than diet must also be considered.

It is important to note that regular exercise may help to slow the rate of aging of the skeleton. Regardless of age, individuals who maintain an active lifestyle have significantly greater bone mass compared to sedentary counterparts, and this benefit is carried into the seventh and even eighth decade of life! In fact, the decline in vigorous exercise with the sedentary lifestyle associated with advancing age closely parallels the age-related loss of bone mass.

It appears that exercise modifies bone metabolism at the point of stress, and that bone deposition is controlled locally by the muscular forces acting on specific bones. Especially beneficial, therefore, is exercise of a weight bearing nature; this includes walking, running, dancing, rope skipping, or activities such as resistance exercise training in which significant muscular force can be generated against the long bones of the body.

A paradox between exercise and bone dynamics has been noted for young women who train intensely and reduce body weight and body fat to a point where the menstrual cycle actually ceases, a condition termed *secondary amenorrhea.* A hormonal imbalance associated with the cessation of menstruation removes estrogen's protective effect on bone, and makes these women vulnerable to calcium loss and a possible decrease in bone mass.

Sodium. How much is enough? The recommended level for sodium intake for adults is between 1100 and 3300 mg per day, or the amount of sodium in ½ to 1½ teaspoons of salt (about 40% of table salt is sodium). For the person consuming the typical Western diet, however, about 4500 mg of sodium or 8 to 12 grams of salt are ingested daily, a value that is 20 times the 500 mg of sodium that the body actually needs. This large sodium intake is primarily due to the heavy reliance placed on salt in processing, curing, cooking, seasoning, and storing of foods. Aside from table salt, common sodium-rich dietary sources are monosodium glutamate (MSG), soy sauce, condiments, canned foods, baking soda, and baking powder.

In general, if sodium intake is low, the hormone *aldosterone* acts on the kidneys to conserve sodium. Conversely, if sodium intake is high, the excess is excreted in the urine and salt balance is maintained at normal levels throughout a wide range of intakes. For certain susceptible individuals, this is not always the case and excessive sodium intake is not regulated. High sodium intake tends to increase fluid volume and significantly elevate blood pressure. This sodium-induced hypertension occurs in about one-third of people suffering from hypertension.

For decades, one first line of defense in the treatment of high blood pressure was to eliminate all excess sodium in the diet. Because sodium is widely distributed naturally in foods, it was easy to obtain the daily requirement without relying on "extra" salt. A reduced sodium intake may favorably lower blood pressure. Although the effectiveness of sodium restriction for controlling hypertension in the general population is not known for sure, it appears that individuals who are "salt sensitive" may respond favorably in reducing their hypertension when dietary sodium is curtailed.

MINERALS AND EXERCISE PERFORMANCE

For individuals who consume the Recommended Dietary Allowance of minerals, there is no evidence that mineral supplementation benefits exercise performance. The proper maintenance of both fluid and electrolyte balance is of critical importance, especially during exercise in warm environments. When sweating excessively, the body loses the electrolytes present in sweat. These conditions impair heat tolerance and exercise performance. If electrolytes, and particularly water, are not replaced, severe dysfunction in the form of heat cramps and heat stroke can occur. The yearly toll of heat-related deaths during spring and summer football practice provides a tragic illustration of the importance of both fluid and electrolyte replacement. Thus, it is prudent for athletes, tunnel and mine workers, and others who sweat profusely during work to increase their normal salt and fluid intake automatically, independent of their thirst, to offset the effects of dehydration. *The crucial and immediate need is to replace the water lost through sweating.*

A 1 liter or 2.2 pound sweat loss is accompanied by a loss of about 1.5 g of salt. These electrolytes can easily be replenished by adding a slight amount of table salt to the fluids ingested or to the normal daily food intake. Thus, ingesting the so-called athletic drinks is of no special benefit in replacing the minerals lost through sweating. In fact, research indicates that most individuals unconsciously consume more salt when the need exists. For fluid losses in excess of 9 to 10 pounds and for prolonged periods of work in the heat, salt supplements may be necessary and can be achieved by adding about ⅓ teaspoon of table salt per quart of water. Although a potassium deficiency may occur with intense exercise in the heat, the appropriate potassium level is generally assured by consuming a diet containing normal amounts of the mineral, or by eating potassium-rich foods such as citrus fruits and bananas. A glass of orange or tomato juice replaces almost all of the calcium, potassium, and magnesium lost in about 3 quarts (6 lb) of sweat.

Water

WATER CONTENT OF THE BODY

Water is the most important environmental substance essential to human life. It makes up about 80% of the liquid substance of all cells. Aside from its excellent temperature stabilizing properties, it dissolves more substances than any other known solvent. Food and oxygen are always supplied in an aqueous solution to the cells, and waste products always leave the cell via this medium. Water is remarkably inert and most substances remain unchanged when dissolved in water. In solution they may remain unaltered within the body until they are needed.

From 40 to 60% of a person's body weight consists of water. Because water makes up about 72% of the weight of muscle tissue and only 20 to 25% of the weight of fat, the differences between individuals in terms of total body water are determined largely by differences in body composition. Therefore, for two individuals of the same body weight, the total body water will be larger for the individual with the greater muscle mass. On the average, men contain relatively less body fat than women. This explains why approximately 55% of men's body weight is water, while only 50% of women's body weight is water. This would amount to 85 pounds of water or 10.2 gallons for a 154-pound man and 65 pounds of water or 7.8 gallons for a 130-pound woman.

The distribution of water in the body is usually described in terms of its location. There are two main water "compartments." One is *intracellular*, referring to fluid inside each cell. The other compartment is *extracellular*, referring to the fluids outside the cells. These include the fluids that make up the plasma of blood and lymph, and a variety of other fluids like saliva, fluids in the eyes, fluids secreted by glands and the intestines, fluids that bathe the nerves of the spinal cord, and fluids excreted from the skin and kidneys. Of the total body water, about 62% is intracellular and 38% is extracellular.

NORMAL WATER BALANCE IN THE BODY

Because a delicate balance is maintained between the body's water intake (gain of water) and water output (loss of water), its water content remains fairly stable from day to day and from month to month (Fig. 1-7).

Water Intake

The water needs of the body are supplied from three sources: (1) from fluids, (2) in foods, and (3) during metabolism.

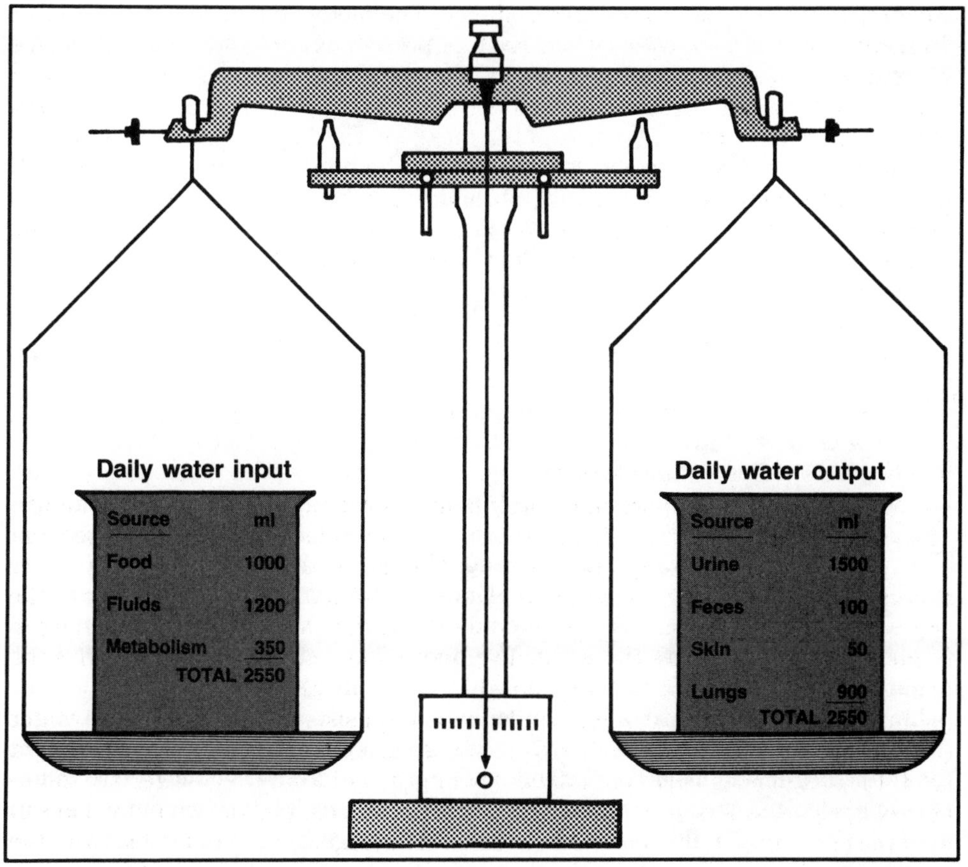
Daily water input
Source ml
Food 1000
Fluids 1200
Metabolism 350
TOTAL 2550
Daily water output
Source ml
Urine 1500
Feces 100
Skin 50
Lungs 900
TOTAL 2550

Figure 1-7. *Water balance in humans.*

FROM FLUIDS This source includes the normal intake of drinking water as well as the water contained in beverages and soups. The adult fluid intake ranges from about 800 to 1600 ml of water each day, with an average of approximately 1200 ml. This amount will vary considerably under certain conditions, especially during exercise and thermal stress, where fluid intake can increase 5 or 6 times above normal. One of the more interesting examples of fluid depletion occurred during a 2-day, 17-hour run across Death Valley, California. A highly conditioned runner ran 55 miles of the 110-mile distance in 125°F heat. The runner lost 30 pounds in body weight during the 2 days. However, with the fluid replacement (salt solution and glucose, including soft drinks and fruit juices), the final body weight loss was only 3 pounds. In terms of fluid depletion, the runner had lost between 3½ and 4 gallons of fluid.

IN FOODS The second source of water is food, mainly fruits and vegetables that have a surprisingly large water content. On the other hand, the amount of water contained in honey, candy, and butter is relatively low.

DURING METABOLISM Water is produced during energy-yielding chemical reactions. For example, when a molecule of sugar is metabolized, energy is released and carbon dioxide and water are produced. The metabolism of 100 g of carbohydrate produces 55 g of water, while 100 g of protein and fat yields 42 and 107 g of water, respectively.

Water Output

There are four ways water is lost from the body: (1) in urine, (2) through the skin, (3) as water vapor in expired air, and (4) in feces.

IN URINE Urine is formed in the kidneys, the two organs located toward the back in the lower abdominal area. The major function of the kidneys is to filter the fluid of the blood and reabsorb essential nutrient materials—such as proteins, minerals, and electrolytes—that otherwise would be lost in the urine. Urine is approximately 96% water. Under normal conditions, urine is continuously formed in the kidneys and is passed to the bladder for storage at the rate of about 1 ml per minute. For an adult, the volume of urine excreted each day ranges from 1000 to 1500 ml (about 1 to 1½ quarts). This volume will vary considerably, however, depending on such factors as temperature, humidity, fluid intake, diet, and level of physical activity.

THROUGH THE SKIN Water is lost through the skin in the form of sweat produced from specialized glands. These sweat glands are very small structures located beneath the skin, and are primarily found on the palms of the hands, soles of the feet, forehead, and underneath the arms. The body's capacity for sweat production is manifested by about 3000 individual sweat glands in 1 square inch of skin on the palm. In total, there are approximately 2.5 million sweat glands distributed throughout the surface of the body. Under normal environmental conditions (not too hot, cold, or humid) 500 to 700 ml of sweat are secreted each day. The volume of sweat secreted through the skin increases dramatically during exercise to help dissipate heat that builds up in the muscles from the energy-producing metabolic reactions.

When the sweat comes into contact with the skin, a cooling effect occurs only as the sweat evaporates. The cooled skin in turn serves to cool the blood that is shunted from the interior toward the surface of the body. The evaporative cooling effect can be demonstrated by placing a few drops of rubbing alcohol on the skin. Because alcohol evaporates more rapidly than water or sweat, the cooling sensation is more pronounced. The process of sweat production and subsequent evaporation provides a refrigeration mechanism to help cool the body and keep body temperature from rising too high. From 8 to 12 liters, or about 25 pounds, of sweat can be produced during prolonged exercise performed in a hot, humid environment. Marathon runners frequently experience fluid losses in excess of 6 quarts (10 to 12 lbs) during competition, a loss that represents between 6 to 10% of body weight.

The relative humidity of the surrounding air is also an important factor that affects the efficiency of the sweating mechanism in temperature regulation. The term *relative humidity* refers to the water content of the air. During conditions of 100% relative humidity, the air is completely saturated with water vapor. Thus, evaporation of fluid from the skin to the air is impossible and this important avenue for body cooling is closed. Under such conditions sweat beads on the skin and eventually rolls off. On the other hand, on a dry day the air can hold considerable moisture, the evaporation of fluid from the skin is quite rapid, and body temperature is more easily controlled.

As Water Vapor Small droplets of water are contained in the expired air during each breath. As a result about 250 to 300 ml of water are eliminated daily as a result of breathing. In furry animals that cannot use evaporative cooling from the skin, water evaporation from the respiratory passages provides the important means of temperature regulation. In these animals, evaporative cooling increases considerably by means of the rapid, shallow breathing called panting.

In Feces Approximately 70% of fecal matter is composed of water, the remainder being nondigestible material, bacteria from the digestive process, and the residues of digestive juices from the intestines, stomach, and pancreas. The daily amount of water eliminated in feces is about 100 ml. Under abnormal conditions like diarrhea or vomiting, water losses may be considerable, ranging from 1500 to 5000 ml.

WATER REPLACEMENT

The loss of body water is the most serious consequence of profuse sweating. The amount of water lost through sweating depends on the severity of physical activity as well as on the environmental temperature and humidity. The most effective defense against the heat is adequate hydration; this is achieved by balancing water loss with water intake.

Adequacy of Rehydration

Changes in body weight before and after exercise should be used to indicate water loss in exercise and the adequacy of rehydration during the subsequent exercise. Coaches often have their athletes "weigh-in" before and after practice and insist that weight loss be minimized by periodic water breaks during activity. In fact, if rehydration were left entirely to the person's thirst, it could take several days to reestablish fluid balance, even after severe dehydration!

Practical Recommendations for Fluid Replacement

Ingestion of "extra" water prior to exercise in the heat provides some protection because it increases sweating during exercise and brings about a significantly lower body temperature during exercise. In this regard, it would be wise to consume 400 to 600 ml (13 to 20 oz) of water 10 to 20 minutes before exercising in the heat. This procedure, however, does not eliminate the need for continual fluid replacement during the exercise. A volume of about 250 ml (8.5 oz) ingested at 10- to 15-minute intervals is probably a realistic goal because larger volumes tend to produce feelings of a "full stomach."

Studies of fluid absorption indicate that cold fluids (5°C; 41°F) are emptied from the stomach at a *faster* rate than fluids at body temperature. *Gastric emptying is retarded when the ingested fluid contains sugar, whether in the form of glucose, fructose, or sucrose!* With intense exercise, even a small amount of carbohydrate slows fluid movement from the stomach into the intestinal tract to be absorbed by the body. From a practical standpoint during exercise in the heat, when the need for water greatly exceeds the need for carbohydrate supplementation, glucose in solution hinders water replenishment. Certainly, drinking commercial preparations such as Gatorade that contain 5% glucose, would significantly retard the replacement of lost fluid during exercise in the heat. In this regard, research is encouraging because the negative effects of sugar molecules on water absorption can be reduced if a glucose polymer solution (glucose units linked together) such as polycose (Ross Laboratories, Columbus, Ohio) is used in formulating the drink. The number of particles in solution with polymerized glucose is greatly reduced, thereby facilitating the movement of water from the stomach to the intestines for absorption. *In terms of health and survival, water replacement is of primary concern during prolonged exercise in the heat.*

Summary

The three major categories of foods are composed of the organic elements carbon, hydrogen, and oxygen. The addition of a fourth element, nitrogen, distinguishes the proteins from carbohydrates and fats. These nutrients differ in form and structure depending on the way their atoms are linked or bonded together. In the carbohydrate molecule, atoms of hydrogen and oxygen are bonded to a chain of 6 carbon atoms in a ratio of 2 hydrogen and 1 oxygen for every carbon. Essentially, the more complex carbohydrates, such as starch and the body's carbohydrate store, glycogen, are formed by the union of numerous simple sugar molecules like glucose. In the body, carbohydrates function as fuel to power the vital functions of all cells. This food is manufactured in plants and consumed in the diet in the form of cereals, fruits, potatoes, and breads. It is now apparent that the fibrous materials contained within plants contribute to proper gastrointestinal functioning and may favorably modify blood cholesterol. With fat, relatively large numbers of carbon and hydrogen atoms are packed within the molecule, with only a small number of oxygen atoms. As with carbohydrates, a major function of dietary fat is to supply energy. This energy is important during long-term exercise when the available stores of carbohydrates (glycogen) are reduced. However, various forms of fat serve additional important biologic and health-related functions. These include blood clotting, hormone synthesis, the protection of vital organs, insulation, and the transport of four important vitamins. Fats are found in meats, fish, poultry, and numerous plants; the greatest portion of fat in the American diet comes from animal sources that are generally high in cholesterol and saturated fats, two dietary compounds that contribute to an increased risk of heart disease if consumed in excess for prolonged time periods. It simply is not the one or two "greasy-type" foods that are consumed every once in a while that pose the problem; it's the long term *habits* of poor quality nutrient intake of high cholesterol and saturated fatty foods that is probably at the heart of the problem.

Protein is crucial to normal growth and function of the body, although the energy derived from this food is usually minimal in relation to the body's total energy needs. Protein compounds make up the contractile elements of the muscle fiber. Other proteins provide structural integrity to bones, skin, and the membranes surrounding cells, as well as to the specific structures within cells. Other protein compounds provide the basic materials for synthesizing hormones, enzymes, and the oxygen-carrying compounds contained within the blood and muscles. The protein within animal and plant cells provides the crucial amino acid building blocks necessary for constructing the body's life-sustaining compounds.

Vitamins are relatively simple organic compounds needed in minute quantities if the normal operation of the body is to proceed smoothly. These substances serve as crucial links in many metabolic reactions. A vitamin deficiency over a relatively long time period can cause serious symptoms, including a variety of skin defects, night blindness, stunted growth, bleeding, metabolic disorders, and eventually death. Vitamins are usually classified according to their solubility; vitamins A, D, E, and K are soluble in fats and oils and the B-complex and vitamin C are soluble in water. *Generally, eating a balanced diet provides adequate quantities of all vitamins.* This requirement does not appear to be increased with exercise.

About 4% of a person's body weight is composed of a group of 22 mostly metallic elements called minerals. These minerals form integral parts of hormones, enzymes, and vitamins, as well as providing the major hardening constituents of bones and teeth. Minerals provide for the movement of water between the fluid compartments of the body and are also responsible for the development of electrical gradients across membranes of nerves to permit neural communication. In most cases the minerals lost through sweating can be replaced in the diet and specific supplementation is not required. The mineral iron is a crucial constituent of the oxygen-carrying compound hemoglobin and also, with the mineral copper, serves important functions in the metabolic reactions that generate energy within the cells. Calcium is an important mineral for the synthesis and maintenance of bone. Adequate intake of calcium throughout life, combined with an active lifestyle, helps to protect against the severe bone loss often observed in later life.

For most people, an excess intake of sodium is excreted in the urine. However, the large sodium content of the American diet contributes to elevation of blood pressure to levels that pose a health risk. For these "salt sensitive" individuals, reducing sodium intake can favorably lower blood pressure. As is the case with vitamins, adequate mineral intake is assured with a well-balanced diet.

Water provides the medium in which all the body processes occur. A delicate balance in the volume and salinity of body fluids is maintained through the regulation of thirst and the output of urine by the kidneys. Normally, an adult drinks about 1.2 liters of water each day. In warm environments, however, water is lost in sweat, requiring an increase in fluid intake. This is especially critical during exercise performed in hot, humid environments where the quantity of fluid lost through sweating can increase to 1 liter an hour or more. Under these conditions, if adequate water is not replenished, the body's ability to regulate temperature will fail and serious injury or death will occur. Cool, plain water, consumed both prior to and at frequent intervals during exercise, is the most effective defense against dehydration.

Additional Reading

American College of Sports Medicine: Position statement on prevention of heat injuries during distance running. *Medicine and Science in Sports and Exercise. 16:*1X, 1984.

Anderson, R.A., Polansky, M.M. and N.A. Bryden: Acute effects on chromium, copper, zinc, and selected clinical variables in urine and serum of male runners. *Biological Trace Element Research. 6:*327, 1984.

Block, G. et al.: Nutrient sources in the American diet: quantitative data from the NHANES II survey. *American Journal of Epidemiology. 122:*13, 1985.

Bogert, L.J. et al.: *Nutrition and Physical Fitness.* Philadelphia, W.B. Saunders Co., 1979.

Boland, R.: Role of vitamin D in skeletal muscle function. *Endocrine Reviews. 7:*434, 1986.

Byers, T. and S. Graham: The epidemiology of diet and cancer. *Advances in Cancer Research. 41:*1–69, 1984.

Cann, C.E.: Decreased spinal mineral content in amenorrheic women. *Journal of the American Medical Association. 251:*626, 1984.

Clement, D.B., and Sawchuck, L.L.: Iron status and sports performance. *Sports Medicine. 1:*65, 1984.

Costill, D.L., Dalsky, G.P. and W.J. Fink: Effect of caffeine ingestion on metabolism and exercise performance. *Medicine and Science in Sports and Exercise. 10:*155, 1978.

Costill, D.L. et al.: Dietary potassium and heavy exercise: effects on muscle, water and electrolytes. *American Journal of Clinical Nutrition. 36:*266, 1982.

Deuster, P.A. et al.: Nutritional survey of highly trained women runners. *American Journal of Clinical Nutrition. 44:*954, 1986.

Dwyer, J.: Vegetarianism. *Contemporary Nutrition. 4,* no. 6, 1979.

Gohil, K. et al.: Vitamin E deficiency and vitamin C supplements: exercise and mitochondrial oxidation. *Journal of Applied Physiology. 60:*1986, 1986.

Goodhart, R.S., and M.E. Shils (Eds.): *Modern Nutrition in Health and Disease,* 6th ed., Philadelphia, Lea & Febiger, 1980.

Gordan, G.S. and C. Vaughan: Calcium and osteoporosis. *Journal of Nutrition. 116:* 319, 1986.

Guthrie, H.A.: *Introductory Nutrition.* St. Louis, C.V. Mosby, 1983.

Hoeg, J.M. et al.: An Approach to the Management of Hyperlipoproteinemia. *Journal of the American Medical Association. 255:*512, 1986.

Joffres, M.R. et al.: Relationship of magnesium intake and other dietary factors to blood pressure: the Honolulu heart study. *American Journal of Clinical Nutrition. 45:*469, 1987.

Lipid Research Clinics Program: The Lipid Research Clinics coronary primary prevention trial results. I. Reduction in incidence of coronary heart disease. *Journal of the American Medical Association. 251:*351, 1984.

Mazess, R.B., Harper, A.E. and H. DeLuca: Calcium intake and bone. *American Journal of Clinical Nutrition. 42:*568, 1985.

McArdle, W.D., et al.: Thermal adjustment to cold-water exposure in exercising men and women. *Journal of Applied Physiology. 56:*1572, 1984.

Mensink, R.P. and M.B. Katan: Effect of monounsaturated fatty acids versus complex carbohydrates on high-density lipoproteins in healthy men and women. *Lancet.* Jan. 17, 122, 1987.

Nickerson, H.J. et al.: Decreased iron stores in high school female runners. *American Journal of Diseases of Children. 139:*1115, 1985.

Palumbo, J.D. and G.L. Blackburn: Human protein requirements. *Contemporary Nutrition. 5,* no. 1, 1980.

Parizkova, J., and V.A. Rogozkin: *Nutrition, Physical Fitness and Health.* Baltimore, University Park Press, 1978.

Percy, E.C.: Ergogenic aids in athletes. *Medicine and Science in Sports. 10:*298, 1978.

Reed, P.B.: *Nutrition: An Applied Science.* St. Paul, West Publishing Company, 1980.

Reiser, R.: A critique of universal diet recommendations for prevention of coronary heart disease. *Contemporary Nutrition. 6*(10), 1981.

Riggs, B.L., and Melton, L.J., III.: Involutional Osteoporosis. *New England Journal of Medicine. 314:*1676, 1986.

Rossignol, A.M.: Caffeine-containing beverages and premenstrual syndrome in young women. *American Journal Public Health. 75:*1335, 1985.

Schaumberg, H. et al.: Sensory neuropathy from pyridoxine abuse.: a new megavitamin syndrome. *New England Journal of Medicine. 309:*445, 1983.

Satabin, P. et al.: Metabolic and hormonal response to lipid and carbohydrate diets during exercise in man. *Medicine and Science in Sports and Exercise. 19:*218, 1987.

Scott, M.L.: Advances in our understanding of vitamin E. *Federation Proceedings. 39:*2736, 1980.

Scrimshaw, N.S. and V.R. Young: The requirements of human nutrition. *Scientific American. 235:*50, 1976.

Shekelle, R.B. et al.: Dietary vitamin A and risk of cancer in the Western Electric study. *Lancet. 2:*1186, November 28, 1981.

Sims, L.: Dietary status of lactating women. *Journal of the American Dietetic Association. 73:*139, 1978.

Suter, P.M. and R.M. Russell: Vitamin requirements of the elderly. *American Journal of Clinical Nutrition. 45:*501, 1987.

Tobian, L.: Dietary salt and hypertension. *American Journal of Clinical Nutrition. 32:*2659, 1979.

Vitovsek, S.H.: Is more better? *Nutrition Today. 14:*10, 1979.

Weinhouse, S.: *The role of diet and nutrition in cancer.* Cancer. *58:*1791, 1986.

Wilcox, A.R.: The effects of caffeine and exercise on body weight, fat-pad weight, and fat cell size. *Medicine and Science in Sports and Exercise. 14:*317, 1982.

Willett, W.C.: Dietary fat and the risk of breast cancer. *New England Journal of Medicine. 316:*22, 1987.

Willett, W.C. and B. MacMahon: Diet and cancer. An overview. *New England Journal of Medicine. 310:*633, 697, 1984.

Williams, M.H.: *Nutritional aspects of human physical and athletic performance.* Springfield, Charles C Thomas, 1976.

Williams, P.T. et al.: Relationship of dietary fat, protein, cholesterol, and fiber intake to atherogenic lipoproteins in men. *American Journal of Clinical Nutrition. 44:*788, 1986.

Winston, M.: Diet and coronary heart disease. *Contemporary Nutrition. 6*(9), 1981.

2

Optimal Nutrition for Exercise and Sport

AN OPTIMAL DIET may be defined as one in which the supply of required nutrients is adequate for tissue maintenance, repair, and growth. The general consensus among nutritionists is that active, exercising men and women do not require additional nutrients beyond those obtained in a balanced diet. For example, people who eat well-balanced meals of meats, cereals, vegetables, fruits, and milk consume more than an adequate supply of vitamins to meet daily needs. Because vitamins can be used repeatedly in metabolic reactions, the vitamin needs of athletes and other active people are generally no greater than the requirements of sedentary people. Also, as the level of energy expenditure increases significantly, the amount of food required increases to maintain body weight. Competitive marathon runners, for example, will consume as much as 5,000 calories daily simply to supply the energy required for their daily training. This increase in food intake in itself will usually increase the intake of vitamins and minerals provided the person maintains a well-balanced diet. *In essence, sound nutrition for an active person is sound human nutrition.* The extra calories required for exercise can be obtained from a variety of nutritious foods of the individual's choice. However, sound nutritional guidelines must be followed in planning and evaluating food intake.

Recommended Nutrient Intake

Figure 2-1 illustrates the caloric contributions of the major food components in a balanced diet recommended for active people.

PROTEIN

As discussed in Chapter 1, the standard recommendation for protein intake is 0.8 g of protein per kg of body weight. This amounts to approximately 12% of the

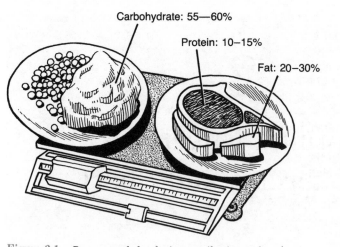
Carbohydrate: 55—60%
Protein: 10–15%
Fat: 20–30%

Figure 2-1. *Recommended caloric contributions of major food components in a balanced diet for active men and women.*

total calories in the average American diet. A person who weighs 170 lb (77.1 kg) would therefore require about 62 g or 2.2 oz of protein daily. This amount of protein is contained in three 8 oz glasses of whole milk and a piece of pizza with beef topping from Pizza Hut, or two lamb chops (10 oz) and a large cup of cream of vegetable soup, or one Burger King Whopper, 2 glasses of whole milk, and 2 scrambled eggs. As you can see, it doesn't require too much food to achieve the daily requirement for protein intake.

It should be noted, however, that the average American consumes more than *twice* the protein requirement. For athletes, many of whom consume considerable quantities of food, the diet may contain more than 3 to 4 times the protein requirement! *There is simply no benefit from consuming excessive protein.* Muscle mass is *not* increased simply by eating high-protein foods. Additional calories in the form of protein are used for energy or converted to fat and stored in the subcutaneous depots. Clearly, one can become fat by eating protein! Furthermore, excessive protein intake may be harmful because the metabolism of large quantities of this nutrient can place an inordinate strain on liver and renal function.

Preparations of Simple Amino Acids. The practice among some weight lifters and body builders of consuming protein in the form of liquids, powders, or pills that have been chemically "predigested" in the laboratory to simple amino acids is a waste of money and may actually be counterproductive in terms of desired outcome. The sales pitch is that the simple amino-acid molecule is absorbed more easily by the body, and in some magical way, becomes available rapidly to facilitate the expected muscle growth brought on by training. *But nothing could be farther from the truth!* Dietary proteins are absorbed by the body when they are part of the more complex di- and tripeptide molecules compared to the simple amino-acid molecule. The intestinal tract is better able to handle protein in its more complex form, whereas a concentrated amino-acid solution draws water into the intestines. This process can cause irritation, cramping, and diarrhea. *Consuming so called "purified amino acids" is NOT the way to add muscle mass.*

FAT

Standards for optimal fat intake have not been firmly established because relatively little is known about the human requirement for this nutrient. The amount of dietary fat varies widely according to personal taste, money spent on food, and the availability of fat-rich foods. For people living in Asia, only about 10% of the energy in the average diet is furnished by fat; in contrast, fat accounts for 40 to 50% of the caloric intake for people living in the United States, Canada, Scandinavia, Germany, and France. Many nutritionists believe that to promote optimal health, fat intake should not exceed 30% of the energy content of the diet. Of this, less than 30% should be in the form of saturated fats. Even this quantity of dietary fat may be too high, especially for those who suffer from gallbladder disease and certain diseases of the cardiovascular system.

To attempt to eliminate "all" fat from the diet, however, may be unwise as well as detrimental to exercise performance. With low-fat diets, it is difficult to increase one's intake of carbohydrate and protein to furnish sufficient energy to maintain a stable body weight during strenuous training. Because the major essential fatty acid, *linoleic acid*, and many vitamins gain entrance to the body through dietary fat, a "fat free" diet could eventually result in a relative state of malnutrition! Fifteen to 25 g of dietary fat on a daily basis is probably the minimal level of fat that should be consumed. It doesn't take long to consume this amount—2 oz of bologna has 16 g, one pork chop has 21 g, and 10 chicken nuggets from McDonalds contain 34 g of fat. If you're the typical American, you consume over 100 g of fat or about 4 oz per day, every day of the year!

CARBOHYDRATE

At this time it is difficult to state precisely how much carbohydrate should be consumed in the diet. Like fat, the prominence of carbohydrates in the diet varies widely throughout the world, depending upon factors such as the availability and relative cost of fat and protein-rich foods. Carbohydrate-rich foods such as grains, starchy roots, and dried peas and beans are usually the cheapest foods in relation to their energy value. In the Far East, carbohydrates (rice) contribute 80% of the total caloric intake, whereas in the United States only about 40 to 50% of the energy requirement comes from carbohydrates. For a sedentary 70-kg person, for example, this amounts to approximately 147 g of carbohydrate per day.

Most evidence suggests there is no health hazard in subsisting chiefly on carbohydrates (starches), provided that the essential amino acids, minerals, and vitamins are also present in the diet. In fact, the diet of the relatively primitive Tarahumara Indians of Mexico is high in complex carbohydrates (75% of calories) and accompanying fiber, and correspondingly low in cholesterol (71 mg/day), fat (12% of calories), and saturated fat (2% of calories). These people are noted for their remarkable physical endurance; they reportedly run distances of up to 200 miles in competitive soccer-type sports events that often last several days! This type of diet may offer health benefits to those who partake of it. Particularly notable among the Tarahumaras is the virtual absence of hypertension, obesity, and death from cardiac and circulatory complications.

If the individual is physically active, the "prudent" diet should contain about 60% of its calories in the form of carbohydrates, predominantly unrefined starches. Because glycogen synthesis is related to dietary carbohydrate, some researchers have recommended increasing the daily intake of carbohydrate to 70% of total calories to prevent the gradual depletion of the body's glycogen stores with successive days of hard training. The specific dietary-exercise techniques for facilitating glycogen storage will be discussed in a following section.

The Four-Food-Group Plan: The Essentials of Good Nutrition

A practical approach to sound nutrition is to categorize foods that make similar nutrient contributions and then provide servings from each category in the daily diet. A key word is *variety.* This can be readily achieved by use of the *Four-Food-Group Plan* (Table 2-1). Adequate nutrition will be assured as long as the recommended number of servings from the variety provided in each group is supplied, and cooking and handling are proper. More of these and other foods can be used as needed for growth, for activity, and for desirable weight. For individuals on meatless diets, a small amount of milk, milk products, or eggs should be included because vitamin B_{12} is only available in foods of animal origin. In fact, if milk and eggs are included in a vegetarian diet ("lacto-ovovegetarian" diet), nutritional quality will be every bit as good as the typical recommended diet that contains meat, fish, and poultry.

Table 2-1. *The Four-Food-Group Plan—the foundation for a good diet.*

FOOD CATEGORY	EXAMPLES	RECOMMENDED DAILY SERVINGS[c]
1. Milk and milk products[a]	Milk, cheese, ice cream, sour cream, yogurt	2[e]
2. Meat and high-protein[b]	meat, fish, poultry, eggs—with dried beans, peas, nuts, or peanut butter as alternatives	2
3. Vegetables and fruits[d]	Dark green or yellow vegetables; citrus fruits or tomatoes	4
4. Cereal and grain food	Enriched breads, cereals, flour, baked goods, or whole-grain products	4

[a]If large quantities of milk are normally consumed, *fortified* skimmed milk should be substituted to reduce the quantity of saturated fats.

[b]Fish, chicken, and high-protein vegetables contain significantly less saturated fats than other protein sources.

[c]A basic serving of meat or fish is usually 100 g or 3.5 oz of edible food; 1 cup (8 oz) milk; 1 oz cheese; ½ cup fruit, vegetables, juice; 1 slice bread; ½ cup cooked cereal or 1 cup ready-to-eat cereal.

[d]One should be rich in vitamin C; at least one every other day rich in vitamin A.

[e]Children, teenagers, and pregnant and nursing women—4 servings.

Table 2-2. *Four daily menus formulated from guidelines established by the Four-Food-Group Plan.*[a]

3 MEALS A DAY	5 MEALS A DAY	6 SMALL MEALS A DAY	3 MEALS, 3 SNACKS
Breakfast ½ cup unsweetened grapefruit juice 1 poached egg 1 slice toast 1 teaspoon butter or margarine ½ cup skim milk tea or coffee, black Lunch 2 ounces lean roast beef* ½ cup cooked summer squash 1 slice rye bread 1 teaspoon butter or margarine 1 cup skim milk 10 grapes Dinner 3 ounces poached haddock* ½ cup cooked spinach tomato and lettuce salad 1 teaspoon oil + vinegar or lemon 1 small biscuit 1 teaspoon butter or margarine ½ cup canned drained fruit cocktail ½ cup skim milk	Breakfast ½ grapefruit ⅔ cup bran flakes 1 cup skim or low-fat milk or other beverage Snack 1 small package raisins ½ bologna sandwich Lunch 1 slice pizza carrot sticks 1 apple 1 cup skim or low-fat milk Snack 1 banana Dinner baked fish with mushrooms (3 oz.)* baked potato 2 teaspoons margarine ½ cup broccoli 1 cup tomato juice or skim or low-fat milk	Breakfast ½ cup orange juice ¾ cup ready-to-eat cereal ½ cup skim milk tea or coffee, black Mid-Morning Snack ⅓ cup low fat cottage cheese Lunch 2 ounces sliced turkey on 1 slice white toast 1 teaspoon butter or margarine 2 canned drained peach halves ½ cup skim milk Mid-Afternoon Snack 1 cup fresh spinach and lettuce salad 2 teaspoons oil + vinegar or lemon 3 saltines Dinner 1 cup clear broth 3 ounces broiled chicken breast* ⅓ cup cooked rice with 1 teaspoon butter or margarine ¼ cup cooked mushrooms ½ cup cooked broccoli ½ cup skim milk Evening Snack 1 medium apple ½ cup skim milk	Breakfast ½ small grapefruit 1 cup cereal, such as Wheaties 1 cup skim milk 3 teaspoons sugar 2 slices toast 2 pats butter 1 tablespoon jelly, coffee or tea Lunch 3 ounces hamburger* 1 bun slice lettuce & tomato 20 french fries 1 medium banana 1 cup milk Dinner 6 ounces baked chicken (no skin)* 1 medium baked potato ½ cup cooked carrots 2 dinner rolls 2 pats butter 1 cup fresh fruit cup 1 cup milk coffee or tea Snacks: (morning, afternoon, evening) 1 sweet roll or doughnut 1 cup fruit juice sandwich 2 slices bread, whole wheat 1 slice ham mustard 1 cup milk
Total Calories: about 1200	Total calories: about 1400	Total Calories: about 1200	Total Calories: about 3000[b]

*Cooked weight.

[a]Each menu provides *all* essential nutrients; the energy or caloric value of the diet can be easily increased by increasing the size of the portions, the frequency of meals, or the variety of foods consumed at each sitting.

[b]3000 kcal diet from *Food in Training*, General Mills, Inc., Minneapolis.

The Four-Food-Group Plan guidelines provide for the necessary vitamin, mineral, and protein requirements even though the energy content of this food intake amounts to only about 1200 calories per day. In terms of average values for adult Americans, the total daily energy requirement is about 2100 calories for women and 2700 calories for men. *Once the basic nutrient requirements are met, the extra energy needs of the active person can be supplied from a variety of food sources based on individual preference.*

Table 2-2 presents examples of three daily menus formulated from the guidelines of the basic diet plan shown in Table 2-1. These menus provide all of the essential nutrients, even though the energy value of each is considerably below the average adult requirement. In fact, these menus can serve as excellent nutritional models for reducing diets. For active individuals whose daily energy requirements may be as large as 5000 calories, all that need be done once the essentials are provided is to increase the quantity of food consumed; this is achieved either by increasing the size of portions, the frequency of meals or snacks, or the variety of nutritious food consumed at each meal.

Computerized Meal Plans

Nutritionists and exercise specialists have applied computer technology in the formulation of well-balanced meals and exercise programs for weight control. The creation of daily menus is based on the Four Food Group Plan and dietary exchange method developed by the Amercian Dietetic Association. Rather than prescribing a particular food plan, the computerized dietary plan allows the person to select the specific foods they will eat from a basic list of the most common foods. Combined with age, weight, height, weight loss desired, and current level of physical activity, the computer prepares three nutritious meals for breakfast, lunch, and dinner for a 14-day period. The menu varies from day to day. The meals are balanced for nutrient intake of carbohydrate, fat, protein, vitamins and minerals, and are designed so the individual can reduce excess weight (fat) at a safe but steady level. The 15 to 18 page printout includes a weight loss curve, daily meal plans, and a beginner, intermediate, or advanced aerobic walk/jog/run, cycle, or swim program. Appendix A shows examples of the nutrition and exercise computer printout, as well as the questionnaire that can be completed and mailed for your own personal use.

Diet and Endurance Performance

The specific nutrient fuel for muscular contraction depends not only on exercise intensity, but also on the duration of the activity and, to some degree, on the fitness and diet of the individual. During continuous, moderate exercise the energy for muscular contraction is provided predominantly from the body's fat and carbohydrate reserves. If exercise continues and glycogen stores in the liver and muscles are reduced, an even greater percentage of the energy for exercise must be supplied by the breakdown of fat. This food nutrient is mobilized from storage sites such as adipose tissue and the liver and delivered via the circulation to the working muscles. However, if exercise is performed to the point where the glycogen stored in specific muscles is severely lowered, the performer may tire easily. Endurance athletes commonly refer to this sensation of fatigue as "hitting the wall." Interestingly, glycogen is reduced *only* in the muscles that are actively involved in performing the exercise. Because enzymes are not present to aid the transfer of glycogen between muscles, the relatively inactive muscles retain their glycogen supply.

Fatigue can occur during prolonged exercise even though sufficient oxygen is available to the muscles and the potential energy from stored fat remains almost unlimited. This is because the relatively small amount of glycogen stored in the muscles becomes depleted. If a solution of glucose and water is ingested at the point of fatigue, exercise may be prolonged for an additional period of time, but for all practical purposes the muscles' "fuel tank" will read empty and continued energy production is severely limited.

CARBOHYDRATE NEEDS IN INTENSE TRAINING

Strenuous endurance training such as distance running, swimming, cross-country skiing, or cycling can bring on a state of fatigue, whereby successive days of hard training become exceedingly more difficult. This "staleness" may be related to a gradual depletion of the body's carbohydrate reserves with repeated strenuous training, even though the person's diet contains the typical percentage of carbohydrate. Figure 2-2 shows that after three successive days of running 16.1 km

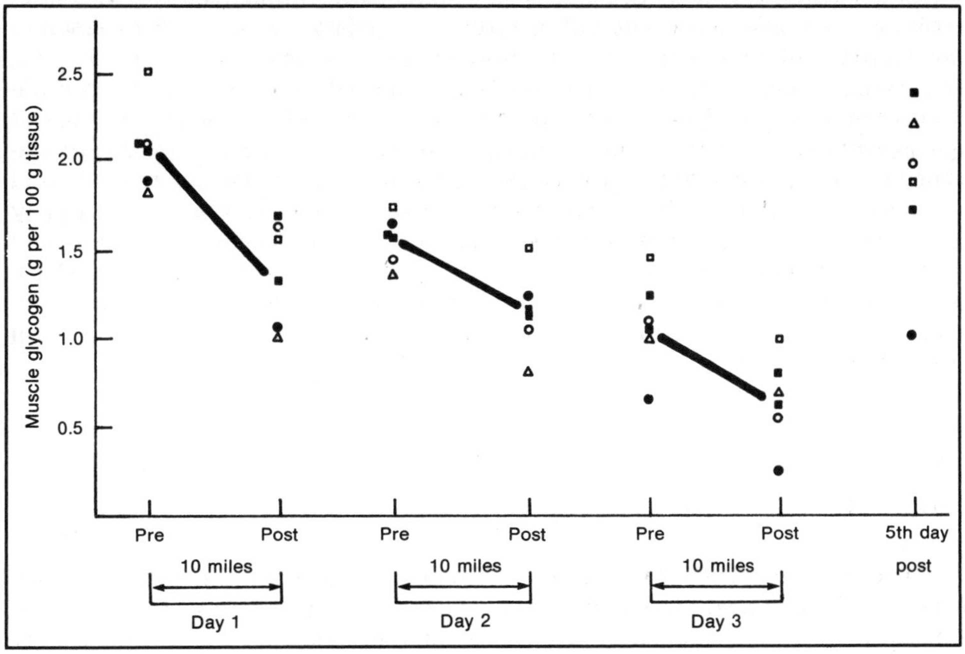
Muscle glycogen (g per 100 g tissue)
2.5
2.0
1.5
1.0
0.5
Pre
Post
Pre
Post
Pre
Post
5th day
post
10 miles
10 miles
10 miles
Day 1
Day 2
Day 3

Figure 2-2. *Changes in muscle glycogen concentration for 6 male subjects before and after each 16.1 km run performed on 3 successive days. Muscle glycogen was measured 5 days after the last run and is referred to as "fifth day post."*

(10 miles) a day, the glycogen in the thigh muscle was nearly depleted. This occurred although the runners' daily food intake contained 40 to 50% carbohydrates. By the third day, the quantity of glycogen used during the run was much less than the first day, with the energy for work supplied predominantly by the body's fat reserves. When dietary carbohydrate was increased to 70% of caloric intake (500 to 600 g/day), glycogen depletion was not evident with hard training.

If glycogen becomes severely depleted, it is not rapidly restored. Although liver glycogen is restored rapidly, at least 48 hours are required to restore muscle glycogen levels after prolonged, exhaustive exercise. From the values displayed in Figure 2-2, some individuals may require more than 5 days to reestablish muscle glycogen levels if the diet contains only a moderate amount of carbohydrate. Unmistakably, if a person performs long-term, strenuous exercise on successive days, daily allowances must be adjusted to permit optimal glycogen resynthesis. *In addition, at least 2 days of rest and high carbohydrate intake must be provided to establish optimal muscle glycogen levels.*

DIET, GLYCOGEN STORES, AND ENDURANCE

In the late 1930s scientists observed that endurance performance improved significantly simply by consuming a carbohydrate-rich diet for 3 days. Conversely, endurance capability was drastically reduced if the diet consisted predominantly of fat. Because of this important relationship between diet and physical performance, researchers have evaluated several possible ways of increasing the glycogen content of muscle. In one series of experiments, subjects consumed three different diets. One diet maintained the normal caloric intake but supplied the major quantity of calories in the form of fat. The second diet was normal and contained the recommended daily percentages of carbohydrates, fats, and proteins. The third diet provided 82% of the calories as carbohydrates. The results showed that the glycogen content sampled from the leg muscles of subjects fed the high-fat diet, the normal diet and the high-carbohydrate diet averaged 0.6, 1.75, and 3.75 g of glycogen per 100 g of muscle, respectively. In addition, the endurance capacity of the subjects varied considerably depending on the diet each consumed in the days *prior* to the endurance test. The endurance capacity of the subjects fed the high-carbohydrate diet was more than three times greater than the endurance capacity of these same subjects on the high-fat diet. *Clearly, these findings emphasize the important role of nutrition in establishing the appropriate energy reserves.* A diet deficient in carbohydrates rapidly depletes muscle and liver glycogen, and subsequently affects performance in intense, short-term anaerobic exercise, as well as in prolonged, submaximal aerobic endurance activities. These observations are important not only for the athlete, but for people who modify their diets and consume less than the recommended quantity of carbohydrate.

Reliance on starvation diets or other potentially harmful practices such as high-fat, low-carbohydrate diets, "liquid-protein" diets, or water diets, is counterproductive for weight control, exercise performance, optimal nutrition, and good health. *Low carbohydrate diets make it extremely difficult from the standpoint of energy supply to participate in quality vigorous physical activity or training.*

Sugary Drinks Before and During Exercise: A Wise Solution?

During exercise. Carbohydrate drinks consumed at regular intervals *during* exercise benefit performance in both moderate and relatively high intensity aerobic exercise. Supplementary carbohydrate helps to maintain blood sugar level and augments the glucose available for use by the exercising muscle. Consequently, muscle glycogen is spared because the ingested glucose is used as fuel to power exercise. During low intensity exercise, the beneficial effect of carbohydrate feeding is negligible because this level of aerobic exercise is fueled mainly by the breakdown of fat with little drain on carbohydrate reserves.

A variety of carbohydrate drinks are commercially available, yet none is more effective than a glucose or sucrose mixture. Sugar drinks usually range between an isotonic 5% solution that can be made by adding 50 g of either glucose, fructose, or sucrose to 1 liter of water, to a 25 to 50% concentrated solution. One practical recommendation is to ingest a strong 50% sugar solution (70 g of sugar in 140 ml of water) 20 to 30 minutes after the start of exercise, followed by less concentrated 10% solutions at 20-minute intervals. Of course, fluid replacement is of prime concern when exercising in warm weather. *In this regard, plain, cool water is the beverage of choice.* If sugar is used it should be in polymerized form (see pages 33–34).

Before exercise. The benefits of sugar drinks occur *only* when they are consumed during exercise. In fact, drinking a strong sugar solution 30 to 60 minutes prior to exercise actually hinders endurance capacity. For example, the riding time of young men and women on an exercise bicycle was reduced nearly 20% when they consumed a 25% glucose solution 30 minutes before exercising, compared to similar exercise preceded by drinking the same volume of water. Concentrated sugar drinks consumed before exercise cause blood sugar to rise dramatically within 5 to 10 minutes. This leads to an overshoot in the release of *insulin* (a hormone that regulates blood sugar) from the pancreas that actually produces a decline in blood sugar *(hypoglycemia)* as glucose moves rapidly into the muscle cells. At the same time, insulin inhibits the utilization of fat for energy. Consequently, carbohydrate is used for energy when exercise begins to a much greater degree than under normal conditions. Thus, glycogen depletion and fatigue occur earlier than would normally be the case.

Carbohydrate Loading: A Way to Increase Glycogen Reserves

Research has shown that a particular combination of diet and exercise can result in a significant "packing" of muscle glycogen. This procedure is termed *carbohydrate loading* and is commonly in vogue among endurance athletes. The end result of this specific dietary modification is an even greater increase in muscle glycogen than would occur with a carbohydrate-rich diet. The classic procedure for carbohydrate loading outlined in Table 2-3 is accomplished as follows: First, the glycogen stores are reduced with a period of relatively long, moderate, continuous, exercise. Second, muscle glycogen is further depleted by maintaining a high-fat, low-carbohydrate diet (60 to 120 g carbohydrate) for several days while continuing a moderate exercise program. Third, the activity level is reduced for the next several days and at the same time, a switch is made to a carbohydrate-rich diet (500 to 600 g carbohydrate). With this procedure, the muscle glycogen increases to a new, higher level. Of course, adequate daily protein, minerals and

Table 2-3. *Two-stage dietary plan for increasing muscle glycogen storage.*

Stage 1—Depletion

Day 1: Exhausting exercise performed to deplete muscle glycogen in specific muscles

Days 2, 3, 4: Low carbohydrate food intake (high percentage of protein and fat in the daily diet) and moderate training

Stage 2—Carbohydrate Loading

Days 5, 6, 7: High complex carbohydrate food intake (normal percentage of protein and fat in the daily diet) with low-level exercise or rest

Competition Day

Follow high-carbohydrate pre-event meal

vitamins, and abundant water must also be part of the daily diet. We should emphasize that if a person eats a normal mixed diet that contains 50% of calories from carbohydrate (instead of the high-fat, low-carbohydrate diet in that segment of the classic carbohydrate loading routine), nearly the same high level of glycogen storage can be achieved.

Because glycogen loading occurs *only* in the specific muscles exercised, the person must engage the muscles involved in their sport. In preparation for a marathon, a 15- or 20-mile run is usually necessary; for swimming and bicycling, 90-minutes of moderately intense submaximal exercise would be required.

The combination of diet and exercise to produce glycogen packing or "supercompensation" should be of considerable interest to the serious endurance athlete whose success depends in part on the magnitude of the body's carbohydrate reserves. *For those who are not endurance athletes, or for those involved in activities less than 75 minutes in duration, normal levels of muscle glycogen are more than adequate to provide the energy to sustain exercise.* Normal levels of glycogen can be assured by ingesting approximately 60% of the daily caloric intake as carbohydrates. If the energy demands of daily exercise are high, as in an intensive exercise-training program, the carbohydrate content of the diet should be increased. Many endurance athletes consume so-called "spaghetti and rice" diets to achieve a high level of carbohydrate intake. A week before the actual competition, they use the preceding three-step exercise and dietary modification program to assure the desired glycogen supercompensation.

It should be noted that the wisdom of repeated bouts of carbohydrate loading has yet to be verified. A severe carbohydrate overload interspersed with periods of high fat or protein intake could pose problems to people susceptible to adult diabetes or heart or kidney disease. For this reason, the less-stringent modified approach to carbohydrate loading is an attractive option.

SAMPLE DIETS FOR CARBOHYDRATE LOADING

Table 2-4 provides an example of meal plans that can be used during carbohydrate depletion (Stage 1) and carbohydrate loading (Stage 2) that precede the endurance event.

The Precompetition Meal

The main purpose of the precompetition or pregame meal is to provide the athlete with adequate food energy and assure optimal hydration. As a general rule, foods that are high in fat and protein content should be eliminated from the diet on the day of competition. These foods are digested slowly and remain in the

Table 2-4. *Sample meal plan for carbohydrate depletion and carbohydrate loading diets preceding the endurance event.*[a]

MEAL	STAGE 1 DEPLETION	STAGE 2 CARBOHYDRATE LOADING
Breakfast:	½ cup fruit juice 2 eggs 1 slice whole-wheat toast 1 glass whole milk	1 cup fruit juice, hot or cold cereal 1 to 2 muffins 1 tbsp. butter coffee (cream/sugar)
Lunch:	6-oz hamburger* 2 slices bread salad 1 tbsp. mayonnaise & salad dressing 1 glass whole milk	2–3-oz hamburger* with bun 1 cup juice 1 orange 1 tbsp. mayonnaise pie or cake
Snack:	1 cup yogurt	1 cup yogurt, fruit or cookies
Dinner:	2 to 3 pieces chicken, fried 1 baked potato with sour cream ½ cup vegetable iced tea (no sugar) 2 tbsp. butter	1–1½ pieces chicken, baked 1 baked potato with sour cream 1 cup vegetable ½ cup sweetened pineapple iced tea (sugar) 1 tbsp. butter
Snack:	1 glass whole milk	1 glass chocolate milk with 4 cookies

*Cooked weight

[a]During stage 1, the intake of carbohydrate is approximately 100 g or 400 calories; in stage 2, the carbohydrate intake is increased to 400 to 625 g or about 1600 to 2500 calories.

digestive tract for a longer time than carbohydrate rich foods that contain similar amounts of energy.

The time of eating the precompetition meal is not too important in terms of exercise performance. Because the main function of the pregame meal is to provide food energy and water, a 3-hour period is adequate for the meal to be digested and absorbed by the body.

Many athletes are psychologically accustomed and even depend on the "classic" pregame meal of steak and eggs. Although this meal may be satisfying to the athlete, coach, and restauranteur, its benefits have never been demonstrated in terms of exercise performance. In fact, a meal actually so low in carbohydrates may impair optimal performance. For one thing, carbohydrates are digested and absorbed more rapidly than either proteins or fats. This food is therefore available for energy faster and may also reduce the feeling of fullness following a meal. Furthermore, a high-protein meal elevates the resting metabolism more than a high-carbohydrate meal. The heat production may place an additional strain on the body's temperature-regulating ability that could be detrimental to exercise performance in hot weather. Concurrently, the breakdown of protein for energy facilitates dehydration because the by-products of amino acid breakdown demand large amounts of water for urinary excretion.

Carbohydrate intake is favored as the main nutrient energy source for intense exercise and is also of crucial importance in prolonged exercise. *The precompetition meal must provide adequate quantities of this nutrient to assure a normal level of blood glucose and sufficient glycogen "energy reserves" for most activities.* This presumes the person has maintained a nutritionally sound diet throughout training.

Summary

Many dietary options are available for obtaining the required nutrients for tissue maintenance, repair, and growth. Within rather broad limits, the nutrient requirements of active individuals engaged in training programs can be achieved with a balanced diet. With well-planned menus, the necessary vitamin, mineral, and protein requirements can be achieved with a food intake of about 1200 calories a day. Additional food can then be consumed to meet the fluctuating energy needs that depend on the daily level of physical activity. The use of a computer to prepare nutritious meals, based on individual food choices, can play an important role in weight management and dietary control programs designed to reduce excess body fat.

The recommended protein intake is 0.8 g of protein per kg of body weight. For the average non-dieting man and woman, this is a liberal requirement and represents about 12 to 15% of the daily total caloric intake. Athletes generally consume 3 times the recommended protein intake. This is because the proportionately greater caloric intake of physically active people usually provides proportionately more protein.

Precise recommendations for fat and carbohydrate intake have not been firmly established. A prudent recommendation is that 20 to 30% of the daily calories be obtained from fats; of this, at least 70% should be in the form of unsaturated fatty acids because excessive intake of saturated fats is related to various diseases, particularly coronary heart disease. For people who are physically active, 50 to 60% of the calories should come from unrefined complex carbohydrates. With the typical American diet, successive days of prolonged, hard training may gradually deplete the body's carbohydrate reserves. This could lead to a training "staleness" because restoration of muscle glycogen may take several days to return to normal following a single session of prolonged exercise.

Sugary drinks consumed prior to exercise hinder long-term endurance capacity. When consumed during exercise, these drinks facilitate performance by maintaining blood sugar levels and perhaps delaying the depletion of liver and muscle glycogen. These drinks, however, have been shown to retard water uptake and could upset the body's fluid balance.

The precompetition meal should include foods that are readily digested, as well as contribute to the energy and fluid requirements of exercise. For this reason, the meal should be high in carbohydrate and relatively low in fat and protein. Clearly, the typical low-carbohdrate "steak-and-eggs diet" does not meet the requirements for optimal pre-event nutrition. Two or 3 hours should be sufficient time to permit digestion and absorption of the pre-event meal.

Additional Reading

Barnett, D.W. and R.K. Conless: The effects of a commercial dietary supplement on human performance. *American Journal of Clinical Nutrition. 40:*586, 1984.

Bentivegna, A. et al.: Diet, fitness and athletic performance. *The Physician and Sports Medicine. 7:*99, 1979.

Blair, S.N. et al.: Comparison of nutrient intake in middle-aged men and women runners and controls. *Medicine and Science in Sports and Exercise. 13:*310, 1981.

Buskirk, E.R.: Some nutritional considerations in the conditioning of athletes. *Annual Review of Nutrition. 1:*319, 1981.

Conlee, R.K.: Muscle glycogen and exercise endurance: A twenty year perspective, In: *Exercise and Sport Sciences Reviews.* Edited by K.B. Pandolf, New York, N.Y., Macmillan Publishing, 1987.

Connor, W.E. et al.: The plasma lipids, lipoproteins, and diet of the Tarahumara Indians of Mexico. *American Journal of Clinical Nutrition. 31:*1131, 1978.

Costill, D.L.: Nutritional requirements for endurance athletes, In: *Toward an Understanding of Human Performance.* Edited by E.J. Burke, Ithaca, N.Y., Mouvement Publications, 1977.

Coyle, E.F., et al.: Muscle glycogen utilization during prolonged strenuous exercise when fed carbohydrates. *Journal of Applied Physiology. 61:*165, 1986.

Girandola, R.N. et al.: Effects of pangmic acid (B-15) ingestion on metabolic response to exercise. *Biochemical Medicine. 24:*218, 1980.

Hickson, J.F. et al.: Nutritional profile of football athletes eating from a training table. *Nutrition Research. 7:*27, 1987.

Horwitt, M.D.: Interpretations of requirements for thiamin, riboflavin, niacin-tryptophan, and vitamin E plus comments on balance studies and vitamin B-6. *American Journal of Clinical Nutrition. 44:*973, 1986.

Katch, F.I. and V.L. Katch: Computer technology to evaluate body composition, nutrition, and exercise. *Preventive Medicine. 12:*619, 1983.

LeBlanc, J. et al.: Enhanced metabolic response to caffeine in exercise-trained human subjects. *Journal of Applied Physiology. 59:*832, 1985.

Lemon, P.W.R. and F.J. Nagle: Effects of exercise on protein and amino acid metabolism. *Medicine and Science in Sports and Exercise. 13:*141, 1981.

Percy, E.C.: Ergogenic aids in athletics. *Medicine and Science in Sports. 10:*298, 1978.

Sherman, W.N., and Costill, D.L.: The marathon: dietary manipulation to optimize performance. *American Journal of Sports Medicine. 12:*44, 1984.

Stare, F.J.: Nutrition-sense and nonsense. *Postgraduate Medicine 67:*147, 1980.

Van Dam, B.: Vitamins and Sports. *British Journal of Sports Medicine. 12:*74, 1978.

3

Energy Systems for Exercise

Part 1. Energy for Exercise

IN AN AUTOMOBILE ENGINE, the proper mixture of gasoline with oxygen ignites to provide the necessary energy to drive the pistons. Various gears and linkages harness this energy to turn the wheels. *Within this framework energy can be viewed as the capacity or ability to do work.* Increasing or decreasing the energy supply either slows down or speeds up the engine. Similarly, the human body must continuously be supplied with its own form of energy to perform its many complex functions. Aside from the energy required for muscle contraction, people expend considerable energy for other forms of biologic work. This includes the energy required for the digestion, absorption, and assimilation of the food nutrients, for the functioning of various glands that secrete special hormones at rest and during exercise, for the establishment of the proper electrochemical gradients along the cell membrane to permit transmission of signals from the brain via the nerves to the muscles, and for the synthesis of new chemical compounds, such as the protein in muscle tissue that becomes enlarged from specialized strength training. The story of how the body maintains its continuous supply of energy begins with the energy currency, ATP.

The Energy Currency, Adenosine Triphospate (ATP)

The trillions of cells in the body do not use the nutrients consumed in the diet for their immediate supply of energy. Instead, an energy-rich compound called *adenosine triphosphate*, or simply *ATP*, is the "fuel" used for *all* the energy-requiring processes within the cell. In turn, the energy in food is extracted to rebuild

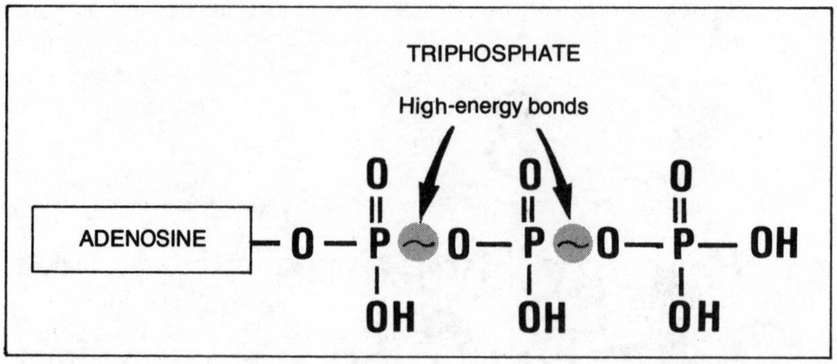
TRIPHOSPHATE
High-energy bonds
ADENOSINE
O — P ~ O — P ~ O — P — OH
O
O
O
OH
OH
OH

Figure 3-1. *Simplified structure of ATP, the energy currency of the cell. The symbol ~ represents the high-energy bonds.*

more ATP. The potential energy stored in the ATP molecule represents chemical energy made in the body as it is needed. As discussed in Chapter 1, molecules are composed of atoms held together by bonds. It is the breaking of these bonds that releases energy. Figure 3-1 illustrates a simplified structure of an ATP molecule.

ATP consists of one molecule of adenine and ribose, called *adenosine,* combined with three phosphates, each consisting of phosphorus and oxygen atoms. A considerable quantity of energy is stored in the ATP molecule at the bonds that link the two outermost phosphate groups with the remainder of the molecule. These bonds, symbolized by ~, represent the high-energy phosphate bonds. When the outermost bond is broken, it releases energy that can be used to power biologic work. The remaining molecule with one high-energy bond is known as *adenosine diphosphate,* or ADP.

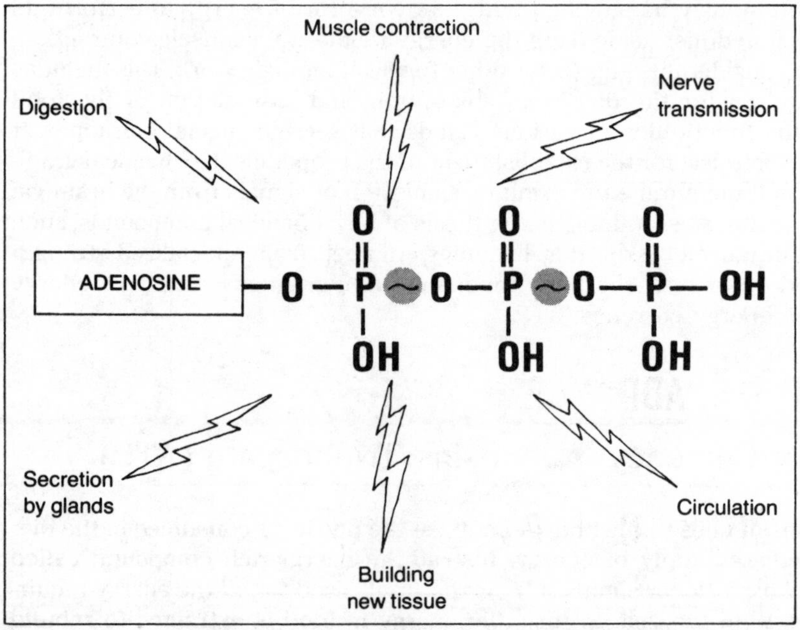
Muscle contraction
Digestion
Nerve transmission
ADENOSINE
O — P ~ O — P ~ O — P — OH
O
O
O
OH
OH
OH
Secretion by glands
Circulation
Building new tissue

Figure 3-2. *ATP is the energy currency for all forms of biologic work.*

The energy released from the breakdown of ATP activates other energy-requiring molecules. For example, the energy from ATP is transferred to the molecules that make up the contractile elements in muscle tissue. Once activated, these elements slide past each other and cause the muscle to shorten. Because the energy released from ATP is harnessed to power all forms of biologic work, ATP is considered the "energy currency" of the cell (Figure 3-2).

Energy-releasing reactions that depend on a constant supply of oxygen are *aerobic.* For example, if the flow of oxygen through the carburetor of an automobile engine is restricted, the energy supply is reduced and the engine will lose power and ultimately stall. This is not the case, however, with the breakdown of ATP. Instead, the ATP molecule releases its energy in the absence of oxygen. This is an *anaerobic* energy-releasing reaction. The capacity to provide energy anaerobically enables the cell to generate energy for immediate use. This immediate energy would not be available if oxygen was required at all times. For this reason we can sprint for a bus, lift considerable weight without taking a breath, and survive submersion under water for more than 1 minute.

The Energy Reservoir, Creatine Phosphate (CP)

Although ATP serves as the energy currency for all cells, its quantity is limited. In fact, only about 3 oz of ATP are stored in the body at any one time. This would provide only enough energy for running as fast as possible for several seconds. Therefore, ATP must constantly be resynthesized to provide a continuous supply of energy. Some of the energy for ATP resynthesis is supplied directly and rapidly by the anaerobic splitting of a phosphate molecule from another energy-rich compound called *creatine phosphate,* or *CP.* This molecule is similar to ATP because a large amount of energy is released when the bond is split between the creatine and phosphate molecules. Figure 3-3 presents a schematic illustration of the release and use of phosphate-bond energy in ATP and CP.

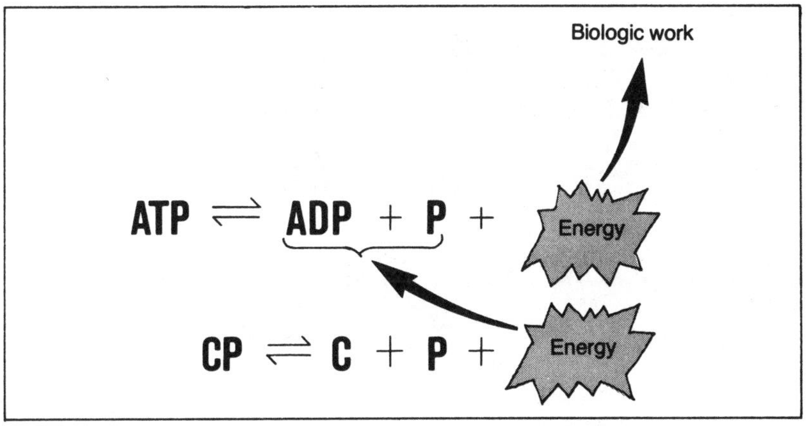
Biologic work
ATP ⇌ ADP + P +
Energy
CP ⇌ C + P +
Energy

Figure 3-3. *ATP and CP are anaerobic sources of phosphate bond energy. The energy from the breakdown of CP is used to rebond ADP and P to form ATP.*

The arrows point in opposite directions to indicate that the reactions are reversible. That is, creatine (C) and phosphate (P) can be joined again to form CP. The same is true for ATP, shown in the top reaction, where the union of ADP and P reforms ATP. The resynthesis of ATP occurs if sufficient energy is available to rejoin an ADP molecule with one P molecule. The breakdown of CP can supply this energy, as is illustrated in the bottom reaction. Cells store creatine phosphate in considerably larger quantities than ATP. Its mobilization for energy is almost instantaneous and does not require oxygen. For this reason, CP is considered the "reservoir" of high energy phosphate.

The energy released from the breakdown of the energy-rich phosphates ATP and CP will sustain all-out exercise such as running or swimming for approximately 5 to 8 seconds. In the 100-yard dash, the body cannot maintain maximum speed for longer than this. During the last few seconds of this sprint race, the runners are actually slowing down, and the winner is the one who slows down least! Thus, the mobilization of energy from the phosphate pool (ATP + CP), and the size of the pool, may be important factors that determine a person's ability to maintain maximum speed over a short distance.

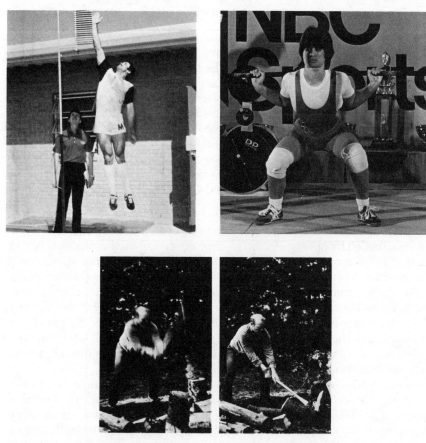

To gain an appreciation of the relative importance of the high-energy phos-

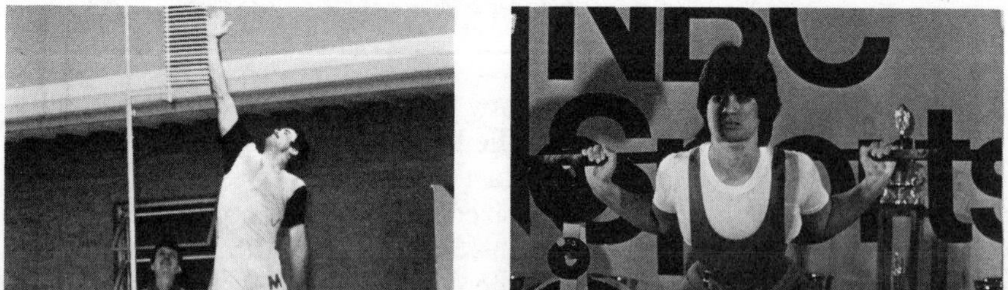

Figure 3-4. ***Importance of the high energy phosphates ATP and CP during physical activity.***

phates in exercise, consider the activities where short but intense bursts of energy are crucial to successful performance. Football, tennis, track and field, golf, volleyball, field hockey, baseball, weightlifting, and wood chopping are but a few activities that may require a maximal effort for up to 8 seconds during the performance (Figure 3-4).

In almost all sports, the capacity of the ATP-CP energy system can play an important role in the success or failure of some phase of the performance. If the all-out effort must continue longer than 8 seconds, or if moderate exercise is to continue for much longer periods, an additional source of energy must be provided for the resynthesis of ATP. If this does not happen, our "fuel tanks" would read "empty" and all movement would cease. *The foods we eat and store in ready access within the body provide the energy to recharge the supply of ATP and CP.*

The identification of the predominant sources of energy required for a particular sport or activity provides the basis for an effective physiologic conditioning program. If one desires an improved capacity for sustained effort such as hiking or distance swimming, for example, it would be unprofitable to train specifically to increase the ATP-CP reserves. On the other hand, a highly conditioned ATP-CP energy system is of considerable importance in sports such as football and baseball.

Energy from Food

As shown in Figure 3-5, the body extracts the potential energy stored within the structure of the carbohydrate, fat, and protein molecules consumed in the diet or stored within the body. *This energy is harnessed for one major purpose—to combine ADP and phosphate to reform the energy-rich compound ATP.*

A flaming steak on an open barbecue is a good illustration of the potential energy stored in food. The heat from the flame ignites the fat in the meat, causing it to suddenly release its stored energy in the form of heat. In the cells of the body, however, the energy is not released suddenly at some kindling temperature and then dissipated as heat. The energy produced by the breaking of chemical bonds is released gradually, at a constant, fairly low temperature through a series of chemical reactions controlled by special *enzymes.* Enzymes regulate the rate or speed of the reactions by helping to bring different molecules together so they interact and bond to one another. Thousands of chemical reactions take place simultaneously within the cell, each governed by a specific enzyme. The end product of the breakdown of foods is the liberation of energy, of which approximately 40% is captured and stored for later use as chemical energy in the bonds of ATP. The remaining energy is dissipated in the form of heat. This is an incredible efficiency compared with machines like the steam engine that transforms its fuel into useful energy with an efficiency of only about 30%.

ATP is made available from food in several ways. The metabolism of glucose illustrates the way the cells extract and capture the chemical energy contained in foods. This example is used for several reasons. First, carbohydrates are the *only* foods that can provide energy anaerobically for the formation of ATP. During heavy, fatiguing exercise where anaerobic reactions must supply a large amount of energy rapidly, carbohydrates are the main contributor to the energy supply. Sec-

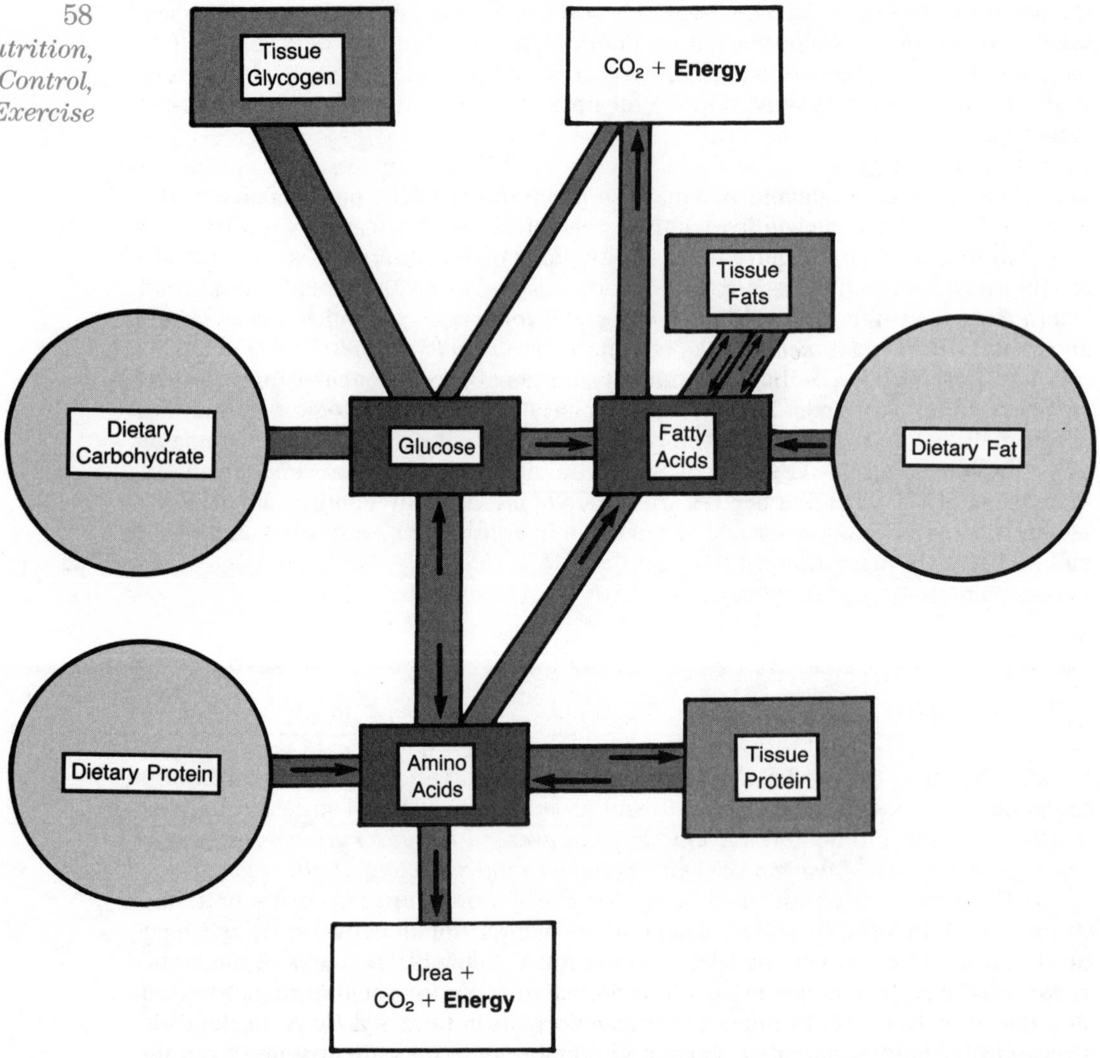
Tissue Glycogen
CO_2 + **Energy**
Tissue Fats
Dietary Carbohydrate
Glucose
Fatty Acids
Dietary Fat
Dietary Protein
Amino Acids
Tissue Protein
Urea + CO_2 + **Energy**

Figure 3-5. *The interlocking pathways of energy generation from the foods ingested or from the body's own resources.*

ond, under conditions of rest and low to moderate levels of exercise in well-nourished individuals, carbohydrates supply between 40 and 50% of the body's energy requirements. Third, during the breakdown of carbohydrates certain chemical compounds are formed so the fat and protein food nutrients can also be degraded or metabolized to supply energy.

ANAEROBIC ENERGY FROM FOOD

When a molecule of glucose enters a cell to be used for energy, it immediately undergoes a series of chemical reactions collectively referred to as *glycolysis*. These reactions do not require oxygen and are thus termed *anaerobic*. As a result of enzyme action, the original 6-carbon glucose molecule is transformed into two

3-carbon molecules of pyruvic acid. The breakdown of glucose to pyruvic acid occurs in the intracellular, watery medium of the cell. Three important aspects to the breakdown of glucose to pyruvic acid occur during glycolysis. First, the bonds that chemically bind the glucose molecule together are broken; second, hydrogen atoms are stripped away from the glucose molecule; and third, two new molecules of ATP are produced.

The extraction of usable energy in the form of two ATP molecules during the anaerobic reactions of glycolysis represents only about 5% of the total number of ATPs produced when the glucose molecule is completely degraded to carbon dioxide and water during subsequent aerobic reactions. Nevertheless, *ATP production during glycolysis is important because it provides a rapid, though limited, source of energy for muscular activity.* The cells' capacity to maintain glycolysis is crucial during physical activities that require a sustained, all-out effort for periods of up to about 60 seconds. The anaerobic energy from glucose can be thought of as a reserve of "rapid" food energy for the resynthesis of ATP. An example of this energy reserve is utilized by the athlete "kicking" the last part of a 1- or 2-mile race, or the basketball team that employs a full-court press during the final minutes of a close game. In other short-duration but high-intensity activities such as a 440-yard run or 100-yard swim, the predominant supply of energy for ATP production also comes from the anaerobic reactions of glycolysis during carbohydrate metabolism.

AEROBIC ENERGY FROM FOOD

Because the anaerobic reactions of glycolysis release only about 5% of the energy contained within the glucose molecule, an additional means must be available for extracting the remaining energy. It is extracted when the pyruvic acid molecules are converted to a form of acetic acid, *acetyl Co-A.* This process releases hydrogen atoms and carbon dioxide. Acetyl Co-A then passes into highly specialized structures within the cell, the *mitochondria.* Think of these structures as the cell's "powerhouses," or "energy factories," where over 90% of the total ATP is produced. Figure 3-6 shows a simplified diagram of the release of hydrogen atoms during the complete breakdown of glucose. In the cell fluid, hydrogen atoms are released as the glucose molecule is degraded to pyruvic acid during glycolysis and during pyruvic acid's subsequent transformation to acetyl Co-A. In the reactions within the mitochondria, carbon and hydrogen atoms are stripped from the molecules of acetyl Co-A. This generates 2 molecules of ATP, 16 additional hydrogen atoms are set free, and 4 molecules of carbon dioxide gas are formed. This "metabolic mill" also extracts hydrogen from fragments of fat and protein (amino acid) metabolism in similar fashion. This aspect of the chemical breakdown of acetyl Co-A is known as the *Krebs cycle.* It was named after the chemist Hans Krebs, who was awarded the Nobel Prize in 1953 for his pioneering studies of these vital metabolic processes.

The freeing of the hydrogen atoms from the basic structures of carbohydrate, fat, and protein during the Krebs cycle is one of the most important chemical events in the cell's energy factory. The right-hand portion of Figure 3-7 shows the transport of hydrogen through another series of chemical reactions. In this system, hydrogen atoms are changed into electrically charged particles. The electrons from hydrogen are passed in "bucket brigade" fashion through a funneling chain of reactions by other special carrier molecules until they reach "the end of the line," where they combine with oxygen to form water. *This process of aerobic metabo-*

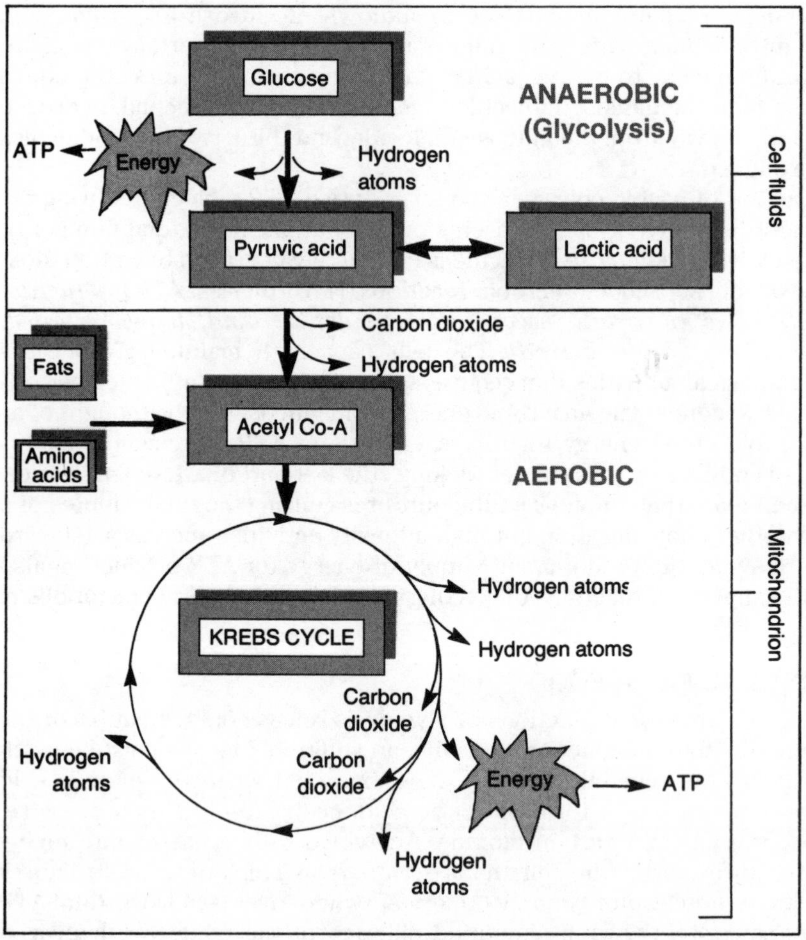
Glucose
ANAEROBIC
(Glycolysis)
ATP
Energy
Hydrogen
atoms
Cell fluids
Pyruvic acid
Lactic acid
Carbon dioxide
Fats
Hydrogen atoms
Acetyl Co-A
Amino
acids
AEROBIC
Mitochondrion
Hydrogen atoms
KREBS CYCLE
Hydrogen atoms
Carbon
dioxide
Hydrogen
atoms
Carbon
dioxide
Energy
ATP
Hydrogen
atoms

Figure 3-6. *The extraction of hydrogen during the complete breakdown of glucose. Note the energy release during glycolysis and Krebs cycle oxidation, and the pathway for the utilization of fats and amino acids at the level of acetyl Co-A pictured above the Krebs cycle during aerobic reactions.*

lism is the most crucial phase of energy metabolism because it is during the transfer of the electrons from hydrogen to oxygen that energy is produced to drive the re-bonding of P to ADP to form ATP. While the rapid release of energy anaerobically from the carbohydrate molecule during glycolysis largely determines maximum exercise performance of short duration, it is one's capacity for the aerobic resynthesis of ATP that is crucial to performance in sustained physical activities lasting beyond 2 minutes in duration.

The diagram of the various pathways of metabolism shown in Figure 3-5 also depicts the possible routes for interconversions between the foods and the possible routes for nutrient synthesis. Excess carbohydrates, for example, provide the fragments for fat synthesis and can also donate the "carbon skeleton" for some protein synthesis. Likewise, some amino acids can be used to synthesize glucose. Because the conversion of carbohydrate to fat is not reversible (notice the one-way

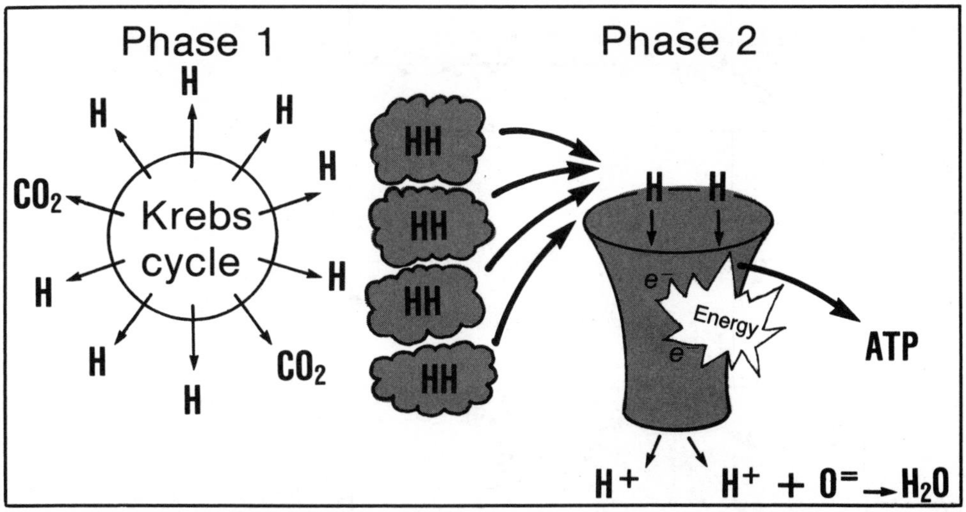
Phase 1
Phase 2
H
H
H
H
CO_2
Krebs cycle
H
H
H
H
H
CO_2
HH
HH
HH
HH
H—H
e⁻
Energy
e⁻
ATP
H+
H+ + O= → H_2O

Figure 3-7. *In the mitochondria, the Krebs cycle generates hydrogen atoms in the breakdown of acetyl-CoA (Phase 1). These hydrogens are then oxidized via the aerobic process of electron transport-oxidative phosphorylation, and significant quantities of ATP are regenerated (Phase 2).*

arrow), fatty acids *cannot* be used to synthesize glucose. Thus, dietary sources of carbohydrate are crucial.

Oxygen Consumption During Exercise

The energy release from anaerobic metabolism is very rapid and does not require oxygen; as such, the total amount of ATP resynthesized in this manner is relatively small. During the aerobic reactions of the Krebs cycle, however, considerable chemical energy stored in the molecules of carbohydrates, fats, and to a lesser degree in proteins, can be released and used effectively to provide a constant supply of ATP. *The aerobic reactions provide by far the major supply of energy to the body.*

STEADY STATE

The curve in Figure 3-8 illustrates the amount of oxygen consumed by the body during a relatively slow jog continued at the same pace for 20 minutes. The usage of oxygen by the cells, referred to as *oxygen consumption*, is indicated on the vertical axis (Y-axis) of the graph; the horizontal or X-axis indicates the progression of time during the exercise period. The quantity of oxygen consumed during any minute can easily be determined by locating a time on the X-axis and its corresponding point for oxygen consumption on the Y-axis. In an attempt to adjust for individual variations in body size on oxygen consumption (that is, bigger people consume more oxygen), oxygen consumption can be expressed in terms of body weight as milliliters of oxygen per kilogram of body weight per minute, or *ml/kg · min*.

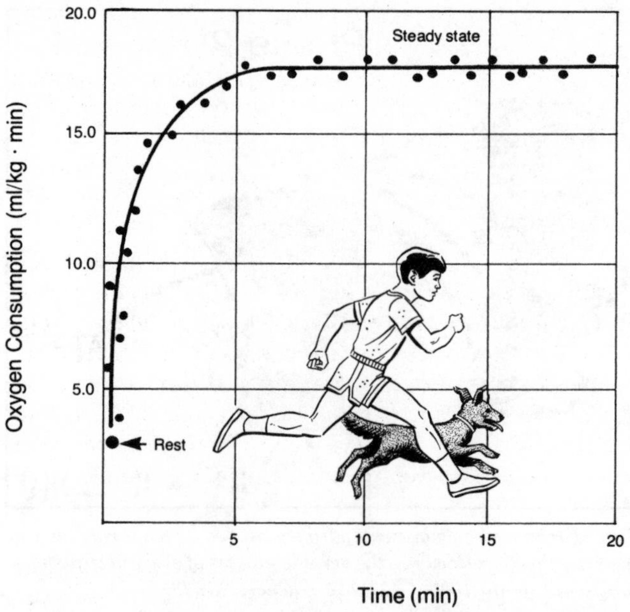

Steady state
Oxygen Consumption (ml/kg · min)
20.0
15.0
10.0
5.0
Rest
5
10
15
20
Time (min)

Figure 3-8. *Time course of oxygen consumption during a continuous jog at a relatively slow pace for 20 minutes. The dots along the curve represent measured values of oxygen consumption determined by the open-circuit method described on pages 98 to 101.*

At rest, the average person's oxygen consumption is between 3 and 4 ml/kg · min (or about 250 ml · min—the equivalent of one-fourth of a liter).

During the first 3 minutes of exercise there is a steep rise in the amount of oxygen consumed above the resting level. The curve then begins to flatten out during minutes 4 and 5 and remains essentially unchanged during the last 14 minutes of jogging. The horizontal or flat part of the curve is referred to as *steady state.* The steady state or plateau in oxygen consumption represents a balance between the energy required by the working muscles and the aerobic energy-releasing reactions. The energy for steady-state exercise is generated predominantly in the slow-twitch muscle fibers (see page 68). Theoretically, once a steady state is attained, exercise could go on indefinitely if the individual had the will power to continue. However, factors other than motivation play an important role in determining the duration of steady-state work. This includes the loss of important body fluids in sweat due to an increase in body temperature and the depletion of essential nutrients, especially blood glucose and glycogen stored in the liver and muscles.

There are many levels of steady state. Steady-state exercise for the athlete might be exhausting for the untrained. For some of us, lying in bed, working around the house, and playing an occasional round of golf represent the spectrum of activity for which adequate oxygen can be supplied to maintain a steady state. The champion marathon runner, on the other hand, can run 26 miles in slightly more than 2 hours and still be in steady state. This 5-minute-per-mile pace is a magnificent accomplishment from the point of view of the many physiologic functions involved. One of the most important of these functions is delivering an adequate supply of oxygen to the exercising muscles. The *delivery* and *utilization* of oxygen are crucial with respect to energy metabolism, especially during activities of relatively long duration. Therefore, the emphasis of physiologic conditioning programs to develop endurance *must* be to improve the transport and utilization of oxygen. Chapter 10 discusses how this is accomplished.

MAXIMAL OXYGEN CONSUMPTION

Consider from the previous example of steady-state exercise that the individual continues to jog at a comfortable pace until a series of six hills is encountered, each steeper than the next. The jogger's goal is to run up each of the hills without slowing down, although it is obvious that with each succeeding hill the task becomes more strenuous. Thus, the amount of energy required, as well as that expended, will increase progressively. In terms of oxygen consumption, the amount of energy released from aerobic reactions increases in proportion to the severity of the exercise. As the hills become steeper, the exercise becomes more severe. Accompanying this increase in exercise intensity is a proportionate and linear increase in oxygen consumption up to a certain limit.

Figure 3-9 illustrates what the curve for oxygen consumption would look like if the jogger were able to run up each hill without slowing down. Oxygen consumption increases and then levels off as the jogger runs up each of the first three hills. This leveling-off of oxygen consumption while running up the first three hills indicates that the runner has reached a progressively higher level of steady state. On the next two hills, the oxygen consumption does not increase by the same amount as it did on the first three hills. In fact, the oxygen consumption does not increase at all during the run up the steepest hill, even though the jogger was just able to

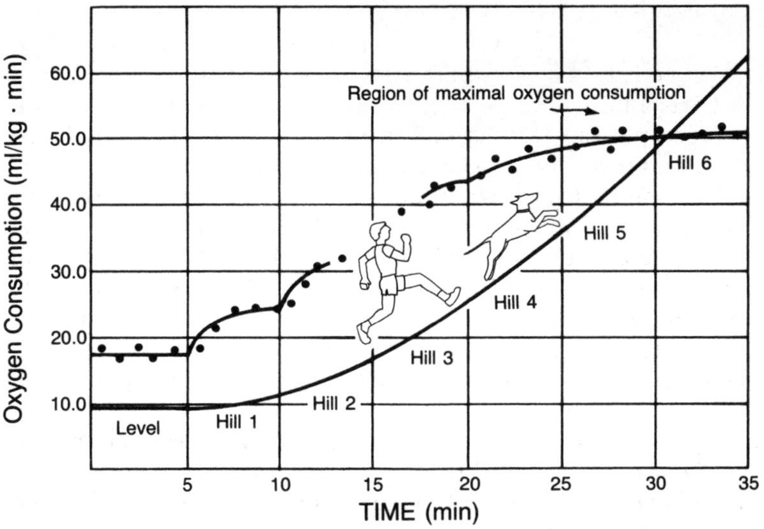
Oxygen Consumption (ml/kg · min)
60.0
50.0
40.0
30.0
20.0
10.0
Region of maximal oxygen consumption
Hill 6
Hill 5
Hill 4
Hill 3
Hill 2
Hill 1
Level
5
10
15
20
25
30
35
TIME (min)

Figure 3-9. *Oxygen consumption while running up hills of increasing slope until the maximal oxygen consumption is reached. This occurs in the region where a further increase in exercise intensity is not accompanied by an additional increase in oxygen consumption. The dots represent the measured values of oxygen consumption during each phase of running up the hills.*

make it to the top! What occurs is that the runner attains his or her maximum capacity to generate energy aerobically and cannot increase it further. The region where the work continues to become more difficult, yet the oxygen consumption fails to increase, is referred to as the *maximal oxygen consumption.* At this region, the runner attained the maximum capacity to deliver and utilize oxygen to the exercising muscles.

If a person exercises at a work intensity above maximal oxygen consumption, as occurred when the jogger ran up the last hill, anaerobic energy-generating reactions must supply the additional energy for this work. This mechanism for energy metabolism predominates because the energy from aerobic reactions is insufficient to meet the total energy demands of the exercise. Because energy can only be supplied maximally from anaerobic sources for about 60 seconds, the runner soon would become exhausted and be unable to continue.

Maximal oxygen consumption is an important factor that determines a person's capacity to sustain high-intensity exercise for longer than 4 to 5 minutes. Figure 3-10 compares the maximal oxygen consumption of male and female athletes with untrained, sedentary persons. The results show that the endurance athletes have nearly twice the aerobic capacity of the sedentary group. The finding

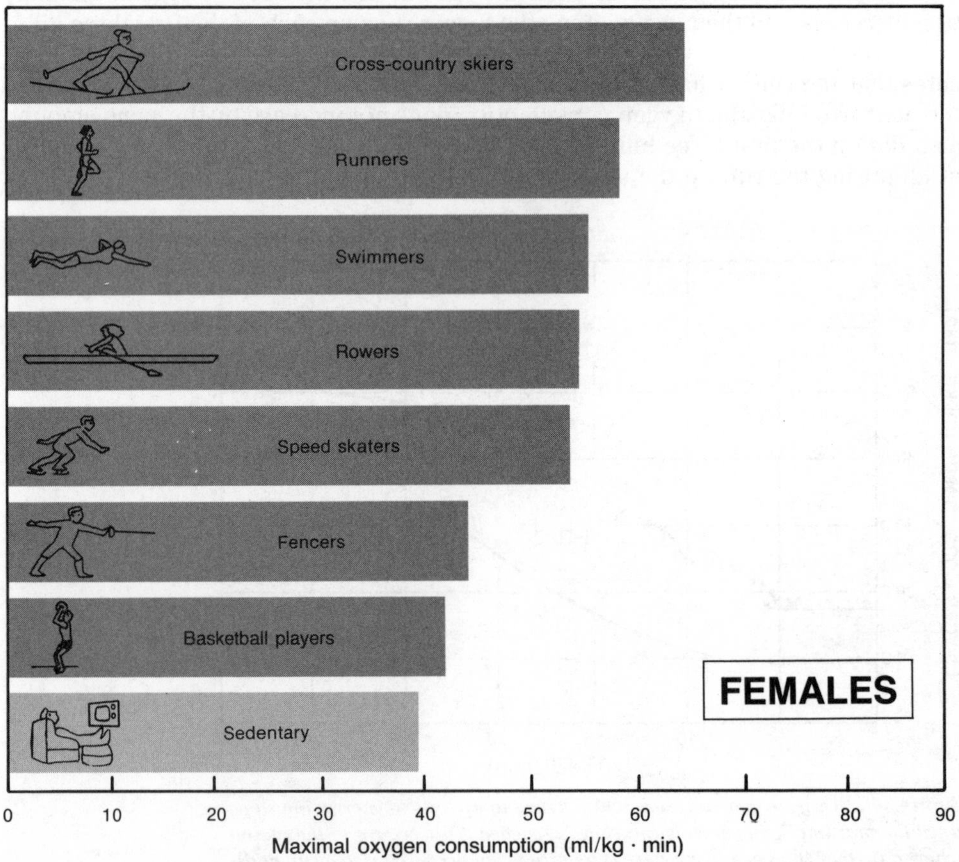
Cross-country skiers
Runners
Swimmers
Rowers
Speed skaters
Fencers
Basketball players
Sedentary
FEMALES
0
10
20
30
40
50
60
70
80
90
Maximal oxygen consumption (ml/kg · min)

Figure 3-10. *Maximal oxygen consumption of male and female olympic-caliber athletes and comparison to healthy sedentary subjects.*

that women have lower maximal aerobic capacities than men of an essentially equal training status occurs to a large extent because women possess more body fat (and less muscle mass) than men. In fact, when the maximal oxygen consumption of women is expressed in relation to "fat-free" body weight, the difference between the sexes becomes smaller. The additional fat tissue, although serving important biologic purposes, acts as "dead weight" in most physical activities.

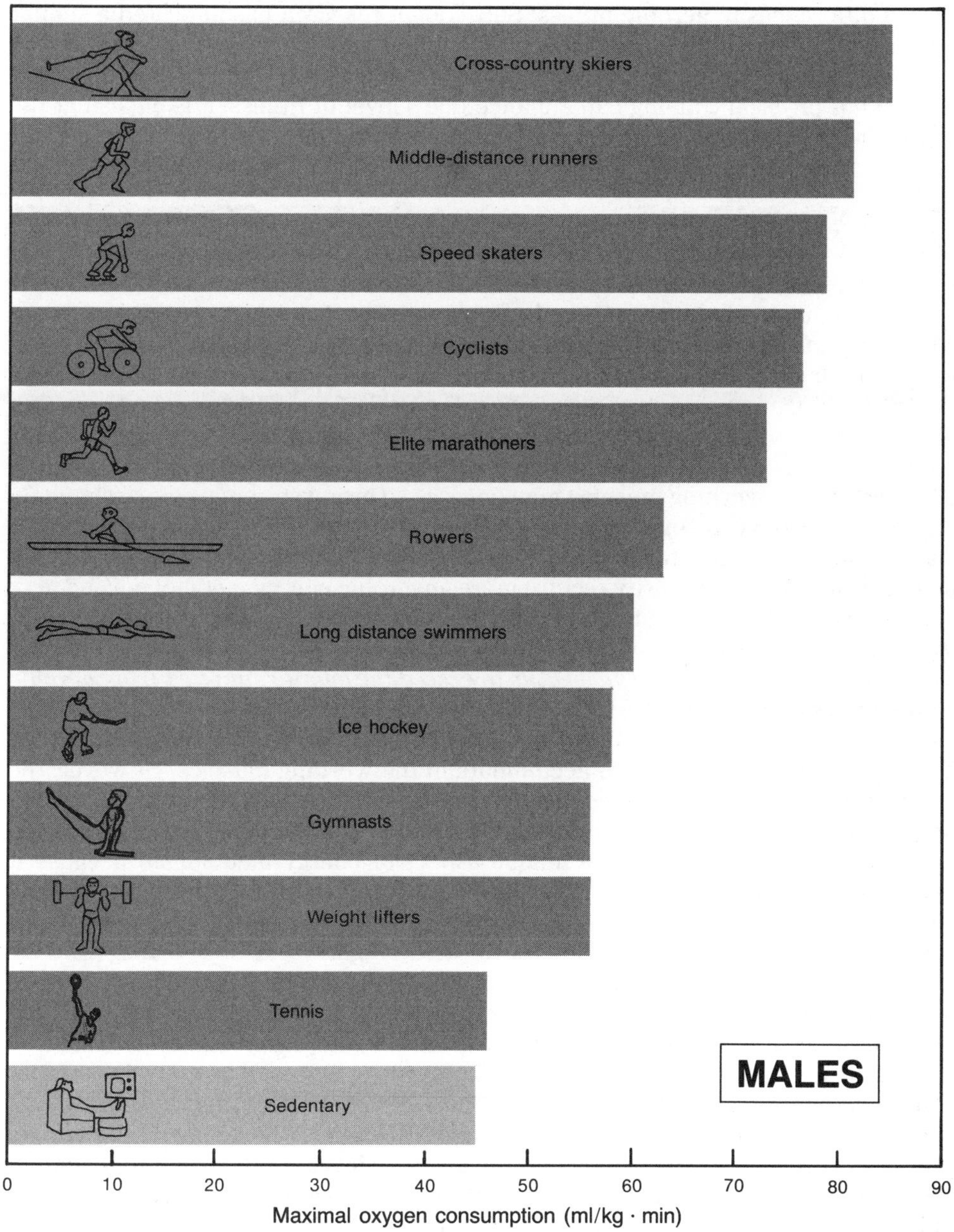
Cross-country skiers
Middle-distance runners
Speed skaters
Cyclists
Elite marathoners
Rowers
Long distance swimmers
Ice hockey
Gymnasts
Weight lifters
Tennis
Sedentary
MALES
0
10
20
30
40
50
60
70
80
90
Maximal oxygen consumption (ml/kg · min)

Figure 3-10. Continued.

Is Fitness Capacity Inherited?

An interesting question concerns whether inherited characteristics influence the values for maximal aerobic capacity presented in Figure 3-10. Although the answer is far from complete, heredity seems to have a profound impact on the differences between individuals in fitness capacity. For example, in one study of 15 pairs of identical twins (same heredity) and 15 pairs of fraternal twins (separate fertilization of two eggs) raised in the same city and whose parents were of similar socioeconomic backgrounds, heredity alone accounted for up to 93% of the observed differences in aerobic fitness! Subsequent research has indicated a similar high degree of hereditability in muscle fiber type, maximum heart rate, anaerobic capacity, as well as the ability to improve fitness with training. While a proper program of physical training can enhance one's level of fitness, it is clear that the *limits* for fitness are also linked to natural endowment.

Lactic Acid

During moderate levels of jogging or slow swimming, the energy demands are adequately met by reactions that use oxygen. In biochemical terms, sufficient ATP for muscular contraction is made available through energy released by the oxidation of hydrogen, mainly in the slow-twitch muscle fibers. Figure 3-8 shows that under these conditions, a steady rate of aerobic metabolism can be maintained for a relatively long time. As the demands for energy become more severe, the supply of oxygen to the working muscles must increase. During strenuous work shown in Figure 3-9, the oxygen consumption reaches a maximum value because the aerobic energy-transferring reactions can no longer increase their energy output. Further increases in exercise intensity require more anaerobic energy metabolism and activation of a larger number of fast-twitch fibers (see page 68). *At about 50 to 55% of the maximal oxygen consumption, the resynthesis of ATP through the anaerobic energy released from glycolysis begins to exceed the energy supplied from aerobic metabolic reactions.* When this occurs, a steady state can not be maintained because more hydrogen is produced than can combine with oxygen to form water. The excess hydrogen begins to accumulate in the working muscles. However, the concentration of hydrogen does not build up significantly because the excess hydrogen atoms combine temporarily with pyruvic acid. The temporary storage of hydrogen with pyruvic acid is a unique aspect of energy metabolism because it allows special carrier molecules to continue to transport hydrogen to combine with the available oxygen. The joining of two excess hydrogen atoms with pyruvic acid forms a new chemical called *lactic acid.* Figure 3-11 shows this process.

The advantage of converting pyruvic acid to lactic acid is that a ready "sump" is provided so the end products of glycolysis can temporarily disappear. Once formed, lactic acid diffuses rapidly from the muscle into the bloodstream and away from the site of the energy-releasing reactions. In this way, glycolysis supplies additional energy anaerobically to resynthesize ATP. Consequently, exercise can continue without an adequate oxygen supply. However, this avenue for extra energy release is only temporary. This is because the level of lactic acid in the blood and muscles increases and the ceiling for aerobic resynthesis of ATP is reached. This causes fatigue to set in and exercise must stop.

Studies of well-trained sprint athletes show they become exhausted after strenuous exercise when the blood lactic acid level is 20 to 30% higher than in

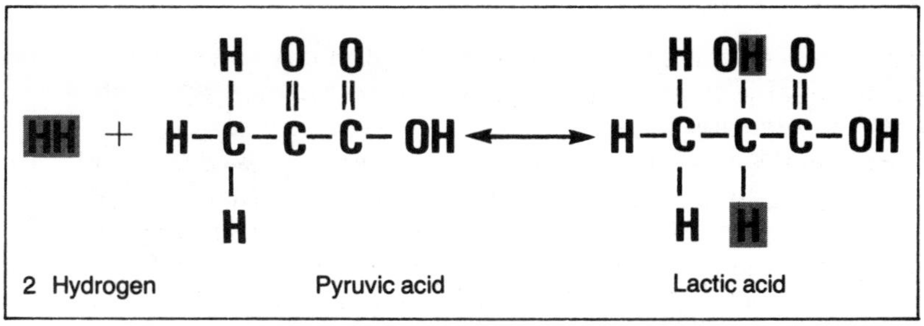
2 Hydrogen
Pyruvic acid
Lactic acid

Figure 3-11. *Excess hydrogen molecules unable to combine with oxygen are passed by special carrier molecules to temporarily combine with pyruvic acid. This forms a new chemical, lactic acid. Note that the reaction is reversible.*

untrained subjects under similar circumstances. *An athlete's ability to tolerate a high level of lactic acid in the blood during competition may account in part for a superior performance, especially in relatively short and intense physical activities.*

Figure 3-12 illustrates the relationship between oxygen consumption and lactic acid formation during light, moderate, and heavy exercise in untrained subjects and endurance athletes. Oxygen consumption is expressed as a percentage of an individual's maximal oxygen consumption. For an untrained person with a maximal oxygen consumption of 40 ml/kg · min, exercise at 50% of maximum would represent an exercise level that required 20 ml/kg · min; for the trained counterpart with a 60 ml/kg · min aerobic capacity, the 50% level would require somewhat greater exercise at 30 ml/kg · min.

During light and moderate levels of exercise, the lactic acid level in the blood remains fairly constant for both groups even though there is an increase in oxygen consumption. Each of the two exercise intensities is maintained in steady state as the ATP for muscular contraction is made available by aerobic metabolism. During exercise that involves approximately 55% of the untrained subjects' maximal oxygen consumption, the lactic acid level in the blood begins to rise. The increase in lactic acid becomes even greater as the exercise becomes more intense and the body cannot meet the additional energy demands aerobically. This pattern is essentially similar for the trained athletes except that the threshold for lactic acid buildup, termed *blood lactate threshold,* occurs at a higher percentage of the athletes' aerobic capacity. This favorable response could be due to the athletes' genetic endowment (type of muscle fiber), or more localized physiologic adaptations that occur with training adaptations (increased capillaries and aerobic enzymes, larger and more numerous mitochondria). Such changes favor less lactic acid accumulation during more intense levels of exercise.

FAST- AND SLOW-TWITCH MUSCLE FIBERS

Biochemists and exercise physiologists are interested in the functional as well as structural differences in muscle fibers. By means of surgical biopsy, small fragments of muscle tissue about the size of a grain of rice are removed and analyzed with chemical and microscopic techniques to determine their specific metabolic characteristics. Two distinct *types* of fibers have been identified in human skeletal muscle. One type is a *fast-twitch* fiber. This fiber generally possesses a high capability for anaerobic metabolism, especially in the production of ATP during the

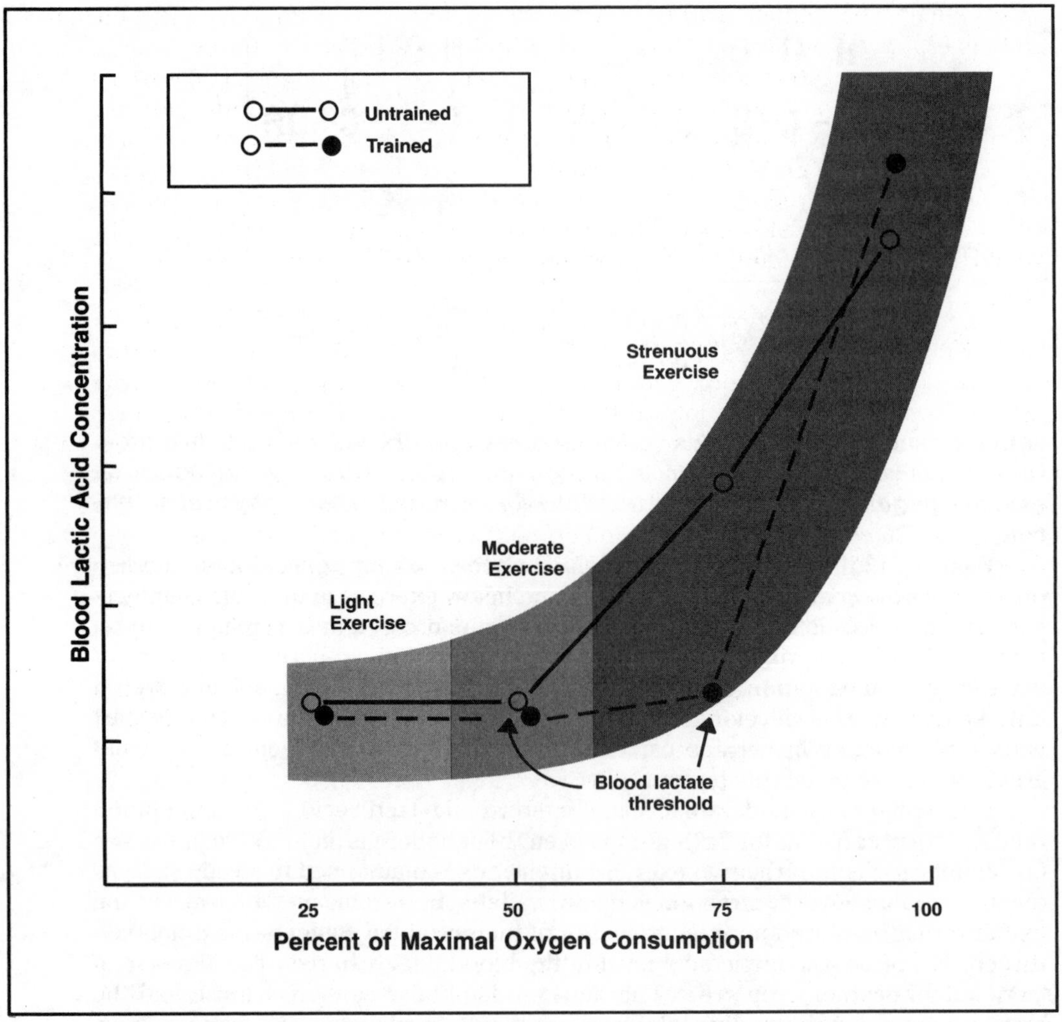
Untrained
Trained
Blood Lactic Acid Concentration
Strenuous Exercise
Moderate Exercise
Light Exercise
Blood lactate threshold
25
50
75
100
Percent of Maximal Oxygen Consumption

Figure 3-12. *Increases in blood lactic acid concentration at different levels of exercise expressed as a percentage of maximal oxygen consumption for trained and untrained subjects.*

initial stages of glucose breakdown in glycolysis. The contraction speed of these fibers is quite rapid. Fast-twitch fibers are activated in short-term, sprint activities, that depend almost entirely on anaerobic metabolism for energy. The metabolic capabilities of the fast twitch fibers are also quite important in the stop-and-go or change-of-pace sports like basketball or field hockey, that at times require rapid energy that only can be supplied by the anaerobic metabolic pathways.

The second fiber type is termed *slow-twitch.* As the name suggests, its contraction speed is half as fast as the fast-twitch fibers. Slow-twitch fibers possess many mitochondria, and a high concentration of the enzymes required to sustain aerobic metabolism. The capacity of slow-twitch fibers to generate ATP aerobically is much greater than for fast-twitch fibers. Hence, slow-twitch fibers become activated in endurance activities that depend almost exclusively on the sustained energy generated by aerobic metabolism. Middle-distance running or swimming, or sports such as basketball, field hockey, or soccer, require a blend of both aerobic and anaerobic capacities, and they activate both types of muscle fibers.

In terms of exercise training and performance, several interesting questions arise concerning fast- and slow-twitch muscle fibers. First, does the distribution of each fiber differ significantly among people, especially those who are successful in various sports? Second, can the metabolic capacity of each fiber be improved through a specific program of physiologic conditioning? Third, can fast-twitch fibers be changed into slow-twitch fibers through aerobic training, and conversely, would an anaerobic conditioning program develop predominantly fast-twitch fibers?

The answer to the first question is a definite yes. The average percentage of slow-twitch fibers in men is about 45 to 50%, but the variation is large. Even within an individual, the distribution pattern of fiber types can vary considerably from muscle to muscle. It seems logical that people with a large proportion of slow-twitch fibers in the leg muscles would be successful in endurance running, while runners with a distribution favoring a predominance of fast-twitch fibers would tend to excel in sprint activities. Muscle biopsies from trained athletes support this contention. Successful endurance runners and cross-country skiers possess between 80 and 90% slow-twitch fibers in their leg muscles, while sprint-type athletes possess a predominance of fast-twitch fibers. As might be expected, athletes who perform in middle-distance events have an approximately equal percentage of the two types of muscle fibers. In an experiment designed to answer the question of whether fiber type can be changed with training, 6 men were trained for 1 hour a day, 4 days a week for 5 months, at an exercise intensity that required 75 to 90% of each subject's maximal oxygen consumption. Muscle biopsies from the leg were obtained and fiber type determinations were made before and after training. Although the work capacity of all subjects increased, training did *not* change the relative distribution of the fast- and slow-twitch muscle fibers in the leg muscles.

In summary, the percentage distribution of muscle fibers differs significantly among people and among the various muscles in the same person. Although the metabolic capacity of both fiber types can be increased through training, it appears that the distribution of these fibers is determined by the genetic code and largely fixed before birth or early in life. The distribution of fiber types probably cannot be changed greatly through physiologic conditioning. It also appears that a certain percentage of each fiber type is associated with success in certain types of sport activities, depending on their specific energy requirements. Although this suggests an obvious genetic predisposition to success in sports and to some degree in conditioning, training *can* improve the metabolic capacity of both slow- and fast-twitch fibers significantly.

Recovery Oxygen Consumption (Oxygen Debt)

After exercise stops, the breathing, pulse rate, and bodily processes do not immediately return to their resting levels. If the exercise is not too strenuous, the recovery period is fast and proceeds unnoticed. If the activity is stressful, like sprinting for a bus or trying to swim 100 yards as fast as possible, the body requires considerable time to return to resting conditions. Recovery from each form of activity is associated to a large extent with the specific metabolic processes involved in that particular form of exercise.

Figure 3-13 shows two curves for oxygen consumption during exercise and recovery. The exercise portion of the top curve is similar to the curve in Figure 3-8 and illustrates the change in oxygen consumption during the transition from rest to moderate, steady-state exercise.

Oxygen consumption during the first 2 to 3 minutes of exercise increases progressively until the body reaches a steady state. At this point, oxygen-consuming reactions supply the energy (oxygen) requirements for exercise. No accumulation of lactic acid in the muscles occurs under these aerobic conditions. Not surprisingly, the oxygen consumption does not increase instantaneously to the

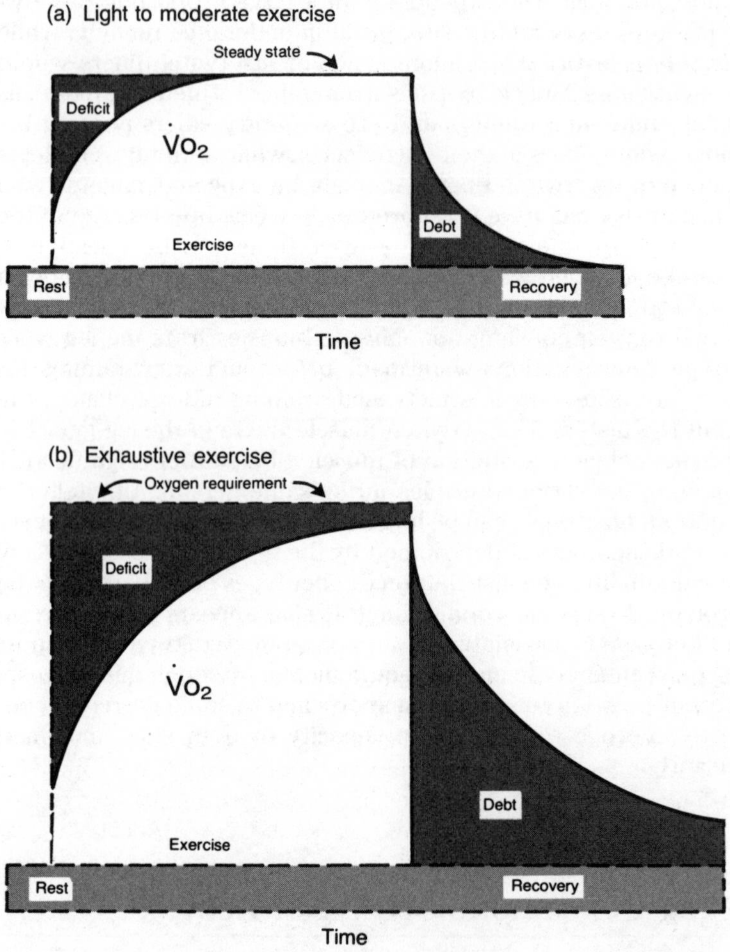
(a) Light to moderate exercise
Steady state
Deficit
$\dot{V}O_2$
Debt
Exercise
Rest
Recovery
Time
(b) Exhaustive exercise
Oxygen requirement
Deficit
$\dot{V}O_2$
Debt
Exercise
Rest
Recovery
Time

Figure 3-13. *Oxygen consumption during and in recovery from (a) light to moderate exercise, steady-state exercise, and (b) exhaustive exercise. There are 2 components to the recovery curve following heavy to exhaustive exercise. The first phase occurs quickly; the second phase is much slower and it can take considerable time to return to resting conditions. Note that in exhaustive exercise, the oxygen requirement of the exercise is* above *the curve of oxygen consumption (symbolized as* $\dot{V}O_2$*).*

steady-state level because the immediate energy for muscular work is always provided directly by the anaerobic breakdown of ATP. Oxygen is used only in subsequent reactions when it combines with the hydrogen atoms released during glycolysis and the reactions of the Krebs cycle. Thus, a temporary "deficit" in oxygen consumption exists during the first few minutes of exercise. The amount of this deficit is shown to the left of the upward trending curve of oxygen consumption. Quantitatively, the deficit represents the difference between the amount of oxygen actually consumed and the amount of oxygen that would have been consumed had a steady state been achieved immediately. The anaerobic energy provided during the deficit phase of exercise represents "borrowed" energy, so to speak, until the steady state is reached. Once exercise stops the deficit is "repaid" at the expense of an elevated oxygen consumption during recovery (labeled as Debt in the figure). During light exercise when steady state is reached quickly, the debt payoff is relatively small and rapid. During the transition from moderate to heavy exercise, on the other hand, the oxygen deficit can be quite large. For exhaustive exercise illustrated in the bottom curve, a steady state cannot be reached and anaerobic reactions provide considerable energy with an accompanying accumulation of lactic acid. The oxygen in excess of the resting value consumed during recovery from exercise, whether it is small from light exercise or large from heavy or exhaustive exercise, is called the *oxygen debt* or more precisely, the *recovery oxygen consumption.* In Figure 3-13, the deficit and recovery oxygen consumption (debt) are indicated by the shaded areas.

The curves of recovery illustrate several important characteristics of oxygen debt. During recovery from light and moderate exercise, oxygen consumption declines rapidly to resting values as soon as exercise stops. One-half the total oxygen debt is repaid within the first 25 to 30 seconds during this "fast" repayment. Within 1 to 2 minutes the oxygen consumption has returned to the resting level. *The extra oxygen consumed in recovery from moderate exercise is associated with the restoration of the ATP and CP high-energy phosphates that were depleted and not resynthesized during the exercise.* A small amount of oxygen is also used to reload the blood with oxygen, and to supply the slightly elevated oxygen demands of the heart and breathing musculature.

In recovery from strenuous exercise, there is a large lactic acid accumulation; this is usually accompanied by an increase in body temperature. In addition to the fast component of the recovery curve of oxygen consumption, there is a second and slower phase termed the "slow" component. Lactic acid during this phase of recovery is reconverted to pyruvic acid and metabolized for energy through the Krebs cycle. Some lactic acid may also be synthesized back to glycogen in the liver. A precise biochemical explanation of the recovery oxygen consumption, especially the role of lactic acid, has not yet been made because the specific chemical dynamics of oxygen debt are still unclear. It is known that the oxygen debt following strenuous exercise becomes larger than the deficit because a considerable amount of oxygen consumed during recovery is not directly related to the level of anaerobic metabolism during exercise. For example, the respiratory muscles require considerably more oxygen for the work of breathing during recovery than at rest. The volume of air moved into and out of the lungs in intense exercise can increase 15 to 20 times above rest, yet still remain elevated for some time in recovery. The heart also works harder and requires a greater oxygen supply during recovery. The elevation of body temperature during exercise also has a direct stimulating effect on metabolic reactions, and hence, a *significant* effect on the recovery oxygen consumption. The blood must also be reloaded with oxygen as it returns from the exercised muscles. In fact, all physiologic systems activated to meet the demands of exercise increase their own particular need for oxygen during recovery.

Some books dealing with exercise imply that lactic acid is a metabolic "waste product." To the contrary, lactic acid is not treated as an unwanted chemical and then excreted from the body. It is a valuable potential source of chemical energy that is retained at relatively high concentrations during intense exercise. When there is sufficient oxygen during recovery, lactic acid is readily converted back to pyruvic acid and used for energy. In this way the body preserves about 90% of the energy in the original glucose molecule for later use as an energy source.

There are important distinguishing features of the fast and slow components of the recovery oxygen consumption. If exercise is not too strenuous so it is performed in steady state, or if it is heavy exercise but of short duration (10 to 15 seconds), lactic acid will *not* accumulate to any appreciable extent. Recovery will be rapid (fast component) and exercise could begin again without the hindering effects of fatigue. If intense exercise must continue beyond a 20-second period—as in basketball, soccer, or hockey—the energy is supplied predominantly from the anaerobic reactions of glycolysis. This occurs at the expense of lactic acid build-up in the blood and exercising muscles. Under these circumstances, recovery takes much longer (slow component) and may not be complete even with short rest periods such as times-out, or even with longer rest periods such as half-time breaks.

Keep Active During Recovery

Lactic acid removal is accelerated by active aerobic recovery exercise. While just about any level of *submaximal aerobic exercise* facilitates the recovery process, the most rapid recovery usually occurs with continuous exercise at a level that can be comfortably maintained. Lactate removal with active recovery is the result of an increased blood flow through the liver, heart, and muscles, because these tissues can use lactate and oxidize it for energy during recovery. If, however, recovery exercise is too intense and performed above the blood lactate threshold, it will be of little benefit and may even prolong recovery by increasing the formation of lactic acid.

The Energy Spectrum of Exercise

The relative contributions of the anaerobic and aerobic energy systems may differ markedly depending on the type of exercise performed. Performances of short duration and high intensity such as the 100-yard dash, 25-yard swim, high jump, volleyball spike, golf swing, or resistance-type exercise, require an immediate energy supply. This energy is provided exclusively from anaerobic sources, specifically the high-energy phosphate compounds ATP and CP stored within the specific muscles activated in the activity. In strenuous exercise that lasts several minutes, the major source of energy comes from the anaerobic process of glycolysis with the resulting formation of lactic acid. Intense exercise of an intermediate duration performed for 5 to 10 minutes as in middle-distance running, swimming, basketball, or soccer, represents a *blend* of metabolic energy demands. Under these conditions, it is desirable to possess a high capacity for both aerobic and anaerobic metabolism. Performances of long duration such as marathon running, distance swimming, cycling, recreational jogging, or hiking require a fairly constant energy supply with little or no reliance on the mechanism of lactic acid production.

Figure 3-14 illustrates the relative contribution of the anaerobic and aerobic energy sources during maximal physical activities of various durations. These data were originally obtained from running and cycling experiments, although they can easily be applied to other activities that involve large muscle groups. For example, a 40- to 60-yard sprint of 5 to 8 seconds would closely approximate a long pass pattern in football, while a 440-yard run of 60 to 70 seconds would be similar in duration to a 100-yard swim.

At one extreme the total energy for exercise would be supplied entirely by anaerobic sources. In middle-distance events or in other intense activities that last from 2 to 4 minutes, the ATP-CP and lactic acid energy systems generate approximately 50% of the energy, while reactions that require oxygen supply the remainder. World-class marathon runners, on the other hand, derive essentially all their energy from aerobic metabolism.

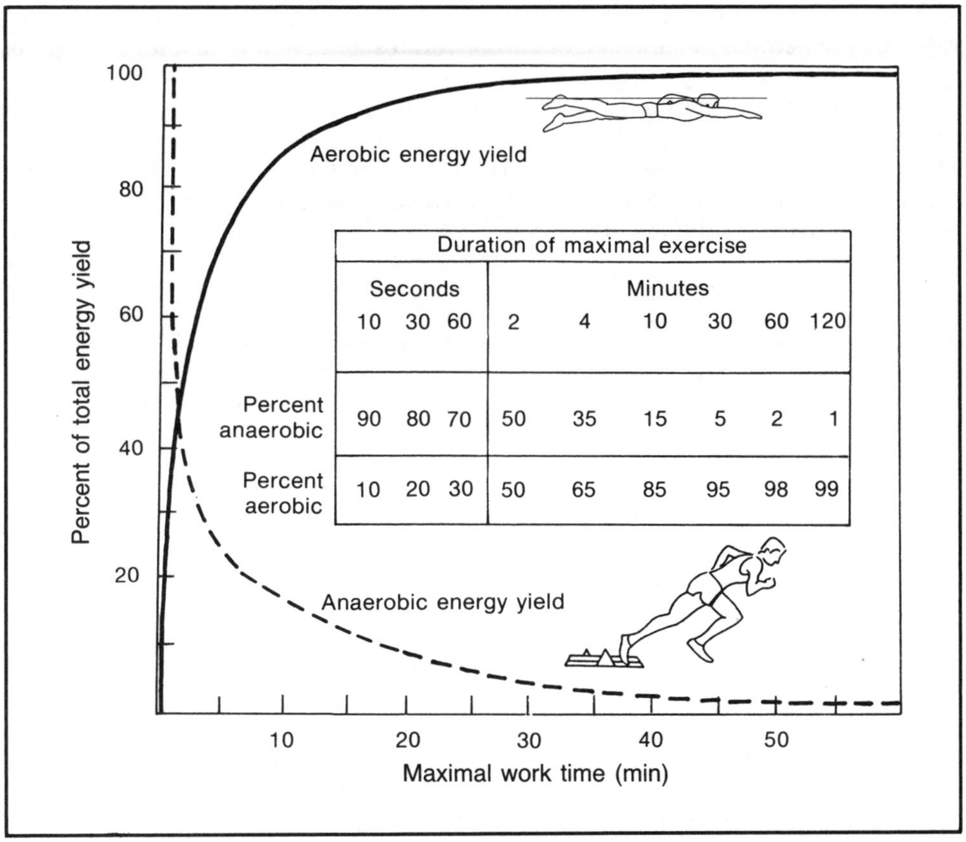
100
80
60
40
20
Percent of total energy yield
Aerobic energy yield
Anaerobic energy yield
Duration of maximal exercise
Seconds
Minutes
10 30 60 2 4 10 30 60 120
Percent anaerobic 90 80 70 50 35 15 5 2 1
Percent aerobic 10 20 30 50 65 85 95 98 99
10
20
30
40
50
Maximal work time (min)

Figure 3-14. *Relative contribution of aerobic and anaerobic energy during maximal physical activity of various durations. It should be noted that 1½ to 2 minutes of maximal effort requires 50% of the energy from aerobic and anaerobic processes.*

An understanding of the energy requirements of various activities provides some explanation why a world record-holder in the 1-mile run is not necessarily a noted distance runner. Conversely, premier marathoners are generally unable to run a mile in less than 4 minutes. As will be discussed in Chapters 9 and 10, *the scientific approach to training is to identify the predominant energy system or systems involved in a given activity, and then to gear training toward the improvement of the energy capacity of that system. Improved capability for energy metabolism will assure improvement in performance.*

Part 2. Ventilation and Circulation: The Oxygen Delivery Systems

Most sport, recreational, and occupational activities require a relatively constant and sustained energy supply. The energy for the resynthesis of ATP is provided by the aerobic metabolism of carbohydrates and fat, and to a minor degree, protein. Unless a steady state can be achieved between exercise energy-yielding reactions and the activity's energy requirements, an anaerobic-aerobic metabolic energy imbalance develops, lactic acid accumulates and fatigue quickly ensues. The ability to sustain physical activity, therefore, depends to a large degree on the capacity and integration of the body's two major oxygen delivery systems, the *ventilatory and circulatory systems.*

Lung Ventilation

LUNG STRUCTURE AND FUNCTION

The lungs provide the surface so oxygen can move from the external environment into the body and carbon dioxide produced in the tissues can exit to the outside. The lung volume of an average-sized adult varies from 4 to 6 liters, or about the amount of air contained in a basketball. If this tissue were spread out like a carpet, it would cover a surface about 35 times greater than the surface area of the person, and would cover half a tennis court! This provides a tremendous interface for the aeration of blood with the environment.

A general view of the structure of the ventilatory system is presented in Figure 3-15. As air moves into the lungs through the nose and mouth, it is filtered, humidified, and adjusted to body temperature. This air conditioning process continues as the inspired air passes down the *trachea* into the *bronchi,* two large tubes that serve as the primary conduits into each of the two lungs. The bronchi further subdivide into many smaller *bronchioles* that conduct the air into the respiratory tract's terminal branches, the *alveoli.* These are the microscopic, thin-walled elastic sacs that serve as the surface for gas exchange between the lungs and the blood.

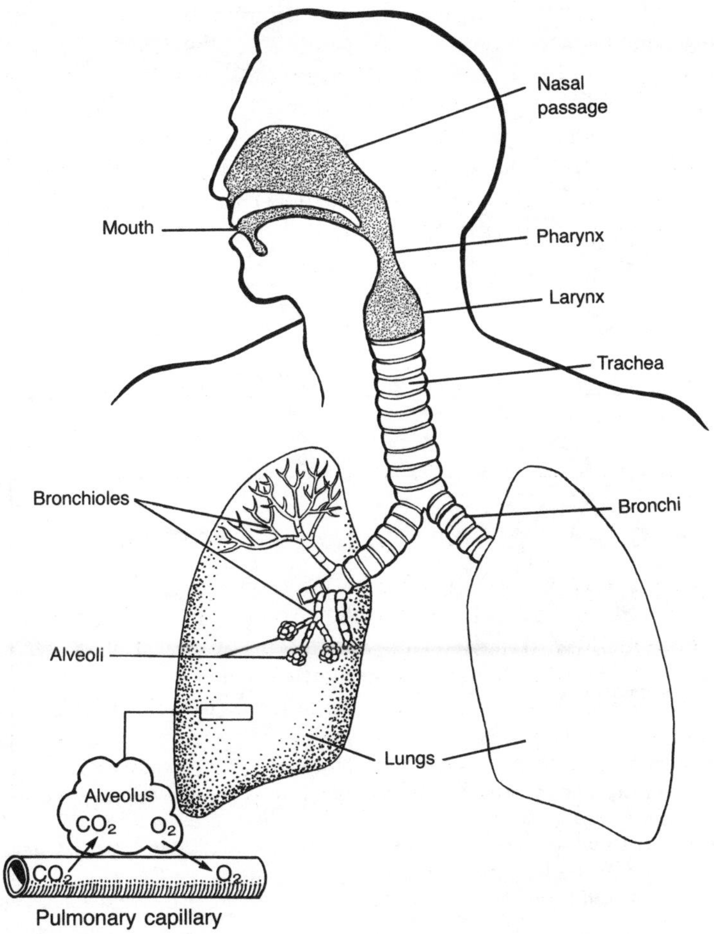
Nasal passage
Mouth
Pharynx
Larynx
Trachea
Bronchioles
Bronchi
Alveoli
Lungs
Alveolus
CO_2
O_2
CO_2
O_2
Pulmonary capillary

Figure 3-15. *A general view of the ventilatory system that shows the respiratory passages, the alveoli, and the function of an alveolus in gaseous exchange.*

Millions of tiny, thin-walled blood vessels, the *capillaries,* lie side-by-side with the alveoli, with air moving on one side and blood on the other. When air is breathed into the lungs, only two thin membranes, that of the alveolus and that of the capillary, provide the barrier to the movement of gases between the internal and external environments.

MECHANICS OF BREATHING

A large, dome-shaped sheet of muscle called the diaphragm serves the same purpose as the rubber membrane attached to the bottom of the jar illustrated in Figure 3-16. This muscle makes an airtight seal that separates the lower chest from the upper abdominal cavity. When air enters the lungs, a process known as *inspiration,* the diaphragm contracts, flattens out, and moves downward toward the abdominal cavity. As a result, the chest cavity enlarges and air rushes in through

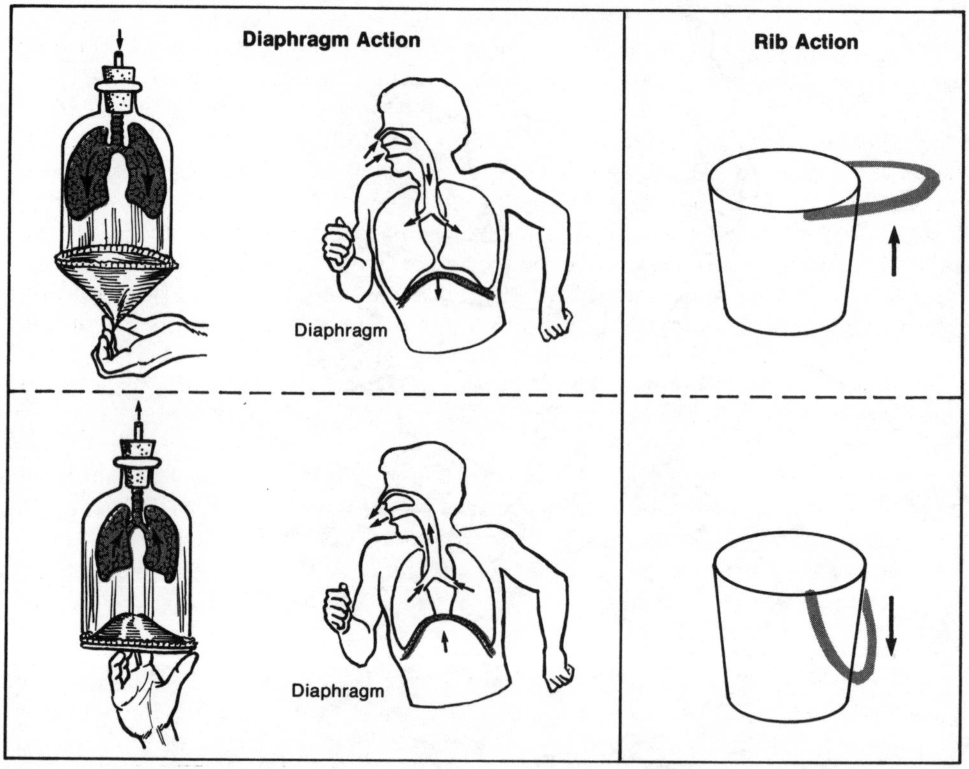
Diaphragm Action
Rib Action
Diaphragm
Diaphragm

Figure 3-16. *Mechanics of breathing. During inspiration, the chest cavity increases in size due to the raising of the ribs and the lowering of the muscular diaphragm. During exhalation, the ribs swing down and the diaphragm returns to a relaxed position. This reduces the volume of the thoracic cavity and air rushes out. The movement of the rubber bottom of the jar simulates the action of the diaphragm and causes air to enter and leave the two balloons; the movement of the bucket handle simulates the action of the ribs.*

the nose and mouth and the lungs inflate. In contrast to the balloons that are attached to the jar, the lungs are not merely suspended in the chest cavity. Rather, the pressure differential between the air within the lungs and the lung-chest wall interface causes the lungs to adhere to the chest wall and literally follow its every movement. *Exhalation*, the process of air movement from the lungs, is predominantly a passive process; during rest and light exercise, it occurs from the relaxation of the inspiratory muscles and the recoil of the stretched lung tissue. This action causes the size of the chest cavity to decrease and air moves out of the lungs.

During vigorous exercise, muscles that act on the ribs and sternum as well as the abdominal musculature, contribute to a rapid change in the dimensions of the chest cavity as airflow within the lungs increases dramatically. Pulmonary ventilation in well-conditioned endurance athletes may increase to 160 to 220 liters of air per minute in response to maximum metabolic demands. Even such strenuous exercise does not tax maximally the athlete's ability to breathe, so a breathing reserve still remains.

Breathe Normally During Exercise

The expiratory muscles play an important role during coughing and sneezing, as well as in stabilizing the abdomen and chest when lifting a heavy object. During a normal breathing cycle, only small changes in pressure within the chest cavity bring about the smooth passage of air within the alveolar chambers. If, however, the *glottis* is closed following a full inspiration, and the expiratory muscles are maximally activated, the pressure increases tremendously within the chest cavity. (The glottis is the narrowest part of the larynx where air passes into and out of the trachea.) A forced exhalation against a closed glottis, termed the *Valsalva maneuver,* occurs commonly in weight lifting and other straining-type activities that require rapid and near-maximal application of force. The increase in pressure during the Valsalva is transmitted through the thin walls of the veins that pass through the chest region. Because venous blood is under relatively low pressure, these veins are compressed and blood flow returning to the heart is greatly reduced. A reduction in venous return can diminish blood supply to the brain and frequently produces dizziness, "spots before the eyes," and even fainting. The best way to prevent these physiologic consequences of straining-type exercise is to *breathe normally throughout an exercise, and refrain from prolonged breathhold when straining to lift a heavy object.*

GAS EXCHANGE IN THE LUNGS

The movement of gas molecules as they enter or leave the lungs and body tissues occurs by the process of *diffusion,* as the gas moves from an area of higher concentration to an area of lower concentration. The exchange of oxygen and carbon dioxide molecules between the lungs and the blood and the subsequent diffusion of these gases at the tissue level, as shown in Figure 3-17, is due entirely to the pressure differentials between the gases in various parts of the body. Because the pressure exerted by the oxygen molecules in the alveoli is considerably greater than in the returning venous blood, oxygen is "forced" through the alveolar membrane into the blood. Carbon dioxide, on the other hand, exists under greater pressure in returning venous blood than in the alveoli. Consequently, the carbon dioxide is driven into the lungs. The process of gas diffusion in the healthy lung is so rapid that an equilibrium of blood gas with alveolar gas takes less than 1 second.

The pressure of oxygen and carbon dioxide gas in the arterial blood differs considerably from the pressure of these gases in the trillions of cells in the body. This is because at the tissue level, oxygen is used continuously during aerobic metabolism to produce an almost equal quantity of carbon dioxide gas. This results in a rapid diffusion of gas between the blood and tissues. Oxygen leaves the blood and moves toward the metabolizing cell, while carbon dioxide flows from the cell to the blood. After leaving the tissues the blood travels in the veins where it is returned to the heart and subsequently pumped to the lungs where diffusion again takes place.

As the demands for energy increase during exercise, large amounts of oxygen diffuse from the alveoli of the lungs into the deoxygenated blood returning from the exercising muscles. Simultaneously, considerable quantities of carbon dioxide produced in the muscles and carried in the blood move into the lungs. Lung ventilation must increase to maintain the proper concentrations of alveolar gases to meet the increased need for oxygen and removal of carbon dioxide. With the proper

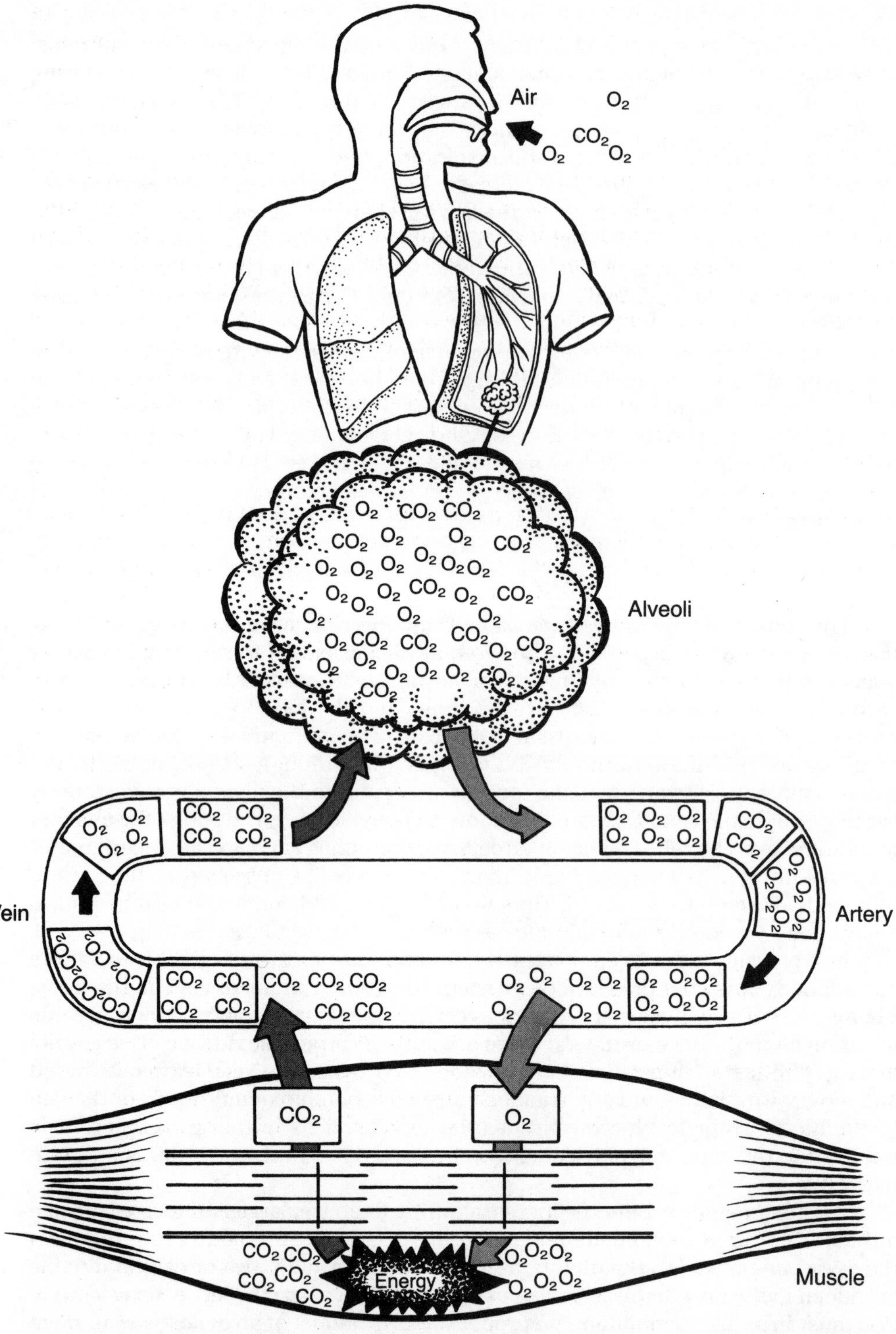
Air
Alveoli
Vein
Artery
Energy
Muscle

Figure 3-17. *Exchange of oxygen and carbon dioxide at rest between alveoli and the blood and the blood and tissues. During exercise, alveolar and arterial oxygen and carbon dioxide values remain almost the same as at rest. In the muscles, however, the increased demands for energy cause the oxygen values to drop precipitously with a corresponding increase in carbon dioxide. Therefore, venous blood will vary considerably in oxygen and carbon dioxide content, depending on the person's level of physical activity.*

adjustment of ventilation to the body's metabolic demands, the composition of alveolar air is kept remarkably constant, even during the most strenuous physical activity.

OXYGEN TRANSPORT

By far, the greatest quantity of oxygen in the blood is carried in "piggyback" fashion by combining with *hemoglobin*, the iron-containing protein compound in the red blood cells. Hemoglobin increases the oxygen-carrying capacity of blood about 65 times above that normally dissolved in the plasma. The iron atoms in each hemoglobin molecule "capture" oxygen molecules loosely and temporarily, thus enabling oxygen to be released in response to the needs of the active tissues. It is the oxygenation of hemoglobin that gives arterial blood its characteristic red color. When the hemoglobin content of the red blood cell decreases significantly, as in certain types of anemia, the quantity of oxygen carried by the blood decreases correspondingly. As discussed in Chapter 1, such a condition could result in reduced performance and early fatigue in activities that depend on a high oxygen supply.

The nature of the adjustment in pulmonary ventilation in the healthy person, as well as the specific chemical characteristics of the hemoglobin molecule, are such that even during vigorous exercise hemoglobin carries nearly its full complement of oxygen. Breathing mixtures of concentrated oxygen, as often practiced by football players during times out, at half-time, or following strenuous exercise, contributes little to the quantity of oxygen already carried in the blood. *Breathing oxygen enriched mixtures may give a psychologic lift, but its contribution to physiologic benefits are trivial at best.*

Of course, as one moves to moderate or high altitude and the barometric pressure falls accordingly, the pressure of oxygen in air is reduced and the hemoglobin molecule is not fully saturated with oxygen. Under these circumstances, oxygen breathing would be of benefit, particularly during endurance exercise at altitude where oxygen delivery is of utmost importance.

LUNG VENTILATION DURING EXERCISE

In the early stages of submaximal exercise, lung ventilation rises rapidly to a steady level similar to the response pattern for oxygen consumption illustrated in Figure 3-8. With each successive increasing level of exercise, efficient adjustments in rate or depth of breathing, or both, bring about a rapid rise in ventilation to a new steady level. The curves in Figure 3-18 illustrate the relationship between pulmonary ventilation and oxygen consumption for both the untrained and trained individual. Each point represents the average value for ventilation achieved for a particular level of oxygen consumption during successive increments of exercise intensity.

During moderate exercise, ventilation volume increases linearly with the quantity of oxygen consumed by the tissues. Because of the increase in ventilation, the pressures of oxygen and carbon dioxide in the alveoli remain at near resting values and there is complete oxygenation of blood flow through the lungs. During vigorous exercise, ventilation volume compared with oxygen consumption increases disproportionately. That is, the amount of air breathed for each quantity of oxygen consumed is greater than during more moderate exercise. If the ability to

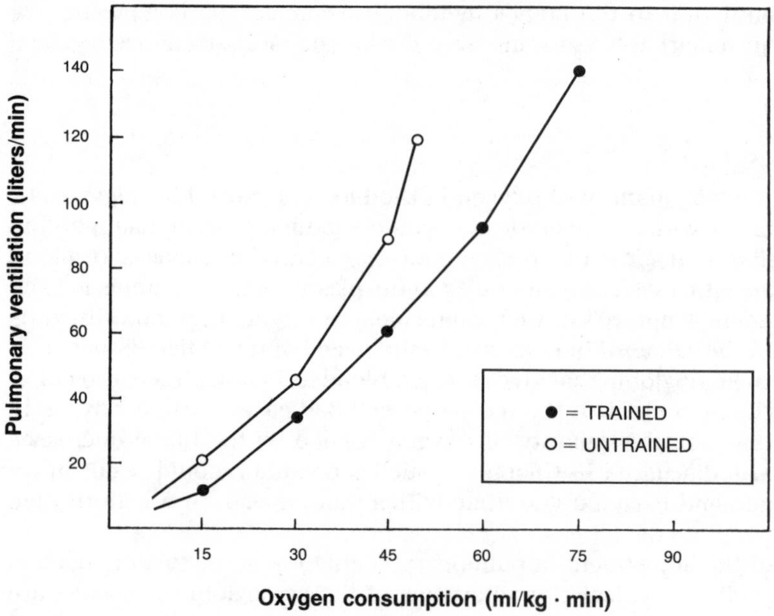
Pulmonary ventilation (liters/min)
140
120
100
80
60
40
20
15
30
45
60
75
90
Oxygen consumption (ml/kg · min)
● = TRAINED
○ = UNTRAINED

Figure 3-18. *Relationship between pulmonary ventilation and oxygen for trained athletes and untrained subjects.*

breathe were inadequate for the metabolic demands, the relation between lung ventilation and oxygen consumption would curve in the opposite direction. Such a curve would indicate a failure of ventilation to keep pace with the oxygen consumption. If such was the case in exercise, we would truly "run out of air." Obviously, this doesn't occur, but overbreathing does during heavy exercise. The shape of the curve relating ventilation to oxygen consumption during exercise of increasing intensity is essentially similar between trained and untrained individuals; an exception is that during any level of submaximal exercise, the ventilation volumes are *lower* for the trained. This adaptation occurs rapidly with training and is beneficial for two reasons: (1) it reduces the fatiguing effects of exercise on the ventilatory muscles, and (2) any oxygen freed for use by the ventilatory muscles becomes available to the exercising muscles.

The lungs of healthy people are more than adequate to maintain proper alveolar gas pressures, even during the most severe exercise when the circulation is stressed to its maximum. For most people, the blood leaving the lungs to flow throughout the body during exercise is loaded with virtually the same amount of oxygen it carries during rest. The bottom line is this—*the capacity to breathe and ventilate the lungs will not limit a healthy person's performance during physical activity.*

EXERCISE AND THE ASTHMATIC

Asthma, a disease that affects about 10 million Americans, is characterized by hyperirritability of the pulmonary airways. For many asthmatics, exercise is a potent stimulus for the airway constriction associated with an asthmatic attack. The movement of large volumes of air during exercise has a cooling effect on the pulmonary system as the incoming air is warmed and humidified. The cooling triggers spasms of the smooth muscle that lines the walls of the respiratory passages, and greatly increases resistance to airflow. This effect becomes apparent during exercise in a cool, dry environment where considerable moisture is lost (with a subsequent cooling effect) from the respiratory passages as the incoming air is air-conditioned. However, the exercise-induced asthmatic response is blunted when exercise is performed in a humid environment where there is little cooling of the airways. That is why walking or jogging on a warm, humid day or swimming in an indoor pool, is usually well-tolerated by asthmatics, whereas exercise in the cool, dry air during outdoor winter sports often triggers an asthmatic attack. For the asthmatic who wants to exercise regularly regardless of environmental conditions, medications are available to limit the degree of airway constriction.

For the normal person, exercise is frequently associated with a dryness in the throat and coughing during the recovery period, especially following exercise in cold weather. Post-exercise coughing results from water loss from the respiratory passages associated with the large air volumes that are inspired and expired during exercise.

CIGARETTE SMOKING

Evidence is now overwhelming that long-term cigarette smoking is highly related to a variety of severe pulmonary and cardiovascular diseases that include emphysema, chronic bronchitis, hypertension, coronary heart disease, and several types of cancer. While these diseases usually take years to become manifest, the immediate effects of smoking are of significance to the exercise enthusiast. The resistance to breathing is increased as much as threefold following 15 puffs on a cigarette and this effect lasts an average of 35 minutes. The residual effect of smoking in vigorous exercise could add significantly to the effect and subsequent oxygen consumption required to maintain adequate ventilation. This reduces the economy of physical activity.

Circulation

The highly efficient ventilatory system is complemented by a rapid transport and delivery system that consists of the blood, the heart, and over 60,000 miles of blood vessels that serve to integrate the body as a unit. The circulatory system serves three important functions during physical activity: (1) to deliver blood to the exercising muscles, where oxygen is exchanged for almost equal amounts of carbon dioxide; (2) to return blood to the lungs where the metabolic gases are exchanged with the ambient environment; and (3) to transport heat, a by-product of cellular metabolism, from the body's core to the skin where it then dissipates to the environment.

THE CARDIOVASCULAR SYSTEM

Figure 3-19 presents a schematic view of the circulatory system. Within the confines of this closed system the force for blood flow is provided by a four-chambered *heart.* The heart, a fist-sized pump, beats about 70 times a minute (100,800 times a day; 36.8 million times a year). At rest, the heart's output of blood is equivalent to 1400 gallons a day, or about 36 million gallons in a lifetime! When this remarkable organ pumps at its maximum capacity during exercise, it puts out more blood than the fluid coming from a household faucet turned wide open.

Figure 3-20 shows the details of the heart as a pump. The two hollow chambers that make up the right side of the heart serve two important functions: (1) to receive oxygen-depleted blood that returns from all parts of the body, and (2) to pump the blood to the lungs for aeration. The left side of the heart receives oxygen-rich blood from the lungs and pumps it into the *aorta,* the main conduit of the

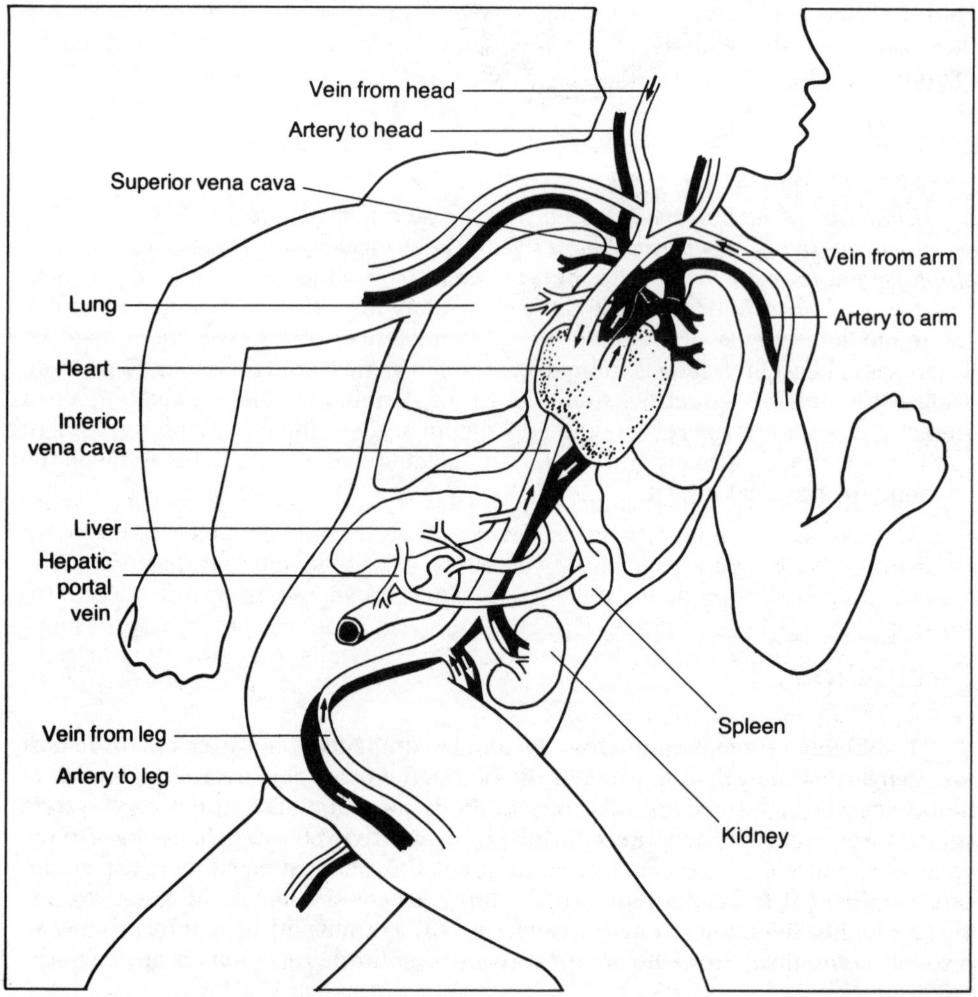
Vein from head
Artery to head
Superior vena cava
Vein from arm
Artery to arm
Lung
Heart
Inferior vena cava
Liver
Hepatic portal vein
Vein from leg
Artery to leg
Spleen
Kidney

Figure 3-19. *General view of the circulatory system. The arterial system is shaded.*

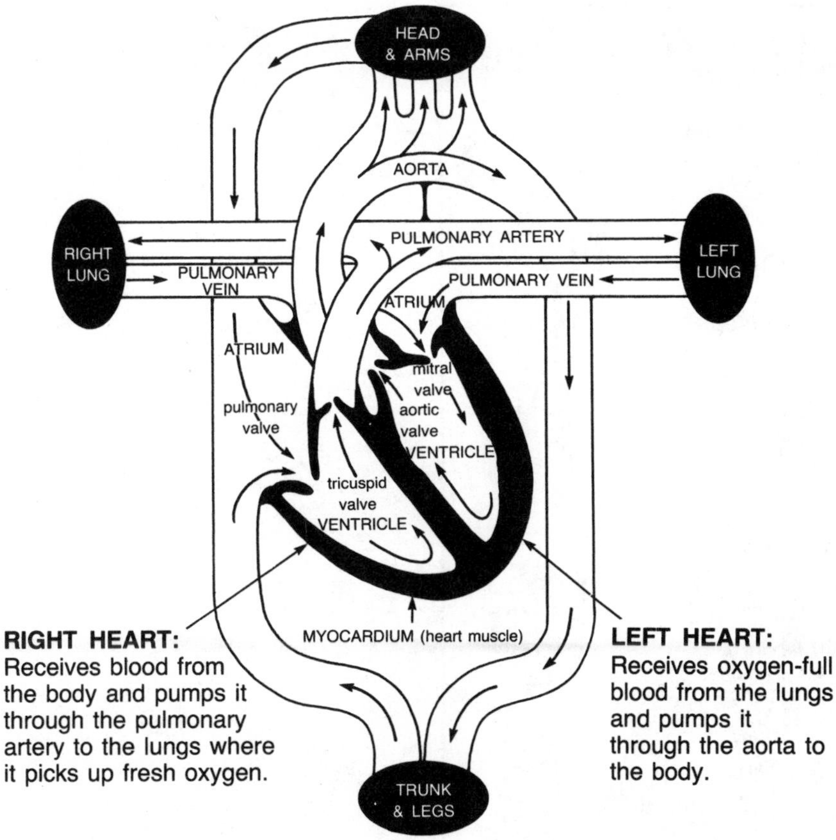
HEAD & ARMS
AORTA
RIGHT LUNG
LEFT LUNG
PULMONARY ARTERY
PULMONARY VEIN
PULMONARY VEIN
ATRIUM
ATRIUM
mitral valve
aortic valve
pulmonary valve
VENTRICLE
tricuspid valve
VENTRICLE
MYOCARDIUM (heart muscle)
RIGHT HEART:
Receives blood from the body and pumps it through the pulmonary artery to the lungs where it picks up fresh oxygen.
LEFT HEART:
Receives oxygen-full blood from the lungs and pumps it through the aorta to the body.
TRUNK & LEGS

Figure 3-20. *The structure of the heart pump.*

arterial system. From it branch other main arterial channels that route oxygen-rich blood to the organs and tissues.

The arterial system eventually branches into smaller blood vessels called *arterioles.* Nerves and local metabolic conditions act on the smooth muscular bands in the arteriole walls and enable these vessels to alter their internal diameter. The dilation and constriction of arterioles allow for the rapid redistribution of blood to and from various body regions. The arterioles end in a network of small blood vessels, called *capillaries,* with microscopically thin walls. *It is only at the capillary level that the exchange of gases and nutrients takes place between the slow-moving blood and the tissues.*

The deoxygenated blood leaves the capillaries, one cell at a time, to enter the *venules* or small veins, and eventually flow into the veins that return the blood to the heart. Spaced at short intervals within the veins are thin, membranous, flaplike valves (Figure 3-21) that permit the one-way flow of blood back to the heart. Because the blood in the veins is under relatively little pressure, they are easily compressed by the smallest muscular contractions or even by minor pressure changes within the chest cavity during the act of breathing. The alternate compression and relaxation of the veins and the one-way action of the valves provides a *"milking"* action for the steady flow of blood from the capillaries into the veins and back to the heart.

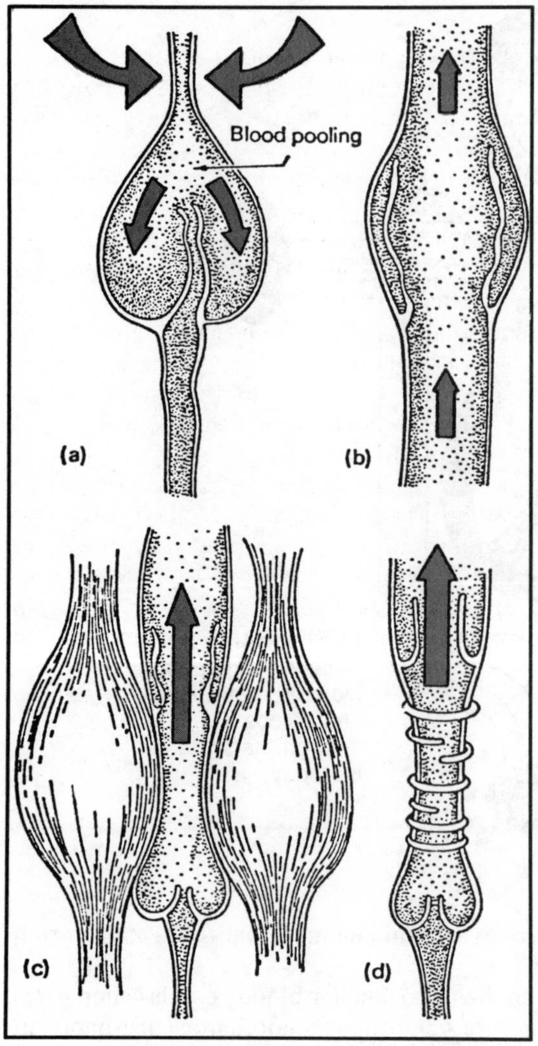
Blood pooling
(a)
(b)
(c)
(d)

Figure 3-21. *Valves in the veins (a) prevent back flow of returning flow, but (b) do not hinder the normal flow very much. Blood can be pushed through veins (c) by nearby active muscle, or (d) by the action of smooth muscle bands.*

During heavy weightlifting or other activities that involve sustained, nonrhythmic muscular contractions, neither the muscle nor ventilatory pumps contribute significantly to venous return. In such situations blood flow to the heart can be impaired to a degree where dizziness and even fainting occur as blood flow to the brain is reduced. Aside from diminishing venous return, such "static" activities also result in a significant but transient increase in arterial blood pressure. *This poses an additional workload for the heart that could be dangerous for those with existing high blood pressure or heart disease.*

BLOOD PRESSURE

With each contraction of the left ventricle a surge of blood enters the aorta, distending it and creating pressure within it. The stretch and subsequent recoil of the vascular wall travels as a wave through the entire system. The wave of pressure can readily be felt as the characteristic pulse in the superficial radial artery on the thumb side of the wrist, temporal artery (side of head at temple), or at the carotid artery along the side of the trachea in the neck ("Adam's apple"). Each site is convenient for counting the heart rate at rest and following exercise because the pulse rate and heart rate are identical in healthy persons. Figure 3-22 illustrates the pulse taken at these three convenient locations.

At rest. At rest, the highest pressure generated by the heart to move blood through a healthy, resilient vascular system is usually about 120 mm Hg during the contraction or *systole* of the left ventricle. As the heart relaxes, the natural elastic recoil of the aorta and other arteries provides a continuous head of pressure to maintain an even blood flow in the arterial system until the next surge of blood is received from the contraction of the heart. During the relaxation phase, or *diastole* of the cardiac cycle, the blood pressure in the arterial system decreases to about 70 or 80 mm Hg. This blood pressure that represents the forces exerted by the blood against the walls of the arteries during a cardiac cycle, is written as 120/80 mm Hg (or stated, 120 over 80). In people with arteries "hardened" by deposits of minerals and fatty materials within the walls, or with an excessive resistance to blood flow in the periphery resulting from kidney malfunction or nervous strain, systolic pressure may increase from 120 to 250 to 300 mm Hg. High blood pressure or *hypertension* imposes a chronic and excessive strain on the normal function of the cardiovascular system. If chronic hypertension is not corrected, it can eventually lead to *heart failure*, where the heart is unable to maintain its pumping ability, or *stroke*, a condition in which brittle vessels burst and cut off the blood supply to vital organs. More will be said about hypertension in Chapter 11.

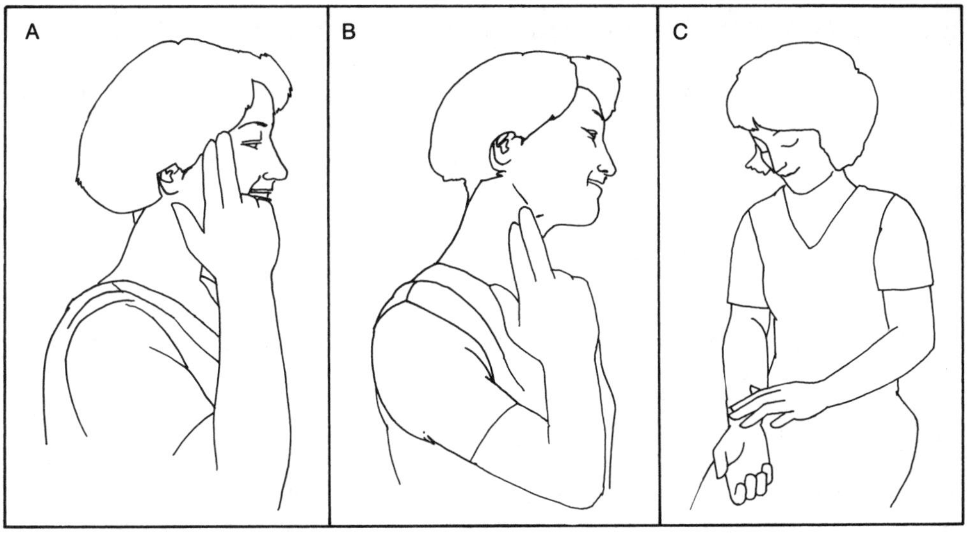
A
B
C

Figure 3-22. *Pulse rate taken at the (A) temporal, (B) carotid, and (C) radial arteries.*

During Exercise. During rhythmic muscular activities such as jogging, swimming, and bicycling, the dilation of blood vessels in the working muscles enhances blood flow through a large portion of the body. The alternate contraction and relaxation of the muscles themselves also provides a significant pumping force to propel blood through the blood vessels and return it to the heart. Increased blood flow during moderate exercise causes systolic pressure to rise rapidly in the first few minutes of exercise and level-off at 140 to 160 mm Hg, while diastolic pressure remains relatively unchanged.

With straining-type exercises such as various forms of resistance exercises (including lifting of barbells), the pressure response is more dramatic as the muscular forces of exercise compress the peripheral arteries and bring about a significant increase in resistance to blood flow. This results in a rapid and often profound elevation in blood pressure. An acute cardiovascular strain could be harmful for individuals who have heart and vascular disease. For these people, more rhythmic forms of moderate exercise are desirable.

Body Inversion

There is a recent popularity in the use of inversion devices by which individuals hang in the upside-down position with the belief that this maneuver can offer relaxation, facilitate a strength-training response, or relieve lower back pain. Although it has yet to be demonstrated with careful research that inverting the body is of any practical or physiologic significance, it is now apparent that it can cause significant increases in blood pressure both at the start and throughout the inversion maneuver. Such observations raise concern as to the possible consequences of inversion for people with high blood pressure, or the wisdom of performing exercise in the upside down position that magnifies the normal rise in blood pressure. Furthermore, only a brief period of inversion doubles the pressure within the eye (intraocular pressure) in healthy young adults. *Clearly, individuals with eye disorders should refrain from prolonged periods of inverted posture.*

CIRCULATORY FUNCTION IN THE TRAINED AND UNTRAINED

The output of the heart pump, referred to as *cardiac output,* is one of the important indicators of the functional capacity of the circulation to meet the demands of aerobic physical activity. Cardiac output is determined by two factors: (1) the rate of the pump's stroke or *heart rate,* and (2) the quantity of fluid ejected with each stroke or *stroke volume.* Thus

Cardiac Output = Heart Rate × Stroke Volume.

The demand for blood flow to the muscles increases in proportion to the severity of the exercise. In relatively sedentary, college-aged males, the cardiac output during strenuous exercise increases about 4 times the resting level to an average maximum of 20 liters or 20,000 ml of blood pumped per minute. Maximal heart rate at this age usually averages 195 beats per minute. Consequently, the "untrained" heart will pump about 103 ml of blood with each beat during maximum exercise. This contrasts with world-class endurance athletes who have maximum cardiac outputs of 35 to 40 liters of blood per minute. For these athletes, maximum heart rate is not appreciably different from the maximum heart rate of sedentary people of similar age. Thus, the stroke volume of the athlete's heart is about 180 ml of blood per beat. *A significantly larger stroke volume is the key factor that enables the endurance athlete to pump more blood each minute than an untrained counterpart.*

Cardiac Output = Heart Rate × Stroke Volume.

At Rest				
Sedentary	5,000 ml	= 70 beats/min	×	71.4 ml
Trained	5,000 ml	= 50 beats/min	×	100.0 ml
Maximum Exercise				
Sedentary	20,000 ml	= 195 beats/min	×	102.6 ml
Trained	35,000 ml	= 195 beats/min	×	179.5 ml

Figure 3-23 a, b, and c illustrates the response of cardiac output, heart rate, and stroke volume, respectively, in relation to oxygen consumption during exercise of increasing severity. The subjects were two groups of men; one group was highly trained endurance athletes, while the other group consisted of sedentary college students measured before and after a 55-day training program designed to improve aerobic fitness.

The researchers observed several important physiologic responses. First, for both trained athletes and students, the cardiac output increased in linear fashion with oxygen consumption throughout the major portion of the work range (Figure 23a). The distinguishing feature between the students and the athletes was a high level of oxygen consumption *and* corresponding cardiac output capacity. In addition, the 35% improvement in aerobic capacity for the students after 55 days of training was accompanied by an almost proportionate increase in maximum cardiac output. Second, the stroke volume of the athletes' hearts was considerably larger than the untrained students' at rest and during exercise (Figure 23c). In addition, the response pattern for stroke volume was similar in both groups during exercise. The increase in stroke volume was greatest when going from rest to light exercise. Thereafter, the increase in stroke volume was quite small. Third, stroke volume increased only slightly from rest to exercise in the untrained men. Thus, the major increase in cardiac output for the untrained subjects was by an increase in heart rate. For the trained athletes, on the other hand, both heart rate and stroke volume increased to augment blood flow to the muscles during exercise. Following 55 days of training, the students' stroke volume (and maximum cardiac output) had increased substantially, but the values were still considerably lower than the stroke volume of the athletes. The degree that both training and genetic factors account for the exceptionally large stroke volumes of successful endurance athletes during maximal exercise is still not resolved. Scientists do generally agree that the ability of the heart trained by exercise to maintain a high stroke volume at rest and during exercise is due to a more forceful contraction that empties the ventricle almost completely with each beat. *Numerous studies have documented that an increase in the heart's pumping capacity occurs in healthy men and women of all ages who undertake vigorous physical conditioning programs.*

Cardiac output is similar at rest and during various submaximum levels of energy expenditure in both sedentary people and those conditioned by exercise.

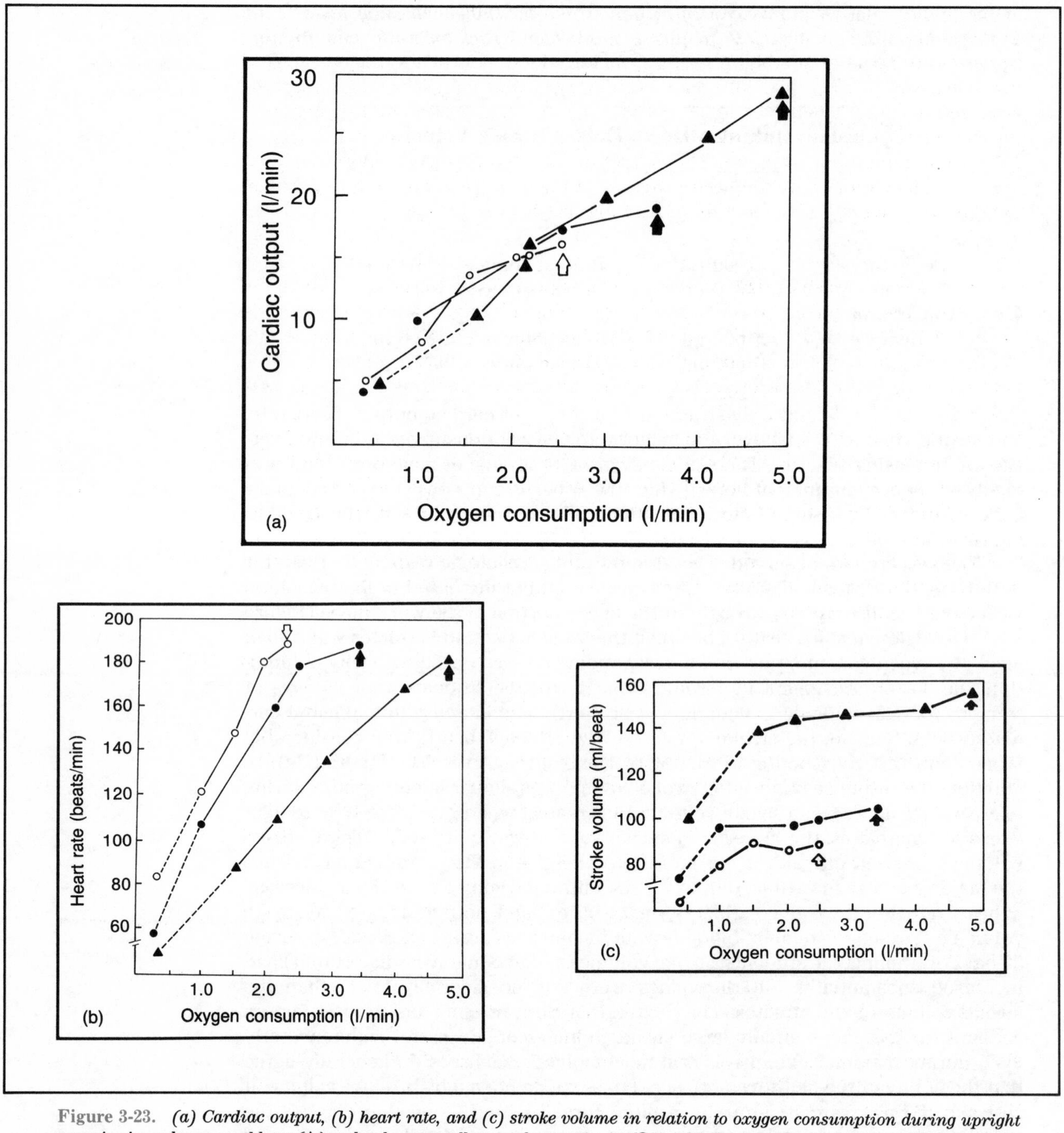

Cardiac output (l/min)
30
20
10
1.0
2.0
3.0
4.0
5.0
Oxygen consumption (l/min)
(a)
Heart rate (beats/min)
200
180
160
140
120
100
80
60
1.0
2.0
3.0
4.0
5.0
Oxygen consumption (l/min)
(b)
Stroke volume (ml/beat)
160
140
120
100
80
1.0
2.0
3.0
4.0
5.0
Oxygen consumption (l/min)
(c)

Figure 3-23. *(a) Cardiac output, (b) heart rate, and (c) stroke volume in relation to oxygen consumption during upright exercise in endurance athletes (▲) and sedentary college students prior to (○) and following (●) 55 days of aerobic training; (⇧, ⬆ = maximal values).*

Consequently, the large stroke volumes of top-flight endurance athletes and the increase in stroke volume of sedentary subjects following an aerobic conditioning program are accompanied by a proportionate reduction in heart rate during submaximal exercise (Figure 3-23b). After training, the same value of cardiac output is achieved during moderate exercise but at a much lower heart rate. It is common for the exercise heart rate to be lowered by 12 to 15 beats per minute during a 12-week conditioning program. The reduction in exercise heart rate provides a practical means for evaluating the progress of physiologic adaptation to physical conditioning. We will discuss this more fully in Chapter 10.

The "Athlete's Heart"

A modest increase in size or *hypertrophy* appears to be a fundamental adjustment of the healthy heart to regular exercise training. There is a greater synthesis of cellular protein as the individual muscle fibers thicken and the contractile elements within each fiber increase in number. The increase in heart size with training is transient in nature and returns to pretraining levels when training intensity is reduced.

A clearer understanding of the changes in heart size and structure with training has been provided by the ultrasonic technique of *echocardiography.* With this approach, sound waves are passed through the heart muscle to provide a "mapping" of the dimensions of the heart muscle itself as well as the volume of its cavities. Different patterns of cardiac enlargement are associated with different types of conditioning. Endurance athletes, for example, who participate regularly in continuous rhythmic exercise that requires a large cardiac output, show normal thickness for the ventricular walls with an enlarged ventricular cavity. The enlarged internal dimensions are certainly in keeping with the development of a large stroke volume that is so beneficial in endurance activities. In contrast, athletes involved in resistance exercise training such as weight lifters, shot putters, or wrestlers who are regularly subjected to acute episodes of elevated arterial pressure caused by straining-type exercises, have normal ventricular volumes but thickened ventricular walls. Undoubtedly, this represents a compensation to the added workload on the left ventricle imposed by training. The consequences are unknown of these apparent differences in training response to long-term cardiovascular health.

Summary

The energy bonded within the food nutrients is not used directly for the performance of biologic work. Instead, the cell harnesses the energy for the resynthesis of its fuel, the high-energy phosphate compound ATP and its "backup" energy supply, CP. Energy from these phosphates is supplied rapidly and anaerobically. However, ATP and CP are stored in limited quantities and consequently must continually be resynthesized. To meet this need, energy is provided through a series of chemical reactions that systematically break down food molecules to simpler form.

Carbohydrates are the only food that provide energy for rebuilding the phosphates anaerobically. In this process, called glycolysis, the glucose molecule is degraded to pyruvic acid. The reactions proceed rapidly and supply the predominant energy for ATP resynthesis during all-out bursts of exercise for durations up to 60 to 90 seconds. If exercise proceeds at a slower tempo but for a longer duration, reactions that require oxygen must generate the energy. In this process of providing aerobic energy, called the Krebs cycle, hydrogen atoms are stripped from fragments of fats, carbohydrates, and to a small degree proteins, and eventually passed to molecular oxygen to form water.

Recent research has identified two types of muscle cells, each with a distinguishing and predominant capacity for energy metabolism. The fast-twitch fiber has a high capacity for anaerobic energy release and is activated during quick bursts of activity. The slow-twitch fibers generate sustained, aerobic energy and are activated in continuous, steady-state work. During such exercise, the oxygen consumption levels off at a point where aerobic metabolism balances the energy demands of the working muscles. If the exercise intensity exceeds a steady-state, the anaerobic reactions of glycolysis must supply the additional energy. Under such conditions of insufficient oxygen supply or utilization, pyruvic acid and hydrogen atoms accumulate and join to form lactic acid. The mechanism of lactic acid production allows the reactions of glycolysis to proceed for a short time before fatigue sets in and exercise must stop. Because the ability to maintain a steady state is so important in long-term exercise, endurance training must be geared toward the improvement of maximal oxygen uptake capacity. Even under conditions of steady-state exercise, however, fatigue will occur if the body's carbohydrate reserves reach low levels, especially muscle glycogen. Thus maintenance of an adequate daily intake of carbohydrates is important for peak physical performance or conditioning.

Although research indicates that a large portion of one's fitness capacity may be genetically determined, the fitness of all individuals can be improved with regular exercise. A key to successful training is to identify the predominant means of energy metabolism required for a desired area of performance, and to train the muscles specifically to augment the capability for that kind of energy output.

Following exercise, the oxygen consumption does not immediately return to the resting level. An elevated oxygen consumption, or oxygen debt, results from a combination of metabolic and physiologic processes caused by the exercise. Recovery is rapid if exercise is moderate and predominantly aerobic, or if intense exercise is brief and stops before lactic acid accumulates. The small oxygen debt is required to reload the blood returning from the exercised muscles, to resynthesize the phosphates used during exercise, and to meet the needs of the slightly elevated bodily functions. Following strenuous exercise, recovery oxygen consumption results from two general factors: (1) the metabolism of lactic acid produced during the anaerobic component of the intense exercise and, perhaps more important, (2) the increased level of bodily function in recovery, including the stimulating effects of an elevated body temperature caused by the exercise. Maintaining a moderate level of physical activity during recovery facilitates the recovery process.

The ventilatory and circulatory systems are crucial in sustaining a high level of aerobic exercise. The lungs provide the surface for gas exchange, while the heart and blood vessels provide a highly efficient delivery system. Under most conditions, the ventilatory system is more than adequate to provide for complete aeration of the blood, even during the most vigorous activities. In healthy men and women, the main factor that limits aerobic performance is the output capability of the heart or the cardiac output (stroke volume × heart rate). The limits for cardiac output are determined largely by the stroke volume of the heart. The changes that occur in heart size and structure consequent to training are associated with specific methods of conditioning (endurance versus strength-type training).

Additional Reading

Appenzeller, O. and R. Atkinson (Eds.): *Sports Medicine.* Baltimore, Urban & Schwarzenberg, 1981.

Banner, A.S., et al.: Relation of respiratory water loss to coughing after exercise. *New England Journal of Medicine. 311:*833, 1984.

Bergh, V. et al.: Maximal oxygen uptake and muscle fiber types in trained and untrained humans. *Medicine and Science in Sports. 10:*151, 1978.

Brooks, G.A.: Anaerobic threshold: review of the concept and directions for future research. *Medicine and Science in Sports and Exercise. 17:*22, 1985.

Bundgaard, A., et al.: Influence of temperature and relative humidity of inhaled gas on exercise-induced asthma. *European Journal of Respiratory Disease. 63:*239, 1982.

Davis, J.A.: Anaerobic threshold: review of the concept and directions for future research. *Medicine and Science in Sports and Exercise. 17:*6, 1985.

Franklin, B.A.: Exercise testing, training and arm ergometry. *Sports Medicine. 2:*109, 1985.

Freedson, P.F., et al.: Intra-arterial blood pressure during graded isometric exercise. *Journal of Cardiac Rehabilitation.* 1987. (In Press)

Goodman, M.N. and N.B. Ruderman: Influence of muscle use on amino acid metabolism. In: *Exercise and Sport Science Reviews.* Vol. 10. Edited by R.L. Terjung. Philadelphia, Franklin Institute Press, 1982.

Gimby, G.: Respiration in exercise. *Medicine and Science in Sports. 1:*9, 1969.

Henritze, J. et al.: Effects of training at and above the lactate threshold on the lactate threshold and maximal oxygen uptake. *European Journal of Applied Physiology. 54:*84, 1985.

Holloszy, J.O., and Coyle, E.F.: Adaptations of skeletal muscle to endurance training and their metabolic consequences. *Journal of Applied Physiology. 56:*831, 1984.

Jones, N.L.: Dyspnea in exercise. *Medicine and Science in Sports and Exercise. 16:*14, 1984.

Karlsson, J., and Jacobs, I.: Onset of blood lactate accumulation during muscular exercise as a threshold concept. I. Theoretical considerations. *International Journal of Sports Medicine. 3:*190, 1982.

LeMarr, J.D., et al.: Cardiorespiratory responses to inversion. *Physician and Sportsmedicine. 11*(11):51, 1983.

Lewis, S.F. et al.: Cardiovascular responses to exercise as a function of absolute and relative workload. *Journal of Applied Physiology. 54:*1314, 1983.

McFadden, E.R., Jr.: Respiratory heat and water exchange: physiological and clinical implications. *Journal of Applied Physiology. 54:*331, 1983.

Rowell, L.B.: Human cardiovascular adjustments to exercise and thermal stress. *Physiological Reviews. 4:*75, 1974.

Rushmer, R.F.: *Cardiovascular Dynamics.* Philadelphia, W.B. Saunders Co., 1976.

Saltin, B.: Metabolic fundamentals in exercise. *Medicine and Science in Sports. 5:*137, 1973.

Saltin, B.: Physiological effects of physical conditioning. *Medicine and Science in Sports. 1:*50, 1969.

Seals, D.R., and Hagberg, J.M.: The effect of exercise training on human hypertension. *Medicine and Science in Sports and Exercise. 16:*207, 1984.

Vogel, J.A. et al.: An analysis of aerobic capacity in a large United States population. *Journal of Applied Physiology. 60:*494, 1986.

Wells, C.L., and Plowman, S.A.: Sexual differences in athletic performance: biological or behavioral? *Physician and Sportsmedicine. 11*(8):52, 1983.

4

Energy Value of Food and Physical Activity

THE GREATEST DEMAND for energy occurs during physical activity. The energy trapped within the chemical bonds of carbohydrates, fats, and proteins is extracted during a series of complex chemical reactions and made available to the cells in the form of energy currency, ATP. Because the three major food nutrients contain energy, and because all bodily functions both at rest and during exercise require energy, it is possible to classify both food and physical activity in terms of a common denominator, *energy*.

Energy Contained in Foods—Calories

A *calorie* is a unit of heat used to express the energy value of food. Although the term is widely used in popular literature, it has a precise scientific meaning. One Calorie (spelled with a capital C), represents the amount of heat necessary to increase the temperature of 1 kg of water, which is slightly more than a quart, by 1°C. A Calorie—or more accurately, a kilocalorie—is abbreviated *kcal.* For example, a McDonalds Big Mac hamburger and regular fries contain about 783 kcal and thus the energy to raise the temperature of about 783 quarts or 196 gallons of water by 1°C. This is indeed a relatively large amount of energy. On the other hand, a boiled egg contains only 80 kcal, or the energy required to increase the temperature of about 80 quarts of water by 1°C.

Measurement of Calories

The energy or kcal value of any food can be measured directly by the amount of heat released from the food when it is burned in an apparatus called a *bomb calorimeter.* This method of directly measuring the energy content of foods is known as *direct calorimetry.*

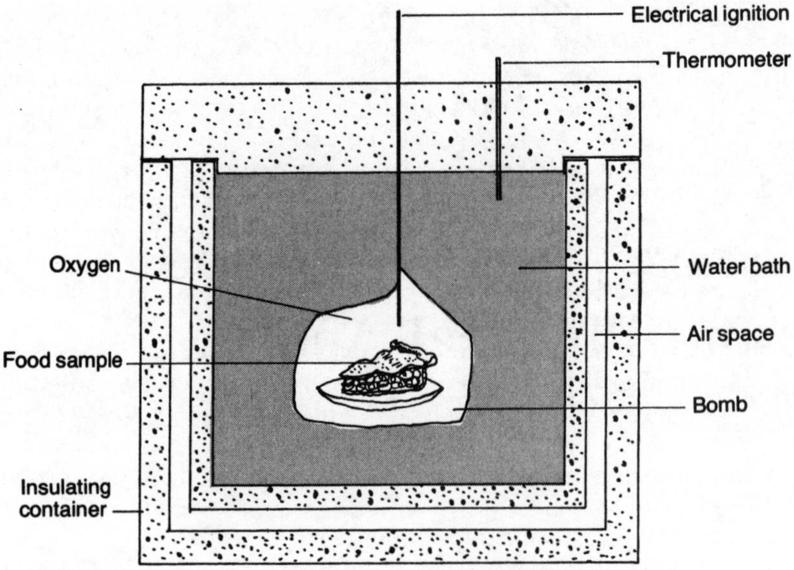
Electrical ignition
Thermometer
Oxygen
Water bath
Air space
Food sample
Bomb
Insulating
container

Figure 4-1. *Determining the caloric value of foods in a bomb calorimeter.*

The bomb calorimeter illustrated in Figure 4-1 works as follows. A weighed portion of food is placed inside a small chamber filled with oxygen. The food is literally exploded and burned in the chamber when an electric current ignites a fuse inside the bomb. The heat released as the food burns is absorbed by a surrounding water bath. Because the calorimeter is fully insulated, no heat escapes to the outside. The precise amount of heat absorbed by the water is determined by measuring the increase in water temperature with a sensitive thermometer. For example, when one 4.7 ounce, 4-inch sector of apple pie is completely burned in the calorimeter, 350 kcal of heat energy are released. This is enough to raise 3.5 kg or 7.7 pounds of ice water to the boiling point.

Caloric Value of Foods

Many laboratories throughout the world have used the bomb calorimeter to determine the energy value of foods. The burning of 1 g of pure carbohydrate yields 4.10 kcal, 1 g of pure protein releases 5.65 kcal, and 1 g of pure fat yields 9.45 kcal. Because most foods in the normal diet consist of various proportions of these three nutrients, the caloric value of a given food such as a hamburger or french fries is determined by the amount of carbohydrate, fat, or protein in an average serving. It is evident from the caloric values for a gram of each nutrient that the energy content of food that contains a considerable amount of fat will be greater than food that is relatively fat-free. As an example, the number of calories in 1 cup of whole milk is 160 kcal, whereas the same amount of skimmed milk contains 90 kcal. If someone who normally consumes 1 quart of milk each day switches to skimmed milk, the quantity of calories ingested each year would be reduced by an amount equal to about 25 pounds of body fat.

When 1 g of carbohydrate or fat is "burned" or metabolized in the cell's energy factory, the body obtains the same value of 4.10 kcal for carbohydrate and 9.45 kcal for fat as did the bomb calorimeter. The energy yield from fat is more than twice that of carbohydrate because of the difference in the structural composition between the two nutrients. As noted in Chapter 1, the chemical formula for a simple carbohydrate is $C_6H_{12}O_6$. There is always a ratio of two hydrogen atoms for each oxygen atom. Fat molecules, on the other hand, contain significantly more hydrogen than oxygen. Palmitic acid, one of the fatty acid constituents of a fat, has the structural formula $C_{16}H_{30}O_2$. Consequently, there are more hydrogen atoms that can be cleaved away during the breakdown of a fat to combine eventually with oxygen to form water and produce energy.

The energy available to the body from the metabolism of protein is less than that released in the bomb calorimeter. In addition to carbon, hydrogen, and oxygen, proteins contain the element nitrogen. Because the body cannot use nitrogen, it combines with hydrogen to form *urea* (NH_2CONH_2) and is excreted in the urine. The elimination of hydrogen represents a loss of potential energy. For this reason, the energy yield from 1 g of protein in the body is 4.35 kcal instead of the 5.65 kcal released during its complete oxidation in the bomb calorimeter.

An important consideration in determining the ultimate caloric yield to the body of the various foods is the efficiency of the digestive processes. Efficiency in this sense refers to the completeness or thoroughness of the breakdown of the foods in the digestive tract, as well as their eventual absorption and elimination as part of the body's various metabolic reactions. Normally about 97% of carbohydrates, 95% of fats, and 92% of proteins are completely digested and absorbed. These average efficiency percentages may vary somewhat depending on the particular foods. This is especially true in the case of protein, where digestive efficiency may vary from a high of 97% with animal protein to a low of 78% for dried legumes. *When the average efficiency of digestion is taken into account, the net kcal value for carbohydrate is 4.0, it is 9.0 for fat, and 4.0 for protein.*

By use of the net kcal values, the appropriate caloric content of any portion of food can be determined as long as its composition and weight are known. Suppose, for example, we wanted to determine the kcal value for one-half cup of creamed chicken. From Appendix A, the weight of this portion size of food is equivalent to 3.5 oz or about 100 g. Based on laboratory analysis of portions made from a standard recipe, the nutrient composition of the creamed chicken is approximately 20% protein, 12% fat, 6% carbohydrate, and the remaining 62% is water. Using these compositional values, the kcal value of the creamed chicken can be determined as follows: Because of the above proportion of nutrients, each gram of creamed chicken will contain 0.2 g of protein, 0.12 g of fat, and 0.06 g of carbohydrate. The net kcal values indicate that 0.2 g of protein contains 0.8 kcal (0.20×4.00), 0.12 g of fat equals 1.08 kcal (0.12×9.00), and 0.06 g of carbohydrate yields 0.24 kcal (0.06×4.00). The total caloric value of 1 g of creamed chicken would therefore equal 2.12 kcal ($0.80 + 1.08 + 0.24$). Consequently, a 100-g serving would have a caloric value 100 times as large, or 212 kcal. These computations are illustrated in Table 4-1. Although this table shows the method for calculating the kcal value of creamed chicken, the same method could be used to calculate the caloric value for a serving of any food. Reducing the size of the portion by half would of course reduce the caloric intake by 50%. Needless to say, if extra fat is added to the preparation of the meal, or if fat-free substitutes are used, the caloric value of the meal will be affected accordingly.

Table 4-1. *Method of calculating the caloric value of a food when its composition of nutrients is known.*

Food: creamed chicken

Weight ½ cup = 3.5 oz = 100 g

Composition:	*Protein*	*Fat*	*Carbohydrates*
1. Percentage	20%	12%	6%
2. Total grams	20	12	6
3. In one gram	0.20 g	0.12 g	0.06 g
Calories per gram:	0.80 (0.20 × 4.00 kcal)	1.08 (0.12 × 9.00 kcal)	0.24 (0.06 × 4.00 kcal)

Total calories per gram: 0.80 + 1.08 + 0.24 = 2.12 kcal

Total calories per 100 grams: 2.12 × 100 = 212 kcal

Fortunately, there is seldom a need to compute the kcal value of foods as shown in the example, because the values have been already determined for almost all foods by the United States Department of Agriculture. What we have done in Appendix A is to present a representative listing of the nutritive value of the more common foods. Included is the weight of an average serving of the food in grams and ounces, the kcal value of the serving, the amount of protein, fat, and carbohydrate present, as well as the quantity of the minerals calcium and iron, and the content of vitamins A and C, thiamin and riboflavin.

For those who have access to a computer based nutritional analysis system, it is unnecessary to calculate the specific nutrient composition of foods. By specifying the portion size, the computer taps its memory for that particular food item and lists the corresponding nutrient composition. In this way, one can determine the total nutrient intake for any diet and compare it with the *Recommended Dietary Allowances* specified by the Food and Nutrition Board. A nutrient analysis is useful to evaluate nutritional status, as well as to compare individuals and groups in terms of their dietary practices. A major drawback with this approach is the large amount of time required to enter the "coded" food items into the computer, as well as the uncertainty regarding portion size. At best, the computerized analysis approach is a first approximation of the "true" nutrient intake, ±10 to 30% even when accurate records are kept.

If you examine Appendix A carefully, you will make a rather striking yet reasonable observation with regard to the energy value of food. Consider for example, five common foods: raw celery, cooked cabbage, cooked asparagus spears, mayonnaise, and salad oil. In order to consume 100 kcal of each of these foods, an individual would need to eat 20 stalks of celery, 4 cups of cabbage, 30 asparagus spears, but only 1 tablespoon of mayonnaise or ⅘ tablespoon of salad oil. The salient point is that a small serving of some foods can have an equal kcal value as large quantities of other foods. Viewed from a different perspective, one would have to consume over 4000 stalks of celery or 800 cups of cabbage to supply the daily energy needs of a fairly sedentary individual, while the same energy would be supplied by ingesting only ⅖ cup of mayonnaise or about 3 ounces of salad oil. The major difference is that foods with a high fat content exist as relatively concentrated sources of food energy and contain little water. On the other hand, foods low in fat or high in water tend to contain relatively little energy. An important concept is that 100 kcal from mayonnaise and 100 kcal from celery are exactly the same in terms of energy. There is no difference between calories from an energy standpoint, a calorie being a unit of heat regardless of the food source. Simply stated, a calorie . . . is a calorie . . . is a calorie. It would be incorrect to consider 100 kcal of mayonnaise as being any more fattening than 100 kcal of celery. The number of calories contained in foods are additive: The more you eat the more calories you consume. If the food has a high concentration of calories as in the case of fatty foods, and you consume even a moderate portion, you will of course consume a relatively large number of calories.

Heat Produced by the Body

DIRECT CALORIMETRY

The amount of heat produced by an animal can be measured in a calorimeter similar to that used to determine the caloric content of food. The human calorimeter illustrated in Figure 4-2 consists of an airtight chamber with an oxygen supply in which a person can live and work for an extended period. A known volume of water is circulated through a series of pipes located at the top of the chamber. Because the entire chamber is well insulated, the heat produced and radiated by the individual is absorbed by the circulating water. The change in water temperature reflects the individual's metabolic energy release for a particular time period. To provide adequate ventilation, the subject's exhaled air is drawn from the room and passed through a series of chemicals that remove the moisture content of the air and absorb carbon dioxide. Oxygen is then added to the air and recirculated through the chamber.

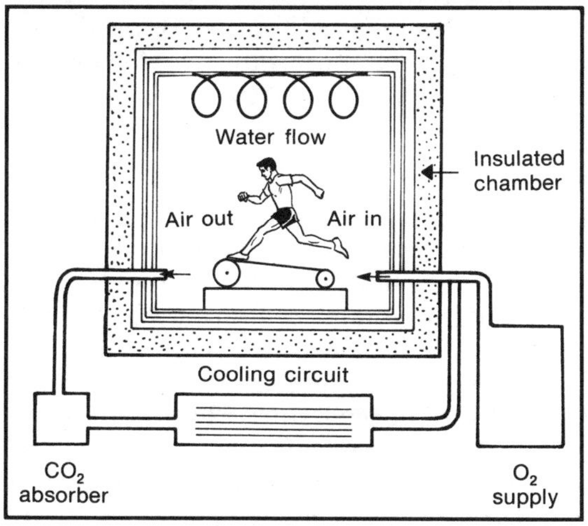
Water flow
Insulated chamber
Air out
Air in
Cooling circuit
CO_2 absorber
O_2 supply

Figure 4-2. *Measuring heat production of the body by direct calorimetry.*

The direct measurement of heat production in humans in a closed chamber is of considerable theoretical importance, yet its use and application are rather limited. The calorimeter is relatively small and quite expensive, accurate measurements of heat production are time-consuming, and its use is generally not applicable for energy determinations during common sport or recreation activities.

INDIRECT CALORIMETRY

All energy-producing reactions in the body depend ultimately on a continual supply of oxygen. By measuring a person's oxygen consumption it is possible to obtain an indirect estimate of energy production. Compared to the direct calorimetric method, the technique of indirect calorimetry is relatively simple, the equipment is much less expensive, and it is highly accurate. There are two methods of indirect calorimetry—(1) *closed-circuit spirometry,* and (2) *open-circuit spirometry.* The open-circuit method is the most widely used technique to measure oxygen consumption, especially during exercise. The subject does not breathe and rebreathe from a prefilled container of oxygen as in the closed-circuit method, but instead inhales ambient air that has a constant composition. Changes in oxygen and carbon dioxide percentage in the exhaled air compared to ambient air in the lungs indirectly reflect the body's constant need to maintain an "energy equilibrium" of the internal processes. Thus, an analysis of two factors, the volume of air breathed and the composition of expired air, provides a relatively simple means to measure the oxygen consumed by the body, and indirectly to infer the energy expenditure.

Oxygen consumption can easily be converted to a corresponding value for energy production. When 1 liter of oxygen is consumed in the burning of a small mixture of carbohydrates, fats, and proteins, approximately 4.82 kcal of heat energy are liberated. This caloric equivalent for oxygen varies only slightly depending on the food mixture. For convenience in calculations, therefore, a value of *5 kcal per liter of oxygen consumed* can be used as an appropriate conversion factor. This amount, 5 kcal, is important because it enables us to determine easily the body's energy production at rest or during steady state exercise simply by measuring the oxygen consumption. There are three common procedures for measuring the rate of oxygen consumption during a variety of physical activities; (1) portable spirometer, (2) meteorologic balloons, and (3) computerized instrumentation.

Portable Spirometer

German scientists in the early 1940s developed a relatively light weight, portable system to determine indirectly the energy expended during various forms of physical activity. The box-shaped apparatus shown in Figure 4-3 weighs only 8 or 9 pounds and is usually carried on the back during the measurement period. The subject breathes through a two-way valve that allows inspiration of ambient air, while the exhaled air passes through a special meter to measure air volume. Samples of the exhaled air are automatically collected in small rubber bags attached to the meter. Oxygen consumption is computed by analyzing the expired air for oxygen and carbon dioxide content. Energy expenditure, expressed in kcal, is then computed from the oxygen consumption. One of the advantages of using the portable spirometer is that it allows the subject considerable freedom of movement during the measurement period. The portable spirometer is useful for measuring

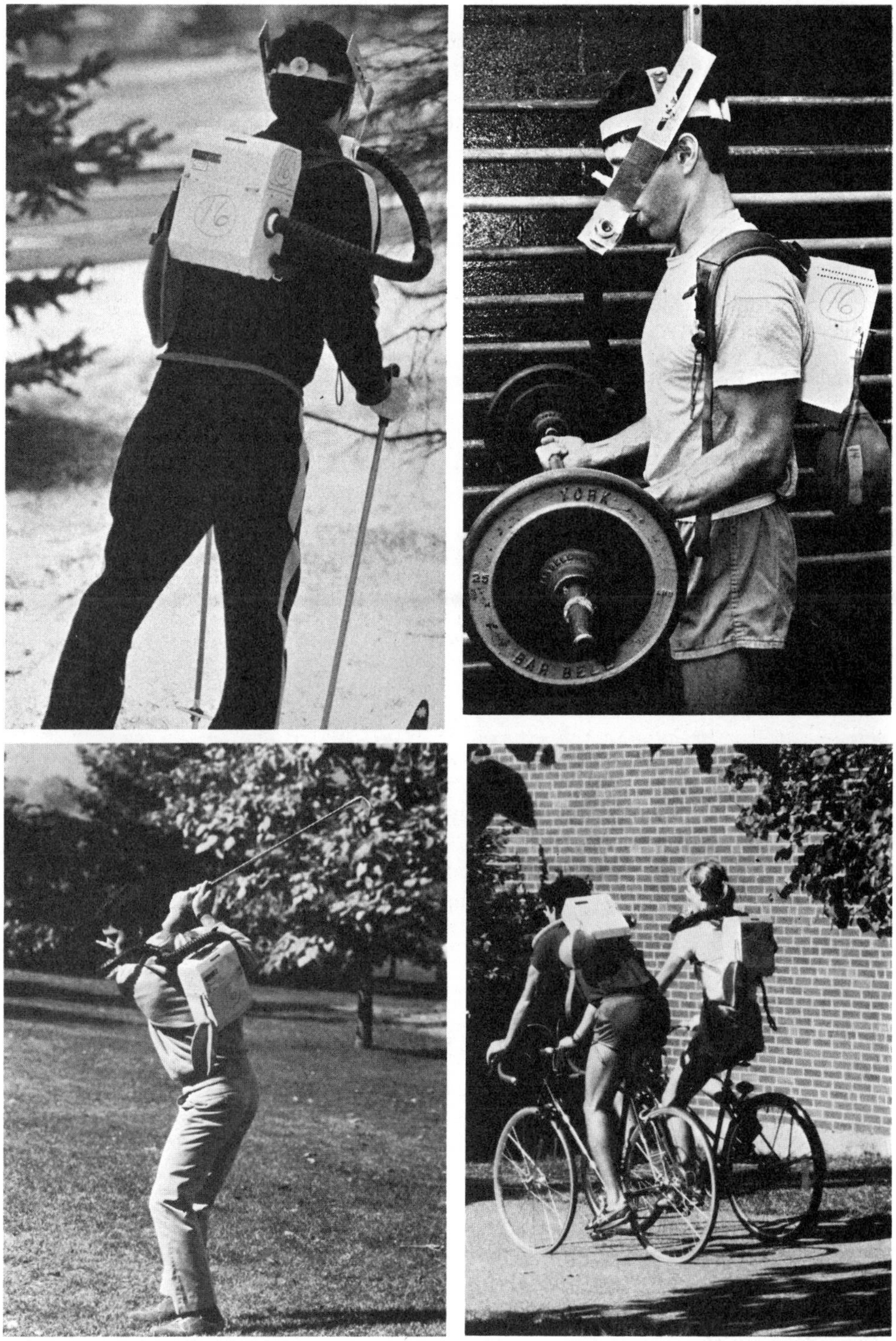
16
YORK

Figure 4-3. *Portable spirometer used to measure oxygen consumption by the open-circuit method during cross country skiing, weight lifting exercise, golf, and leisure cycling.*

energy expenditure for activities that do not require intense and sustained physical efforts. The portable spirometer was used to estimate the energy expenditure for most of the recreational and household activities listed in Appendix B.

Meteorologic Balloons

The subject shown in the left in Figure 4-4 is walking on a motor-driven treadmill. While exercising, the subject wears a special headgear with a two-way breathing valve. The subject breathes ambient air in through one side of the valve and exhales it from the valve into meteorologic balloons. The air is then sampled and analyzed for its oxygen and carbon dioxide composition. Energy expenditure is calculated from oxygen consumption just as it was when using the portable spirometer.

As can be seen in the right side of Figure 4-4, oxygen consumption is being measured during stationary cycle ergometer exercise.

Computerized Instrumentation

Recent advances in computer and microprocessor technology enable the exercise scientist to efficiently and accurately measure metabolic and cardiovascular response to exercise. A computer is interfaced with at least three instruments: (1) a system to continuously sample the airflow from the subject; (2) a meter to record the volume of air flow, and (3) oxygen and carbon dioxide analyzers to measure the concentration of the gas mixture. The computer is preprogrammed to perform all of the necessary calculations based on the electronic signals it receives from the instrument. A printed or graphic display of the subject's data can occur simultane-

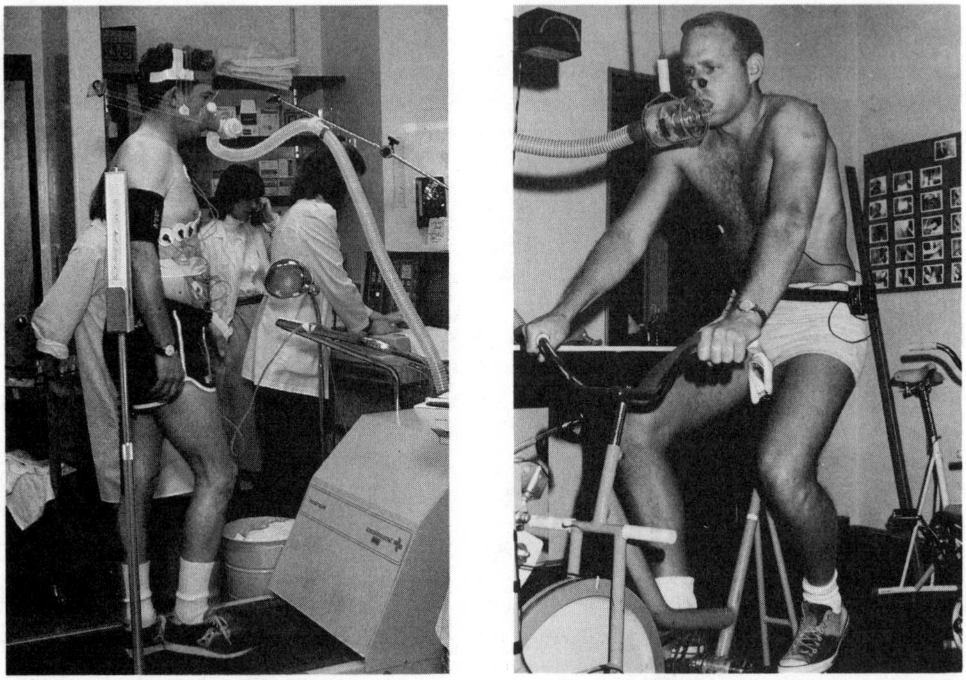

Figure 4-4. *Measurement of oxygen consumption by open-circuit spirometry during treadmill and cycle ergometer exercise.*

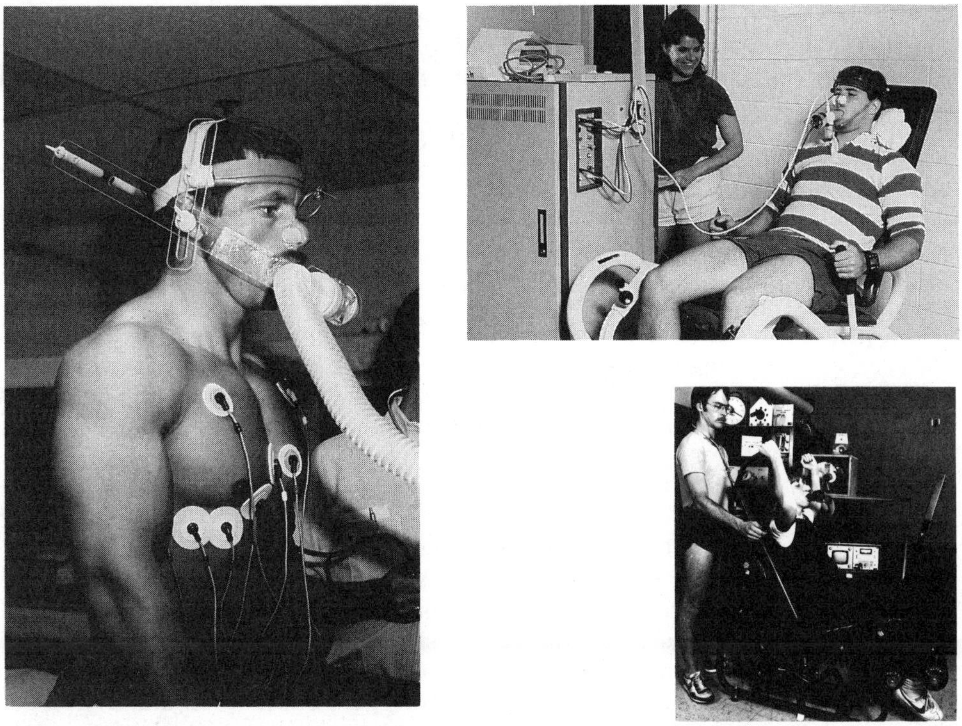

Figure 4-5. *Data collection using computerized instrumentation during hydraulic resistance exercise and at rest prior to exercise.*

ously during exercise and recovery. More advanced systems include automated blood pressure, heart rate, and temperature monitors, as well as preset instructions to regulate the speed, duration, and workload of treadmills, bicycle ergometers, and other exercise devices. The computerized metabolic measurement systems currently in use make it possible to rapidly collect, measure, and analyze a vast amount of physiologic information for a wide variety of work and performance tasks. Figure 4-5 shows examples of the computerized approach during data collection of metabolic and physiological response during hydraulic resistance exercise, and at rest just prior to maximal treadmill exercise in a world champion body builder.

Basal Metabolic Rate

For each individual there is a minimum level of energy required to sustain the body's vital functions in the waking state. This energy requirement, or *basal metabolic rate* (BMR), is usually determined by measuring oxygen consumption under fairly stringent and standardized laboratory guidelines. No food is eaten for at least 12 hours prior to the measurement so no increase will occur in the energy required for the digestion and absorption of foods. Abstaining from food in this manner is referred to as the *post-absorptive state.* In addition, no undue muscular exertion should have occurred for at least 12 hours prior to the determination of BMR. During the test, the subject lies in a dimly lit, temperature-controlled room. After lying quietly for 30 to 60 minutes, the subject's oxygen consumption is measured for a 6- to 10-minute period.

The measurement of BMR under strictly controlled laboratory conditions provides a convenient method for studying the relationship between metabolic rate and body size, gender, and age.

INFLUENCE OF BODY SIZE ON RESTING METABOLISM

A general rule is that when individuals of different body size are compared with respect to resting or basal energy metabolism, the value for energy expenditure is usually expressed in terms of *surface area* and not body weight. The results of numerous experiments have provided data on average values of BMR per unit surface area in men and women of different ages.

The data in Figure 4-6 reveal that the average BMR is *not* equal between the genders, but is 5 to 10% lower in women than in men at all ages. The lower BMR of women can be attributed to their larger percentage of body fat and smaller muscle mass. When the BMR is expressed per unit of *fat-free* or *lean body weight,* the observed gender differences become less apparent. While this observation may be of some theoretical importance, the curves shown in Figure 4-5 still describe the BMR in men and women adequately. From ages 20 to 40, average values for the BMR are 38 kcal per square meter of surface (m^2) per hour for men, and 35 kcal per m^2 per hour for women. If you desire a more precise estimate of the BMR, you can obtain the actual average value for a given age directly from the curves. By using these values for heat production in conjunction with the appropriate value for surface area, it is easy to compute the approximate resting heat production in kcal per minute, and convert this to the total kcal requirement per day. The nomogram in Figure 4-7 provides a simplified method for computing surface area based on height and weight.

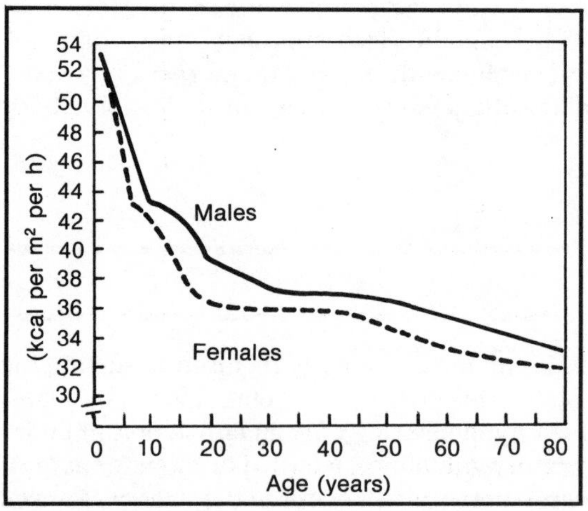
(kcal per m² per h)
54
52
50
48
46
44
42
40
38
36
34
32
30
Males
Females
0
10
20
30
40
50
60
70
80
Age (years)

Figure 4-6. ***Resting metabolic rate as a function of age and gender.***

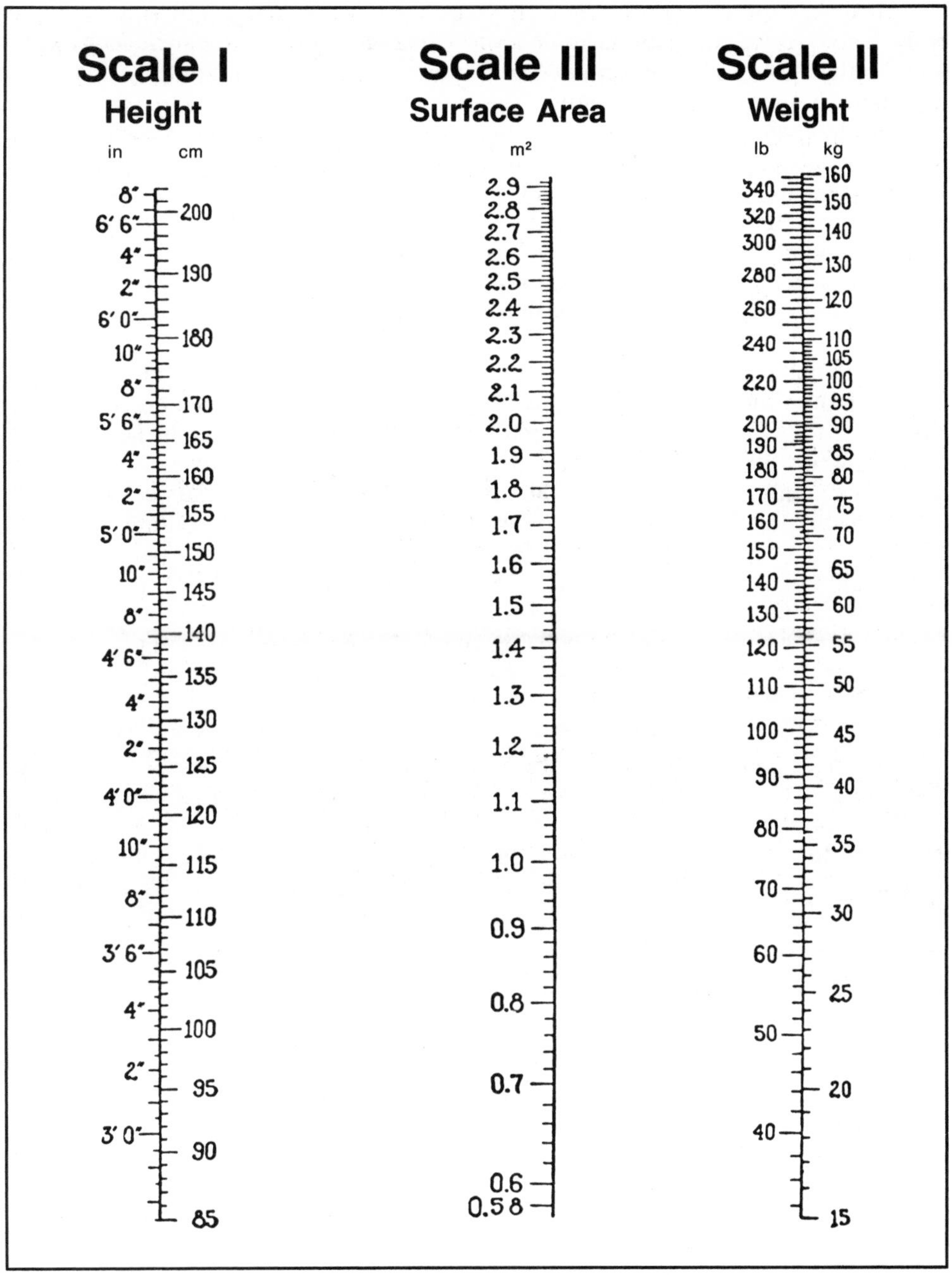
Scale I
Height
in cm
Scale III
Surface Area
m²
Scale II
Weight
lb kg

Figure 4-7. *Nomogram to estimate body surface area from height and weight.*

To determine surface area with the nomogram, locate height on Scale I and weight on Scale II. Connect the two points with a straight edge or piece of thread. The intersection at Scale III gives the surface area expressed in square meters (m^2). For example, if height is 6 feet, and weight is 180 pounds, surface area according to Scale III on the nomogram would be 2.04 square meters.

To determine the approximate heat production or kcal requirement of the body during resting conditions, multiply the average kcal per unit surface area per hour by the surface area determined from the nomogram. Then multiply this by 24 to obtain an estimate of the resting energy requirement on a 24-hour basis. For a 22-year-old man whose surface area is 2.04 square meters, the minimum daily caloric requirement would be 38 kcal/m^2/h × 2.04 m^2 × 24 h, or 1860 kcal per day. Values calculated in this manner will usually be within 10% of the kcal value per day had the BMR been measured under strict laboratory conditions. Computing the minimum daily energy requirements based on age and surface area gives a much more dependable estimate than simply using the average population value for daily resting energy expenditure, that for men and women ranges from about 900 to 1900 kcal/day.

Another method for determining the daily resting energy expenditure would be to compute the caloric equivalent of the total volume of oxygen consumed for basal functions during a 24-hour period. We pointed out in a previous section that approximately 5 kcal of energy are expended for each liter of oxygen consumed during the combustion of a mixed diet. Because the value for oxygen consumption during resting or basal conditions ranges from about 160 to 290 ml/min (average 0.235 liter/min or 235 ml/min), an average value for energy output per minute at rest would be 1.18 kcal (0.235 × 5 kcal). Because there are 1440 minutes in a day, the daily resting energy expenditure would theoretically equal 1700 kcal (1,440 × 1.18 kcal). This value is only a rough approximation because it does not correct for differences in body size such as surface area, body weight, or lean body weight.

Dietary-Induced Thermogenesis

For most people, food has a stimulating effect on energy metabolism that is due mainly to the energy requiring processes of digesting, absorbing, and assimilating the various nutrients. This *dietary-induced thermogenesis* can vary between 9% of the total calories for meals high in carbohydrates to 17% for high-protein meals. It also appears that exercising after eating augments an individual's normal *thermic response* to food intake. This certainly would support the wisdom of "going for a brisk walk" after eating, especially for those interested in weight loss.

The calorie-burning effect of protein ingestion has been used by some to argue for a high-protein diet for weight reduction. They maintain that with a meal high in protein, fewer calories are ultimately available to the body compared to a meal of similar caloric value that consists mainly of fat or carbohydrate. Although this point may have some validity, many other factors must be considered in formulating a sound weight loss program—not to mention the potentially harmful strain on liver and kidney function that could result from excessive protein intake. For one thing, well-balanced nutrition requires a blend of carbohydrate, fat, and protein as well as appropriate quantities of vitamins and minerals. In addition, if exercise is used in conjunction with food restriction for weight loss, it is important to maintain carbohydrate intake to power exercise and conserve the lean tissue that is often lost through dieting.

Research now indicates that individuals who have poor control of body weight often have a blunted thermic response to eating. Undoubtedly over a period of years, this could contribute to considerable accumulation of body fat. The important point, however, is that if a person is physically active, the thermogenic effect represents only a small portion of the total daily energy expenditure.

Energy Metabolism during Physical Activity

An understanding of the energy required for maintaining bodily functions in resting conditions provides a frame of reference to evaluate not only the minimum demands for energy, but also the potential to increase the daily metabolic output. According to numerous surveys, about one-third of a person's time is spent in resting activities like those specified in the test of BMR. The remaining 16 to 18 hours are devoted to a wide range of physical activities. Consequently, the total amount of energy expended during a day can be considerably greater than the basal requirement, depending of course on the type and duration of physical activity performed.

Researchers have measured the energy expended during such varied physical activities as brushing teeth, cleaning house, mowing the lawn, walking the dog, driving a car, playing Ping-Pong, bowling, dancing, swimming, sawing, and even walking on the moon. The portable spirometer shown in Figure 4-3 has been used extensively for determining the energy requirements of most daily chores and sport activities, while the balloon and computer techniques have provided an accurate means for measuring the oxygen consumed in activities such as cycling, swimming, skiing, running, rowing, and resistance training.

Consider an activity like rowing continuously at 30 strokes a minute for 30 minutes. If the oxygen consumption averaged 2 liters per minute, then in 30 minutes the rower would consume 60 liters of oxygen. Because the utilization of 1 liter of oxygen produces about 5 kcal of energy, the researcher can make a reasonably accurate estimate of the energy expended. In this instance, the body generated 300 kcal (60 liters × 5 kcal) to power the exercise. All this energy cannot be attributed solely to the requirements of rowing because the 300 kcal value also includes the normal resting energy requirement during the 30 minutes. By knowing the exerciser's size (weight = 180 pounds; height = 6 feet) surface area can be computed from the nomogram in Figure 4-6. This value for surface area, 2.04 square meters, when multiplied by the average BMR for age (38 kcal/m/h × 2.04 m), gives the resting energy production per hour. This amounts to approximately 78 kcal per hour, or 39 kcal in 30-minutes. Based on this computation, the *net energy expenditure* required solely for the exercise can be determined. This is equal to the total energy expenditure of 300 kcal *minus* that required for resting metabolism. This results in a net energy expenditure of rowing of approximately 261 kcal. The net kcal values for other activities would be computed in similar fashion.

Some investigators have made measurements of the daily rates of energy expenditure for men and women who work in a variety of industrial occupations. They do this by determining the time spent in each activity during the day, and the energy expended for each activity. To calculate the total daily energy expenditure, the time spent in a particular activity is multiplied by the energy cost of the activity. An accurate assessment of the time spent in activities is kept by diary, and energy expenditure is measured with the portable spirometer shown in Figure 4-3. Because it is impractical to carry the spirometer constantly day after day, frequent observations are made for a representative time period. For the miner listed in Table 4-2 who spent 12 hours during the week loading coal, the energy cost of this task ranged from 5.5 to 7.2 kcal per minute. For purposes of computation, a mean value of 6.3 kcal per minute was used to represent the average energy cost for this

Table 4-2. *Energy expenditure of a coal miner in 1 week.*

ACTIVITY	TIME SPENT IN 1 WEEK (H)	(MIN)	RATE OF ENERGY EXPENDED (KCAL/MIN)	ENERGY IN 1 WEEK (KCAL)
Sleep				
1. In bed	58	30	1.05	3690
Nonoccupational				
1. Sitting	38	37	1.59	3680
2. Standing	2	16	1.80	250
3. Walking	15	0	4.90	4410
4. Washing and dressing	5	3	3.30	1000
5. Gardening	2	0	5.00	600
6. Cycling	2	25	6.60	960
Work				
1. Sitting	15	9	1.68	1530
2. Standing	2	6	1.80	230
3. Walking	6	43	6.70	2700
4. Cutting	1	14	6.70	500
5. Timbering	6	51	5.70	2340
6. Loading	12	6	6.30	4570
Total	168 h	0 min		26,460
Average daily energy expenditure				3780

Source: Data of R.C. Garry et al., "Expenditure of energy and the consumption of food by miners and clerks," Medical Research Council, Report No. 289, Her Majesty's Stationery Office, Fife, Scotland, 1955.

time period. The total of 26,460 kcal expended during the 1-week period averaged 3780 kcal per day. This value includes the energy expended during the 8-hour work shift, the energy cost of an 8-hour sleeping period, as well as the remaining 8-hour period spent in non-occupational activities.

Ballet Exercise for Aerobic Fitness and Weight Control

Ballet is one of the most complex and highly developed systems of dance that has become a popular art form with an increasing number of professional dancers. In addition, large numbers of nonprofessional "recreational" dancers and exercise enthusiasts engage in ballet dancing to develop and maintain physiologic fitness and as a means for weight control. While other forms of exercise, both athletic and occupational, have been extensively studied in terms of energy expenditure, little information is available on the metabolic and cardiovascular responses to ballet training. This prompted researchers to study this art form that combines a blend of diverse, simple movements that alternate rapidly with bursts of dynamic complex movements. To quantify the caloric cost and cardiovascular response in ballet, 15 professional male and female dancers from the American Ballet Theatre were studied during actual ballet class work. Each 1-hour class consisted of 28 minutes of supported dance movements or *barre* exercise, and 32 minutes of center floor exercises that were unsupported, free dance combinations similar to those seen on stage. The method of open circuit spirometry with the balloon technique was used to measure oxygen consumption during the floor exercise. Simultaneously, heart rates were monitored by means of radio telemetry. The net caloric expenditure for an entire ballet class averaged only a modest 300 kcal per hour for men and 200 kcal for the women,—this reflects a relatively inefficient exercise method for burning calories. The non-endurance nature of ballet was further substantiated by maximal oxygen uptakes for these elite dancers that were only slightly higher than values for untrained men and women. It can be concluded that standard ballet exercise and training provides a moderate stimulus to enhance aerobic capacity. In terms of its caloric-burning efficiency, it would take a woman approximately eighteen 1-hour class sessions to burn the calories in a pound of adipose tissues. The same number of calories could be burned in half the time with a program that includes vigorous running, rowing, cycling, or swimming.

Energy Cost of Recreation and Sport Activities

The energy requirements of a group of sport and recreational activities is presented in Appendix B. Table 4-3 lists several examples to illustrate the large variation in energy cost that occurs with participation in various forms of physical activity.

Table 4-3. *Gross energy cost for a selected group of recreation and sport activities.*

	KG	50	53	56	59	62	65	68	71	74	77	80	83
ACTIVITY	LBS	110	117	123	130	137	143	150	157	163	170	176	183
Volleyball		2.5	2.7	2.8	3.0	3.1	3.3	3.4	3.6	3.7	3.9	4.0	4.2
Nautilus		4.6	4.9	5.2	5.5	5.8	6.0	6.3	6.6	6.8	7.1	7.4	7.7
Cycling, leisure		5.0	5.3	5.6	5.9	6.2	6.5	6.8	7.1	7.4	7.7	8.0	8.3
Tennis		5.5	5.8	6.1	6.4	6.8	7.1	7.4	7.7	8.1	8.4	8.7	9.0
Swimming, slow crawl		6.4	6.8	7.2	7.6	7.9	8.3	8.7	9.1	9.5	9.9	10.2	10.6
Touch football		6.6	7.0	7.4	7.8	8.2	8.6	9.0	9.4	9.8	10.2	10.6	11.0
Hydraulic resistance exercise		6.6	7.0	7.4	7.8	8.2	8.6	9.0	9.4	9.7	10.2	10.5	10.9
Skiing, uphill racing		13.7	14.5	15.3	16.2	17.0	17.8	18.6	19.5	20.3	21.1	21.9	22.7

Source: Data from Appendix B.

Note: Energy expenditure is computed as the number of minutes of participation multiplied by the kcal value in the appropriate body weight column. For example, the kcal cost of one hour of tennis for a person weighing 150 pounds is 444 kcal (7.4 kcal × 60 min).

Notice, for example, that volleyball requires about 3.6 kcal per minute, or 216 kcal per hour for a person who weighs 157 pounds. The same person will expend more than twice this amount of energy, or 546 kcal per hour, while swimming the crawl. Viewed somewhat differently, 25 minutes of swimming the crawl will require about the same number of calories as participating in recreational volleyball for 1 hour. If the pace of the swim or volleyball game is increased, the energy expenditure will also increase proportionally.

Body size plays an important role with respect to the energy requirements during exercise, just as was the case with BMR. Heavier people generally expend more energy to perform the same activity than people who weigh less. This is because energy expenditure during weight bearing exercise increases in direct proportion to body weight. The relationship between body weight and oxygen consumption is so high that energy expenditure during walking or running can be predicted from body weight with almost as much accuracy compared to the actual measurement of oxygen consumption.

In non-weight-bearing exercise like stationary cycling, on the other hand, there is little or no relationship between body weight and the energy cost of exercise. A practical application of these findings is that walking and other forms of weight-bearing exercise provide a substantial caloric expenditure for heavier people. Notice in Table 4-3 that if a person weighing 183 pounds plays tennis or volleyball, the total expenditure of energy in kcal is considerably greater than for a lighter person who participates in the same activity. When caloric cost is expressed in terms of body weight, that is, kcal per minute per kg of body weight (kcal/min/kg), the difference in caloric cost between subjects of different sizes is considerably reduced. When energy expenditure is expressed in this manner, the differences between men and women during exercise are relatively small. Keep in mind, however, that although the average energy requirement in playing tennis may be approximately 0.109 kcal/min/kg, regardless of race, gender, or body weight, the *total* energy or calories expended by the heavier person is considerably more than by the lighter player. Appendix B presents a more complete list of the gross energy expended in relation to body weight during household, recreational and sport, and occupational and industrial activities. These figures represent average values that can vary considerably depending on skill, pace, and fitness level.

HOW TO USE APPENDIX B

Refer to the column that comes closest to your present body weight. Multiply the number in this column by the number of minutes you spend in an activity. Suppose an individual weighs 137 pounds and spends 30 minutes playing a casual game of billiards. To determine the kcal cost of participation, multiply the caloric value of 2.6 kcal obtained in Appendix B by 30 to obtain a total energy expenditure of 78 kcal. If the same individual does aerobic dance for 45 minutes, the energy expended would be calculated as 6.4 kcal × 45 min or 288 kcal.

Daily Rates of Average Energy Expenditure

A committee of the United States Food and Nutrition Board proposed various norms to represent average rates of energy expenditure for men and women living in the United States. These standards apply to males and females who have occupations that could be considered somewhere between sedentary and active, and who participate moderately in recreational activities like weekend swimming, golf, and tennis. As shown in Table 4-4, the average daily energy expenditure is 2700 kcal for men and 2100 kcal for women between the ages of 23 and 50. As can be noted in the bottom part of the table, about 75% of the average man's and woman's day is spent in relatively sedentary activities. This predominance of daily physical *inactivity* has prompted some sociologists to refer to the modern-day American as *Homo sedentarius,* a term that is probably all too appropriate. A survey by the President's Council on Physical Fitness and Sports revealed that for 36% of American men and 51% of American women, walking was the most prevalent form of exercise, regardless of occupation or race. It is probably a fair estimate that only about 50% of adult American men and women engage in physical activities that require an energy expenditure much above the resting level!

Table 4-5 summarizes data on the daily rates of energy expenditure for people with different occupations from Scotland; data are also included for Swiss peasants and English army cadets. The number in each group varied from 10 to 30, and the subjects were studied during a 1-week period. Although the average rate of energy expenditure increased for each occupational group as presented from top to bottom in the table, there was considerable individual variation within a particular group. The variability was attributed to differences in time spent outside of work, especially the time devoted to recreational pursuits. Differences in the type of work done within each specific profession were also considered important. One

Table 4-4. *Average daily rates of energy expenditure for men and women living in the United States.*

	AGE, YEARS	WEIGHT, LBS.	HEIGHT, IN.	KCAL
Men	15–18	134	69	3000
	19–22	147	69	3000
	23–50	154	69	2700
	51+	154	69	2400
Women	15–18	119	65	2100
	19–22	128	65	2100
	23–50	128	65	2000
	51+	128	65	1800

AVERAGE TIME SPENT DURING THE DAY FOR MEN AND WOMEN

ACTIVITY	TIME, HOURS
1. Sleeping and lying	8
2. Sitting	6
3. Standing	6
4. Walking	2
5. Recreational: sports or exercises	2

Source: Data from Food and Nutrition Board, National Research Council, *Recommended Dietary Allowances,* 8th rev. ed., National Academy of Sciences, Washington, D.C., 1974. (Also Pub. 1146, 1964.)

Table 4-5. *Daily rates of energy expenditure grouped according to occupation.*

OCCUPATION	ENERGY EXPENDITURE, KCAL/DAY		
	AVERAGE	MINIMUM	MAXIMUM
Men			
Elderly retired	2330	1750	2810
Office workers	2520	1820	3270
Coal mine clerks	2800	2330	3290
Laboratory technicians	2840	2240	3820
Older industrial workers	2840	2180	3710
University students	2930	2270	4410
Building workers	3000	2440	3730
Steel workers	3280	2600	3960
Army cadets	3490	2990	4100
Older peasants (Swiss)	3530	2210	5000
Farmers	3550	2450	4670
Coal miners	3660	2970	4560
Forestry workers	3670	2860	4600
Women			
Older housewives	1990	1490	2410
Middle-aged housewives	2090	1760	2320
Laboratory assistants	2130	1340	2540
Assistants in department store	2250	1820	2850
University students	2290	2090	2500
Factory workers	2320	1970	2980
Bakery workers	2510	1980	3390
Older peasants (Swiss)	2890	2200	3860

Source: Data from J.V.G.A. Durnin and R. Passmore, *Energy, Work and Leisure*, Heinemann Educational Books, London, 1967.

elderly retired man was almost as active as the least energetic of the coal miners and forestry workers. His rate of energy expenditure was therefore much higher than the average for his group.

Classification of Work

All of us at one time or another have done some type of physical work that we would classify as exceedingly "difficult." This might be walking up a long flight of stairs, shoveling a driveway full of snow, running uphill to catch a bus, loading and unloading furniture on a truck, digging a deep trench to fix an underground pipe, skiing through a blizzard, or climbing a steep mountain. There are several factors to consider in rating the difficulty of a particular task. One is the amount of *time* it takes, the other is the *intensity* of the effort. Both of these factors may vary considerably. For example, two people of the same body size could expend an equal amount of energy to perform the same task. One might exert extreme effort

Table 4-6. *Five-level classification of physical work based on intensity of effort.*

WORK CATEGORIES	MEN KCAL/MIN	MEN METS	WOMEN KCAL/MIN	WOMEN METS	ACTIVITIES
Light	2.0–4.9	1.6–3.9	1.5–3.4	1.2–2.7	Walking; reading a book; driving a car; shopping; bowling; fishing; golf; pleasure sailing.
Moderate	5.0–7.4	4.0–5.9	3.5–5.4	2.8–4.3	Pleasure cycling; dancing; volleyball; badminton; calisthenics.
Heavy	7.5–9.9	6.0–7.9	5.5–7.4	4.4–5.9	Ice skating; water skiing; competitive tennis; novice mountain climbing; jogging.
Very Heavy	10.0–12.4	8.0–9.9	7.5–9.4	6.0–7.5	Fencing; touch football; scuba diving; basketball game; swim (most strokes).
Unduly Heavy	12.5–>	10.0–>	9.5–>	7.6–>	Handball; squash; cross-country skiing; paddleball; running (fast pace).

over a short period, while the other could exert less effort over a longer period. An example might be climbing several flights of stairs. The first person could run the stairs at maximum speed, expending 15 kcal of energy. The second person moved more leisurely and took 2 minutes to climb the stairs, yet still expended 15 kcal of energy. The basic difference in achieving the 15 kcal output was the time factor, or more accurately, the intensity of work.

Several systems have been proposed for rating the difficulty of work in terms of intensity. The system we use classifies work into categories designated as light, moderate, heavy, very heavy, and unduly heavy.

The five-level classification system presented in Table 4-6 is based on the energy required by untrained men and women to perform different tasks. The amount of energy that corresponds to a particular work level is expressed as kcal per minute and *METS,* a MET being defined as a multiple of the resting metabolism. *One MET is equivalent to an average resting energy expenditure or oxygen consumption.* Physical work performed at 2 METS requires twice the resting metabolism, 3 METS is three times the resting energy expenditure, and so on. Also listed in the table are caloric equivalents and examples of activities that correspond generally to the different intensities of work effort.

Additional Reading

Behnke, A.R.: The relation of lean body weight to metabolism and some consequent systematizations. *Annals of the New York Academy of Sciences. 56:*1095, 1953.

Calloway, D.H. and E. Zanni: Energy requirements and energy expenditure of elderly men. *American Journal of Clinical Nutrition. 33:*2088, 1980.

Cohen, J.L., et al.: Cardiorespiratory responses to ballet exercise and the $\dot{V}O_2$max of elite ballet dancers. *Medicine and Science in Sports and Exercise. 14:*212, 1982.

Consolazio, C.F., R.E. Johnson, and L.J. Pecora: *Physiological Measurements of Metabolic Functions in Man.* New York, McGraw-Hill Book Co., 1963.

Cunningham, J.J.: A reanalysis of the factors influencing basal metabolic rate in normal adults. *American Journal of Clinical Nutrition. 33:*2372, 1980.

Dowdy, D.B., et al.: Effects of aerobic dance on physical work capacity, cardiovascular function and body composition of middle-aged women. *Research Quarterly for Exercise and Sport. 56:*227, 1985.

Garry, R.C., et al.: Expenditure of energy and the consumption of food by miners and clerks. *Medical Research Council,* Report No. 289. Fife, Scotland, Her Majesty's Stationery Office, 1955.

Girandola, R.N., and F.I. Katch: Effects of physical training on ventilatory equivalent and respiratory exchange ratio during weight supported, steady-state exercise. *European Journal of Applied Physiology. 35:*119, 1976.

Kannagi, T., et al.: An evaluation of the Beckman Metabolic Cart for measuring ventilation and aerobic requirements during exercise. *Journal of Cardiac Rehabilitation. 3:*38, 1983.

Kashiwazaki, H., et al.: Correlations of pedometer readings with energy expenditure in workers during free-living daily activities. *European Journal of Applied Physiology. 54:*585, 1986.

Katch, V., et al.: Basal metabolism of obese adolescents: age, gender and body composition effects. *International Journal of Obesity. 9:*69, 1985.

McArdle, W.D. et al.: Metabolic and cardiovascular adjustment to work in air and water at 18, 25, 33°C. *Journal of Applied Physiology. 40:*85, 1976.

McArdle, W.D., et al.: Aerobic capacity, heart rate, and estimated energy cost during women's competitive basketball. *Research Quarterly. 42:*178, 1971.

Montoye, H.L. and H.L. Taylor: Measurement of physical activity in population studies. *Human Biology. 56:*195, 1984.

Passmore, R., and M.H. Draper: The chemical anatomy of the human body. *In Biochemical Disorders in Human Disease,* 2d ed., R.H.S. Thompson and E.J. King (Eds.), London, Churchill, 1964.

President's Council on Physical Fitness and Sports: *National Adult Physical Fitness Survey.* Washington, D.C., May, 1973.

Rothwell, N.J. and M.J. Stock: Regulation of energy balance. *Annual Review of Nutrition. 1:*235, 1981.

Snellen, J.W.: Studies in human calorimetry. In: *Assessment of Energy in Health and Disease.* Columbus, Ohio, Ross Laboratories, 1980.

Town, G.P., et al.: The effect of rope skipping rate on energy expenditure of males and females. *Medicine and Science in Sports and Exercise. 12:*295, 1980.

Wilmore, J.H., Davis, J.A. and A.C. Norton: An automated system for assessing metabolic and respiratory function during exercise. *Journal of Applied Physiology. 40:*619, 1976.

PART II
Body Composition and Weight Control

AN EXCESS ACCUMULATION of body fat is undesirable for a variety of reasons. From a health standpoint, medical problems exist in which obesity or "overfatness" is considered a risk factor, and for which a reduction in excess fat is desirable. These problems include certain types of heart disease, high blood pressure, impaired carbohydrate and fat metabolism, joint, bone, and gall bladder diseases, diabetes, asthma, and various lung disorders. Being too fat is also often accompanied by changes in personality and behavior patterns often manifested as depression, withdrawal, self-pity, irritability, and aggression.

The first step in formulating an intelligent program of weight control is to appraise body size objectively. It is possible to be heavy and even overweight according to height-weight charts, yet possess only a moderate amount of body fat. Many athletes, for example, are quite muscular but are otherwise lean in terms of their overall body composition. For such people a program of dietary modification or exercise for purposes of weight control may be unnecessary. Such an approach would be prudent, however, for others who may be 10 to 15 pounds "overfat." Of even greater importance is the need for effective weight control among the increasingly large segment of the population afflicted with "creeping obesity." During the adult years, both body weight and body fat can increase insidiously to the point where the amount of body fat exceeds even the most liberal limits for normalcy. It is at this point that the health-related aspects of obesity become a serious concern. Unfortunately, the correction of adult-acquired obesity through dietary intervention or exercise is much more difficult than its early prevention.

The chapters that follow deal with topics relevant to body composition, obesity, and weight control. Chapter 5 discusses the underlying rationale for the evaluation of body composition in terms of body fat and lean body weight. In Chapter 6, we define the term "overweight" in terms of the acceptable limits of body fat for a particular age range for men and women. We discuss the interrelated factors often associated with obesity, as well as the efficacy of diet and exercise as a treatment for the overfat condition. Chapter 7 deals with weight control. We discuss the question of weight loss and weight gain within the framework of the "energy balance equation." In addition, a strategy is presented for quantifying food intake, and incorporating exercise and caloric restriction to achieve a desired rate of weight loss. Chapter 8 is concerned with the application of the principles of behavior modification, with emphasis on weight reduction by means of dietary modification and increased energy expenditure through vigorous physical activity.

5

Evaluation of Body Composition

IN THE EARLY 1940s, Dr. Albert Behnke, a U.S. Naval physician and foremost authority on body composition, made detailed measurements of the size, shape, and structure of 25 professional football players, many of whom had achieved All-American status while in college. According to the military standards at that time, a person whose body weight was 15% above the "average weight-for-height," as determined from insurance company statistics, was designated as overweight and rejected by the military. When these overweight standards were applied to the football players who ranged in weight from 170 to 260 pounds, 17 players were classified as too fat and unfit for military service. However, a more careful evaluation of each player's body composition revealed that 11 of the 17 overweight players actually had a relatively low percentage of body fat. The players' excess weight resulted primarily from their large muscular development.

These data were among the first to illustrate clearly that the popular height-weight tables provide little information about the composition or quality of an individual's body weight. A football player may indeed weigh much more than some "average," "ideal," or "desirable" body weight based on height-weight tables, but more than likely, these athletes are not excessively fat or in need of reducing their body size. The extra weight consists of a considerable amount of muscle mass. Thus, the term "overweight" refers only to body weight in excess of some standard, usually the average weight for a specific height. The use of height-weight tables can be quite misleading for the person who actually wants to know how "overfat" he is.

During the past 50 years, many laboratory procedures have been developed to analyze the body in relation to its three major structural components–fat, muscle, and bone. Some of the procedures are time-consuming and require the use of sophisticated, expensive laboratory equipment, whereas other procedures are fairly simple and inexpensive. In this chapter, we will analyze the gross composition of the body and present the rationale underlying the various direct and indirect methods for quantitatively partitioning the body into the two basic compartments of *body fat* and *lean body weight.* In addition, a simple method is presented for determining body composition in terms of percent body fat, pounds of fat, and lean body weight.

Gross Composition of the Human Body

The three major structural components of the human body include muscle, fat, and bone. Because there are marked gender differences in body composition, a convenient basis for evaluation and comparison is to employ the concept proposed by Dr. Behnke of the reference man and reference woman. Figure 5–1 depicts the gross composition for a reference man and woman in terms of muscle, fat, and bone. This theoretical model is based on the average physical dimensions obtained from detailed measurements of thousands of individuals who were subjects in large-scale anthropometric and nutrition-assessment surveys.

The reference man is taller by 4 inches, heavier by 29 pounds; his skeleton weighs more (23 vs. 15 lbs); and he has a larger muscle mass (69 vs. 45 lbs.) and lower total fat content (23.1 vs. 33.8 lbs.) than the reference female. These sex differences exist even when the amount of fat, muscle, and bone are expressed as a percentage of body weight. This is especially true for body fat that represents 15% of the total body weight for the reference man, and 27% of the total body weight of the reference woman. The concept of reference standards does not mean that men and women should strive to achieve the body composition of the reference models, nor that the reference man and woman are in fact "average." The models provide a useful frame of reference to compare different individuals in terms of their body composition.

Essential and Storage Fat

The total amount of body fat exists in two depots or storage sites. The first depot, termed *essential fat,* is the fat stored in the marrow of bones as well as in the heart, lungs, liver, spleen, kidneys, intestines, muscles, and lipid-rich tissues throughout the central nervous system. This fat depot is required for normal physiologic functioning. In the female, essential fat also includes gender-specific or gender-characteristic fat. It is not at all clear whether this fat depot is expendable or serves as reserve storage. The mammary glands and pelvic region are probably primary storage sites for this fat, although the precise quantitative amounts are unknown. In one experiment, the contribution of breast weight to the body's total fat content was estimated to be no higher than 4% for women who varied in body fat content from 14 to 35%. This must mean that sites other than the breasts contribute a larger proportion of gender-specific fat (perhaps in the lower body region that includes the pelvis and thighs).

The other major fat depot, the *storage fat,* consists of fat that accumulates in adipose tissue. This nutritional reserve includes the fatty tissues that protect the various internal organs from trauma, as well as the larger subcutaneous fat volume deposited beneath the skin surface. Although the proportional distribution of storage fat in males and females is similar (12% in males, 15% in females), the total

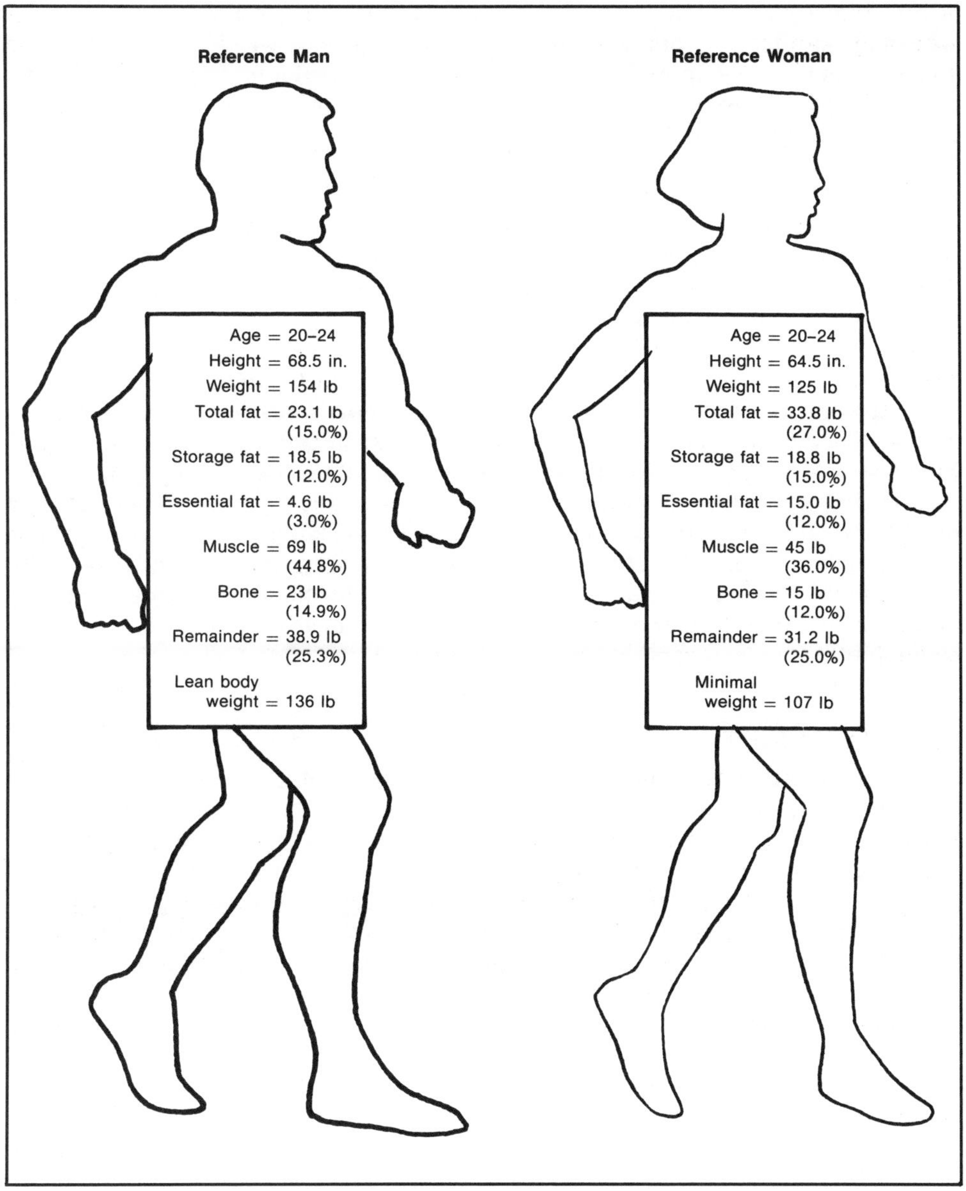
Reference Man
Reference Woman
Age = 20–24
Height = 68.5 in.
Weight = 154 lb
Total fat = 23.1 lb (15.0%)
Storage fat = 18.5 lb (12.0%)
Essential fat = 4.6 lb (3.0%)
Muscle = 69 lb (44.8%)
Bone = 23 lb (14.9%)
Remainder = 38.9 lb (25.3%)
Lean body weight = 136 lb
Age = 20–24
Height = 64.5 in.
Weight = 125 lb
Total fat = 33.8 lb (27.0%)
Storage fat = 18.8 lb (15.0%)
Essential fat = 15.0 lb (12.0%)
Muscle = 45 lb (36.0%)
Bone = 15 lb (12.0%)
Remainder = 31.2 lb (25.0%)
Minimal weight = 107 lb

Figure 5-1 *Body composition of a reference man and woman.*

quantity of essential fat in females, that includes the gender-specific fat, is four times higher than in males. More than likely, the additional essential fat is biologically important for child-bearing and other hormone-related functions.

MINIMAL STANDARDS FOR LEANNESS

There seems to be a biologically lower limit beyond which a person's body weight cannot be reduced without impairing health status. This lower limit in men is referred to as lean body weight and is calculated as body weight minus the weight of storage fat. For the reference man, the lean weight is equivalent to 136 lbs; this includes approximately 3% or 4.1 lbs essential fat. This amount of fat presumably is a lower limit, and any encroachment into this reserve may impair normal physiologic function or capacity for exercise. Similar low values of body fat have also been obtained for champion male athletes in various sports. The body fat content of world-class, male marathon runners ranges from about 4 to 8%. This is only slightly more than the quantity of essential fat that apparently cannot be reduced. The low fat content and body weight for these exceptional athletes reflect, to some degree, a positive adaptation to the prolonged, severe requirements of distance training. A low quantity of body fat permits a more effective transfer of metabolic heat during high intensity exercise, and reduces the quantity of excess weight that the athlete must transport while running. Low values for body fat have also been obtained for other athletes. In our studies of professional football players (1975-1978 New York Jets; 1976-78 Dallas Cowboys; 1979-1980 Miami Dolphins and New Orleans Saints), values of fatness as low as 1.0% of body weight have been recorded for several defensive backs. This corresponds to the body weight with essentially no storage fat.

Considerable individual differences also are found in the lean body weight of different athletes, with values ranging from a low of 106 pounds in some jockeys to a high of 240 to 250 pounds in All-Pro football defensive linemen and Olympic champion discus throwers and power lifters.

MINIMAL WEIGHT (WOMEN)

In contrast to the lower limit of body weight of males that includes 3% essential fat, the lower limit of body weight for the reference female includes 12% essential fat (essential fat plus gender-specific fat). This theoretical limit for minimal weight for the reference woman is equivalent to 107 pounds. In general, the leanest women in the population do not have body fat levels below about 10 to 12% of body weight. This probably represents the lower limit of fatness for most women in good health. The concept of minimal weight in females that incorporates about 12% essential fat is equivalent to lean body weight in males that includes 3% essential fat in adipose tissue.

It should be emphasized that the concept of female minimal weight is based on theoretical considerations, with little actual data. In carefully conducted experiments, values lower than 10% body fat are rarely reported. Data from female distance runners constitute an exception, where a value of 5.9% body fat was reported for one runner who weighed 52.6 kg.

Underweight and Thin

The terms underweight and thin are not necessarily synonymous. In some cases, in fact, they describe physical characteristics that differ considerably. In one study, for example, the structural characteristics of apparently thin females were compared with women who appeared normal in size as well as women who appeared obese. The objective of the research was to determine if body frame size (as measured by bone widths) differed among the three groups.

The results were unexpected. While the thin appearing women were indeed relatively low in body fat, 18.2% compared with 25% body fat for the "normal" size women and 32% for the obese group, there were no differences in the average structural dimensions between the three groups! What this meant was that for women of approximately the same height, there was no such thing as a predominantly small, medium, or large frame size as defined by four trunk and four extremity bone widths. Thus, appearing thin or skinny does not necessarily mean that skeletal frame size is diminutive or that the body's total fat content is excessively low.

Does Low Body Fat Trigger Amenorrhea?

Some researchers have suggested that females with a low percentage of body fat suffer from amenorrhea or disruption of the normal menstrual cycle. Harvard researcher, Dr. Rose Frisch, considers the body weight at 17% fat as the critical body weight, and she says reducing below this weight triggers hormonal and metabolic disturbances that can affect the menses. The critical weight hypothesis proposes that the onset of menstrual function necessitates maintaining a fat level above 17% of body weight and that 22% body fat is the level required to maintain a normal cycle. Although the lean-to-fat ratio does appear to be important, other factors must be considered because there is ample evidence that females who are below 17% body fat have normal menstrual cycles and maintain a high level of physiologic capacity.

A report of women in the U.S. Military Academy at West Point demonstrated that participation in a rigorous physical training and exercise program markedly affected previously normal menstrual patterns. Eighty-six percent of the 70 freshman women in 1976, who averaged 19% body fat, had normal menstruation before entering West Point, but within 2 months of starting the program, 73% reported discontinued menstruation. After 6 months, 42% experienced irregularities. After 15 months, 7% had still not resumed their normal periods. This same pattern was observed for the 1977 and 1978 freshman classes. Other recent studies have shown that from one-half to one-third of female athletes have abnormal menstrual functions. Strenuous physical training per se, and perhaps the accompanying psychologic stress, can affect menstrual patterns, independently of the level of body fat. Conversely, there are currently many outstanding female athletes (long distance runners, gymnasts, body builders) who have normal menses with no disruption of their cycles during intensive training and competition, and who compete at a body fat level in the range of 8 to 13%.

In a study from one of our laboratories, 30 female athletes and 30 non-athletes, all below 20% body fat, were compared for menstrual cycle regularity, irregularity, and amenorrhea. Four of the athletes and 3 non-athletes, who ranged in body fat from 11 to 15%, had regular cycles, while 7 athletes and 2 non-athletes had irregular cycles or were amenorrheic. For the total sample (fat range from 11 to 20%), 14 athletes and 21 non-athletes had regular cycles, respectively. These data corroborate previous findings, and lead us to reject the hypothesis of a critical fat level of 17% that is related to the female reproductive cycle. If a critical fat level does exist, it may be specific for each woman and probably changes throughout life. The complex interplay of physical, hormonal, nutritional, psychologic, and environmental factors on menstrual function must be considered. The exercise-associated disturbances in menstrual function can be reversed with changes in life style without serious consequences. What is not known, however, is the effect sustained amenorrhea may have on the reproductive system. Certainly, detailed studies of reproductive function of athletes in and out of training will provide more definitive answers relative to this important topic. Failure to menstruate or cessation of the normal cycle should be evaluated by a gynecologist/endocrinologist because it may reflect an underlying and significant medical problem.

Female Body Builders

During the late 1970s, body building for females gained widespread popularity throughout the United States as women aggressively pursued this previously male dominated sport. As more women undertook the rigorous demands of training with weights, competition became more intense and the level of achievement increased markedly. Because success in body building is based on a "slim" and lean appearance, complemented by a well-defined musculature, interesting questions were raised with regard to body composition. How lean are such competitors, and does their presumably low level of body fat disrupt normal menstrual function?

The results of one study of the body composition of 10 competitive female body builders revealed that these athletes were quite lean, averaging 13.3% body fat (range from 8.0 to 18.3%) with an average lean body weight of 46.6 kg. Their body weight averaged 53.8 kg, height 160.8 cm, and age 27.1 years. With the exception of champion gymnasts who also average about 13% body fat, the body builders were shorter in height by 3 to 4%, lower in body weight by 4 to 5%, and possessed 7 to 10% less total weight of body fat compared with other top female athletes. The most striking compositional characteristic of the female body builders was their dramatically large lean-to-fat ratio of 7:1 (weight of the lean mass relative to the weight of the fat mass) in comparison to 4.3 to 1 for other female athletic groups. Figure 5-2 illustrates the remarkable muscular development of four champion female body builders.

As more data become available on other aspects of female body builders, such as strength and fatigue levels and cardiorespiratory and hormonal functions, a more complete picture will emerge regarding the physiologic consequences of both short and long term participation in the sport of body building. It is interesting to note that menstrual function was normal in 8 of 10 body builders in the previously mentioned study where percent body fat ranged from 8 to 18%.

Common Laboratory Methods to Assess Body Composition

The fat and lean components of the human body have been determined by two general procedures. One procedure measures body composition directly by chemical analysis. The second approach assesses body composition indirectly with hydrostatic weighing or with simple circumferences or fatfold measurements. While direct methods form the basis for indirect techniques and are useful in animal research and for human cadaver analysis, the use of indirect procedures enables the scientist to assess the body composition of living people with relative accuracy.

CHEMICAL MEASUREMENT

CHEMICAL ANALYSIS. Although there has been considerable research dealing with the direct measurement of body composition in various species of animals,

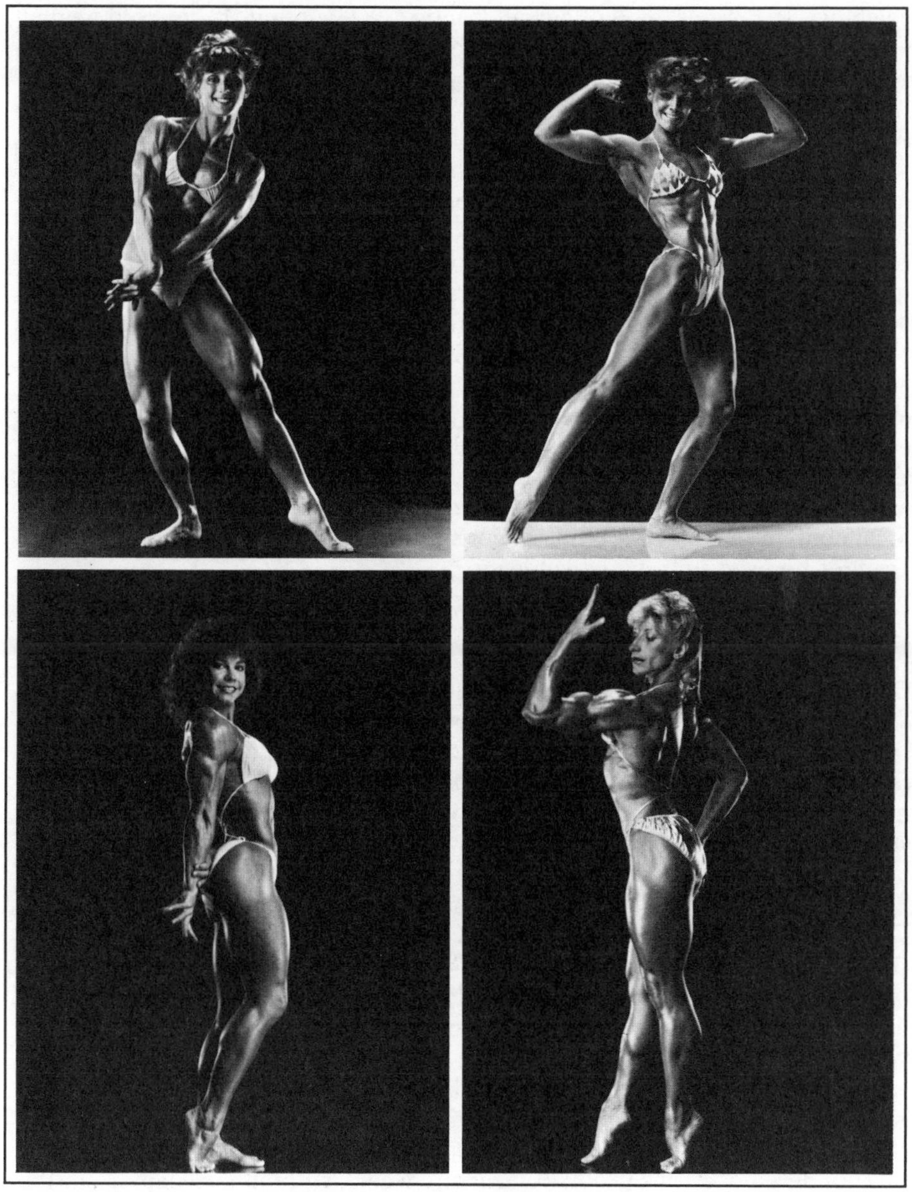

Figure 5-2. *Four champion female body builders. Photos courtesy of Joe Weider, Photo Library and Muscle and Fitness Magazine; Photo credit to John Balik (photographer).*

relatively few studies have employed precise chemical techniques to analyze human fat content. Such analyses are time-consuming and tedious, require highly specialized laboratory equipment, and involve many ethical and legal problems in obtaining cadavers for research purposes. For these reasons, only a few analyses of human cadavers have been made during the past 100 years. In 1863, detailed dissections were made of a 33-year-old man, a 22-year-old woman, and an 18-year-old boy, who died in an accident. Prior to 1980, chemical analyses had been made of only 7 cadavers. Of those seven, one subject, a 46-year-old male, 5 feet, 6 inches tall, weighing 118 pounds, died of a skull fracture. A 99-pound, 42-year-old woman committed suicide by drowning, whereas the other 5 male subjects, aged 25, 35, 41, 48, and 60, died of circulatory diseases.

Since 1980, a large scale cadaver study was completed on a group of older men and women (average age 74 years, range 55 to 94 years). A wealth of new information is now available on tissue morphology and structural characteristics, but unfortunately the results pertain to this older age sample. Consequently, it is difficult to pinpoint by direct chemical analysis the compositional structure of an "average" subject. This is particularly true in terms of body fat that exhibits extreme variability between individuals of the same gender, regardless of height or body weight.

Data from animal studies and the limited number of human cadaver studies reveal that the weight of the dry, fat-free skeleton remains remarkably constant, even when large variations exist in the percentage of total body fat.

While the fat content varies considerably, the composition of the skeletal mass and lean tissues remains relatively invariable. The constancy of these tissues has enabled researchers to develop mathematical equations to determine the body's fat and lean percentages. This is indeed fortunate, as the direct method for determining the fat content of cadavers, while of considerable theoretical importance, obviously cannot be used with living subjects.

INDIRECT ASSESSMENT

The following section presents two indirect procedures to assess body composition. The first procedure describes Archimedes' principle as applied to hydrostatic weighing. With this method, percent body fat is computed from body density (the ratio of body weight to body volume). The second procedure involves the prediction of body fat from circumference or girth measurements. This method is of practical significance because body fat can be predicted both simply and accurately.

Body Volume Determination

About 2000 years ago the Greek mathematician Archimedes discovered a basic principle that is currently applied in the evaluation of body composition. An itinerant scholar of that time described the interesting circumstances surrounding the event:

> King Hieron of Syracuse suspected that his pure gold crown had been altered by substitution of silver for gold. The King directed Archimedies to devise a method for testing the crown for its gold content without dismantling it. Archimedes pondered over this problem for many weeks without succeeding, until one day, he stepped into a bath filled to the top with water and observed the overflow of water. He thought about this for a moment, and then, wild with joy, jumped from the bath and ran naked through the streets of Syracuse shouting "Eureka! Eureka! I have discovered a way to solve the mystery of the King's golden crown."

Archimedes reasoned that a substance such as gold must have a volume proportionate to its weight, and the way to measure the volume of an irregular object such as the crown was to submerge it in water and collect the overflow. Archimedes took a lump of gold and silver, each having the same weight as the crown, and submerged each in a container full of water. To his delight he discovered that the crown displaced more water than the lump of gold and less than the lump of silver.

What this meant was that the crown was indeed composed of silver and gold as the King had suspected.

Essentially, what Archimedes evaluated was the specific gravity of the crown (ratio of the weight of the crown to the weight of an equal volume of water) compared to the specific gravities for gold and silver. Archimedes probably also reasoned that an object submerged in water must be buoyed up by a counterforce that equals the weight of the water it displaces. This buoyancy force helps to support an object in water against the downward pull of gravity. Thus, the object is said to lose weight in water. Because the object's loss of weight in water equals the weight of the volume of water it displaces, we can redefine specific gravity as the ratio of the weight of an object in air divided by its loss of weight in water. Thus,

$$\text{Specific gravity} = \frac{\text{Weight of an object in air}}{\text{Loss of weight in water}}$$

or

(weight in air minus weight in water)

In practical terms, suppose the crown weighed 5.0 pounds in air, and when weighed underwater, it weighed 0.29 pounds less or 4.71 pounds (Figure 5–3). The specific gravity of the crown would then be computed by dividing the weight of the crown (5.0 pounds) by its loss of weight in water (0.29 pounds). This results in a specific gravity of 17.24. Because this ratio is considerably different than the specific gravity of gold (19.3), we too can conclude: "Eureka! Eureka! the crown is a fraud!"

The physical principle Archimedes discovered can be applied directly to the assessment of body composition in humans. This is achieved by determining the

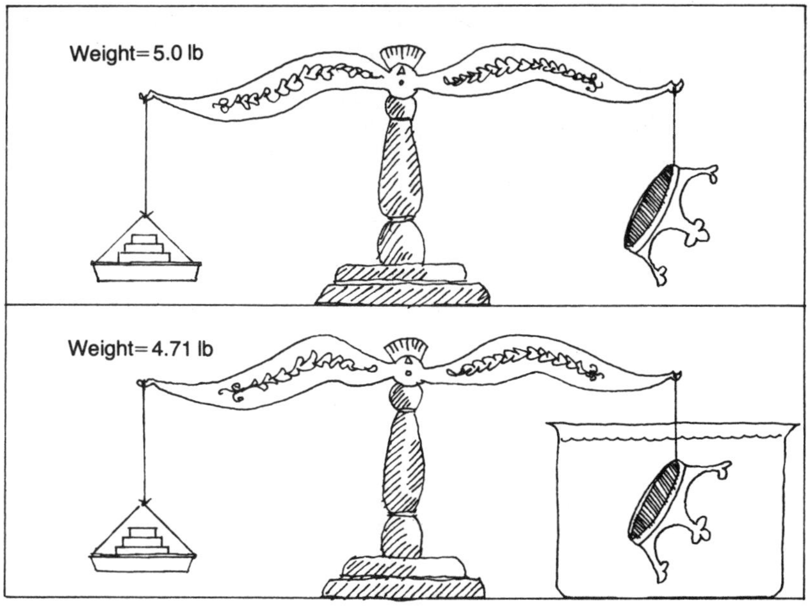
Weight=5.0 lb
Weight=4.71 lb

Figure 5-3. *Archimedes' solution for determining the gold content of the king's crown.*

volume of the body by water submersion in relation to the total body mass. Because density is mass per unit volume, one can compute the body density once the mass and volume are known.

Density of the Human Body For illustrative purposes, suppose a subject weighs 50 kg as measured on a conventional scale, and 2 kg when submerged completely underwater. According to Archimedes' principle, the buoyancy or counterforce of the water must equal 48 kg. The loss of weight in water of 48 kg is exactly equal to the weight of the displaced water. Because the density of water at any temperature is known, we can compute the volume of water displaced. In this example, 48 kg (48,000 g) of water would equal a volume of 48 liters or 48,000 cc (1 g water = 1 cm^3, in volume or $1\ g \cdot cc^{-1}$, at 39.2°F). If volume was measured at the cold water temperature of 39.2°F, no density correction would be necessary. In practice, however, researchers use warmer water and apply the appropriate density value for water. The density of the subject, computed as weight ÷ volume, would be 50,000 g (50 kg) ÷ $48{,}000\ g \cdot cc^{-1}$ or $1.0417\ g \cdot cc^{-1}$. This particular value for body density is midway between the value of $0.90\ g \cdot cc^{-1}$ for fat extracted from adipose tissue and $1.10\ g \cdot cc^{-1}$ for fat-free tissue. Once body density has been determined, the next step is to determine the amount of fat that corresponds to that value.

Computing Percent Body Fat from Body Density The relative percentages of fat in the human body can be estimated with a simple equation that incorporates density. This equation was derived from the theoretical premise that the densities of fat and fat-free tissues remain relatively constant (density of fat = $0.90\ g \cdot cc^{-1}$; density of fat-free tissue = $1.10\ g \cdot cc^{-1}$) even with large variations in total body fat. Thus, the proportions of the fat and lean components can be determined from an algebraic expression that relates these proportions to the density of the whole body. The following equation is used to compute percent body fat by incorporating the determined value of body density.

$$\text{Percent body fat} = \frac{495}{\text{Body density}} - 450.$$

The value of body density of 1.0417 g/cm determined for the 50 kg subject in the previous example can now be substituted in the equation for percent body fat as follows:

$$\text{Percent body fat} = \frac{495}{1.0417} - 450 = 25.2\%\ \text{fat}.$$

Thus, 25.2% of 12.6 kg or the 50 kg body weight is fat. The remaining 37.4 kg is lean body weight. For simplicity, we will use the term lean body weight, although we realize that by subtracting out the total body fat yields a remainder that is "fat-free." The calculation of lean body weight in males includes the essential fat; in females, the minimal weight also includes the essential fat.

The weight of fat is calculated by multiplying body weight by percent fat.

$$\text{Fat weight (kg)} = \frac{\text{Body weight (kg)} \times \text{Percent fat}}{100}$$

$$= 50 \text{ kg} \times 0.252$$
$$= 12.6 \text{ kg.}$$

Lean body weight is calculated by subtracting the weight of fat from body weight.

$$\text{Lean body weight (kg)} = \text{Body weight (kg)} - \text{Fat weight (kg)}$$

$$= 50 \text{ kg} - 12.6 \text{ kg}$$
$$= 37.4 \text{ kg.}$$

The determination of body weight and the calculations for body density, percent body fat, and lean body weight are quite simple. The more difficult task is the accurate assessment of body volume and thus body density. Body volume is conveniently measured by the procedure of hydrostatic weighing.

Hydrostatic weighing (also referred to as underwater weighing) computes body volume as the difference between body weight measured in air and weight measured during water submersion. In other words, body volume is equal to the loss of weight in water with the appropriate temperature correction for the water's density. Figure 5-4 illustrates two common procedures for measuring body volume by underwater weighing. The left side of Figure 5-4 shows the procedure in a laboratory setting; the other procedure was done under field conditions using an existing therapy pool at a physical fitness training facility of a professional football team.

A diver's belt is first secured around the waist to insure that the subject does not float toward the surface during submersion. While seated with the head out of the water, the subject makes a forced maximal exhalation as the head is lowered underwater. The breath is held for about 5 seconds while the underwater weight is recorded directly from an accurate scale, or electronically by the use of a force transducer and appropriate instrumentation. Eight to twelve repeated weighings are made to insure that a dependable underwater weight score is obtained. This amount of practice is given because there is a predictable "learning curve" in making a forced exhalation during submersion. Without practice, a lower underwater weight score would translate into a higher estimate of body fat. Even with repeated weighings, a small volume of air, the residual lung volume, still remains in the lungs. This air volume is measured for each subject just before or during the underwater weighing and its buoyant effect subtracted in the calculation of body density. The temperature of the water is also recorded to correct for the density of water at the weighing temperature.

Let us now put theory into practice by showing the sequence of steps used to compute body density, percent fat, pounds of fat, and lean body weight. The sub-

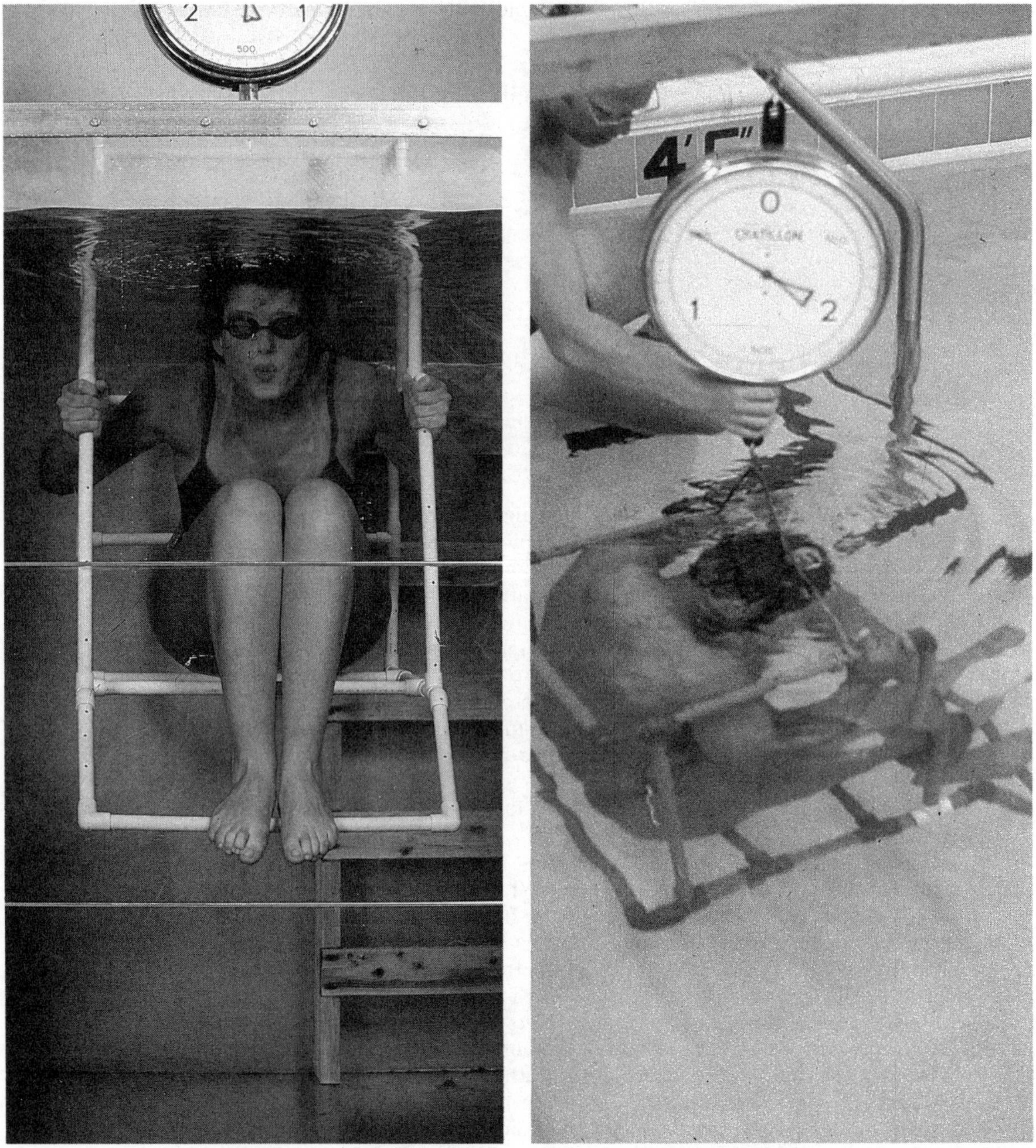
2
1
500
0
CHATILLON
1
2

Figure 5-4. *Left. Measuring body volume in the laboratory by the seated underwater weighing method. The subject is submerged in a 5′ × 5′ × 5′ stainless steel tank with plexiglass front. A heater maintains water temperature at 98°F, and a filtration system maintains water purity. A 9 kg, 10 g autopsy scale hangs above the tank to which the lightweight (1.5 kg) tubular plastic chair support is suspended. Right. The autopsy scale was suspended from a beam above the therapy pool. A similar chair was used in both situations, and the same procedures were followed in obtaining an underwater weight score.*

jects are two professional football players, an offensive guard, and a quarterback. For each player we made the following measurements:

	Offensive guard	Quarterback
Body weight	110 kg	85 kg
Underwater weight	3.5 kg	5.0 kg
Residual lung volume	1.2 liters	1.0 liters
Water Temperature correction	0.996	0.996

Because the loss of weight in water is equal to volume, the body volume of the offensive guard is 110 kg − 3.5 kg = 106.5 kg or 106.5 liters; for the quarterback, body volume is 85 kg − 5.0 kg = 80.0 kg or 80 liters. Dividing body volume by the water temperature correction factor of 0.996 increases the volume slightly for both players, from 106.5 liters to 106.9 liters for the offensive guard and from 80.0 liters to 80.3 liters for the quarterback. Because the residual lung volume also contributes to buoyancy, we must now subtract this volume from the body volume. When this is done, the body volume of the offensive guard becomes 105.7 liters (106.9 liters − 1.2 liters); for the quarterback, body volume is 79.3 liters (80.3 liters − 1.0 liters). Body density is then computed as weight ÷ volume. For the offensive guard, body density is 110 kg ÷ 105.7 liters = 1.0407 kg/liters or 1.0407 $g \cdot cc^{-1}$. For the quarterback, body density is 85.0 ÷ 79.3 = 1.0719 $g \cdot cc^{-1}$.

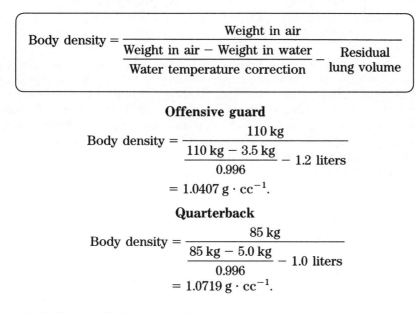

$$\text{Body density} = \frac{\text{Weight in air}}{\dfrac{\text{Weight in air} - \text{Weight in water}}{\text{Water temperature correction}} - \text{Residual lung volume}}$$

Offensive guard

$$\text{Body density} = \frac{110\text{ kg}}{\dfrac{110\text{ kg} - 3.5\text{ kg}}{0.996} - 1.2\text{ liters}} = 1.0407\ g \cdot cc^{-1}.$$

Quarterback

$$\text{Body density} = \frac{85\text{ kg}}{\dfrac{85\text{ kg} - 5.0\text{ kg}}{0.996} - 1.0\text{ liters}} = 1.0719\ g \cdot cc^{-1}.$$

Percent body fat is calculated as follows:

$$\text{Percent fat} = \frac{495}{\text{Density}} - 450$$

Offensive guard

$$\text{Percent fat} = \frac{495}{1.0407} - 450$$
$$= 25.6\%$$

Quarterback

$$\text{Percent fat} = \frac{495}{1.0719} - 450$$
$$= 11.8\%$$

The total weight of the body is calculated as follows:

$$\text{Weight of fat} = \frac{\text{Body weight} \times \text{Percent fat}}{100}$$

Offensive guard

$$\text{Weight of fat} = 110\text{ kg} \times 0.256$$
$$= 28.2\text{ kg.}$$

Quarterback

$$\text{Weight of fat} = 85\text{ kg} \times 0.118$$
$$= 10.0\text{ kg.}$$

Lean body weight is calculated as follows:

$$\text{Lean body weight (LBW)} = \text{Body weight} - \text{Weight of fat}$$

Offensive guard

$$\text{LBW} = 110\text{ kg} - 28.2\text{ kg}$$
$$= 81.8\text{ kg.}$$

Quarterback

$$\text{LBW} = 85\text{ kg} = 10.0\text{ kg}$$
$$= 75.0\text{ kg.}$$

This analysis of body composition clearly illustrates that the offensive guard possesses more than twice the percentage of body fat than the quarterback (25.6% versus 11.8%) and almost 3 times as much total fat (28.2 kg versus 10.0 kg). On the other hand, lean body weight, which provides a good indication of muscle mass, is also larger for the guard than for the quarterback. Although the offensive guard is 25 kg heavier than the quarterback, similar differences in body composition can also be demonstrated for people of the same body weight, especially between physically active and sedentary people. Results such as these demonstrate clearly that the crucial aspect of body composition evaluation is to determine the fat and lean components of the body, and not to rely solely on body weight as an index of "acceptability" regarding body size and shape.

Prediction of Body Fat from Circumference Measurements

Hydrostatic weighing is one of the most accurate indirect methods to assess the body's fat content. However, proper measurement with this technique requires equipment and facilities not normally available in a doctor's office, hospital, physical education department, or health spa. Thus, alternative but simple procedures to predict body fatness have been developed. One of these procedures is to measure the girth or circumferences at selected sites on the body. It is easy to take circumferences with a cloth measuring tape and accuracy can be achieved with a minimum of practice. Appendix C presents a description of procedures for using the circumference method to predict body fat in young and older men and women. You can use Appendix C to answer the question, "How fat am I?" Once you have an estimate of fatness, you can compute your total weight of fat (referred to as absolute fat weight), lean body weight, and "desirable" body weight (based on a desired level of body fat).

MEASUREMENT OF SUBCUTANEOUS FAT BY THE FATFOLD TECHNIQUE. Approximately one-half of the body's total fat content of young adults is located in the tissues beneath the skin. The feasibility of measuring this subcutaneous fat was suggested by anthropologists at the end of World War I. By 1930, researchers developed a pincer-type caliper that enabled them to measure this fat at representative sites on the body with relative accuracy. The caliper works on the same principle as the micrometer used to measure the distance between two points. The procedure for measuring fatfold thickness is to firmly grasp, with the thumb and forefinger, a fold of skin and subcutaneous fat away from the underlying muscular tissue following the natural contour of the fatfold. The pincer arms of the caliper exert constant tension at their point of contact with the skin. The thickness of the double layer of skin and subcutaneous tissues can then be read directly from the caliper dial. The procedure for taking the fatfold measurements, as well as the precise location of the fatfold sites, must be standardized if results are to be reliable and used for comparative purposes.

There are two ways to use fatfolds. The first is to add the scores from the various measurements and use this value as an indication of the relative degree of fatness among subjects. The sites most commonly measured are at the back of the right, upper arm (referred to as the triceps), the fatfold measured just below the inside border of the right scapula (subscapula), the vertical fold measured just above the hipbone (supra-iliac), the vertical fold measured 1 inch to the right of the umbilicus (abdomen), and the vertical fold measured at the midline of the thigh, two-thirds the distance from the knee cap to the hip. The sum of fatfolds can be used to reflect changes in fatness before and after a physical conditioning or weight reduction program.

A second way to use fatfolds is in conjunction with the mathematical equations that have been developed to predict body density or percent body fat. These equations are often quite useful in ranking or ordering individuals within a group in terms of relative fatness. The equations are *population specific,* in that they accurately predict fatness in samples of subjects similar to those on which the equations were derived.

Although the fatfold technique has been widely used in the fields of physical education, nutrition, and medicine, it presents a major drawback in that the person taking the measurements must have considerable expertise with the proper techniques to obtain consistent and accurate fatfold values. When fatfolds are measured for research purposes, for example, the investigator has usually had experience taking several thousand measurements and is quite consistent in duplicating values for the same subject made on the same day, on consecutive days, or even weeks apart. In such cases, the fatfold technique can provide a useful means for body composition evaluation.

New Indirect Procedures for Assessment of Body Composition

There are alternate indirect procedures that enable the researcher to gain valuable information about body composition. One technique makes use of ultrasonic technology to measure fat and muscle thickness at selected body sites. A second technique converts the fat thickness at three sites from an upper arm x-ray to an accurate estimate of percentage body fat. A third procedure, called computerized axial tomography scanning, creates images of fat distribution within the body. A fourth procedure, bioelectrical impedance, attempts to measure the resistivity to the flow of an electrical current passed between two parts of the body, with subsequent conversion to percent body fat. Although this procedure has gained in popularity in some fitness centers and health spas, there is little confirming evidence of the validity of the procedure. In addition, the cost of the impedance meter and accompanying software seems prohibitively high ($3000 to $6000) in relation to other indirect techniques such as fatfolds or girths that are not only inexpensive, but give more valid results.

ULTRASOUND

A lightweight, portable ultrasound meter is used to measure the distance between the skin and fat-muscle layer, and between the fat-muscle layer and bone. The ultrasound meter operates by emitting high frequency sound waves that penetrate the skin surface. The sound waves pass through adipose tissue until they reach the muscle layer, where the sound waves are then reflected from the fat-muscle interface to produce an echo that returns to the ultrasound unit. The time for sound wave transmission through the tissues and back to the receiver is converted to a distance score and displayed on a light emitting diode (LED) scale.

With ultrasound, we have evaluated the pattern of fat gain and loss on the trunk and extremities in athletes and in obese and normal weight non-athletes before and after sports and exercise training. Figure 5-5 shows the ultrasound meter for recording fat and muscle thickness. The use of ultrasound for "mapping" muscle and fat thickness at various sites on the body, and estimating total body fat is a useful and valid technique for assessment of body composition.

X-RAY

Figure 5-6 illustrates a procedure for determining an individual's body fat content. A standard x-ray picture is taken of the right upper arm. The thickness of

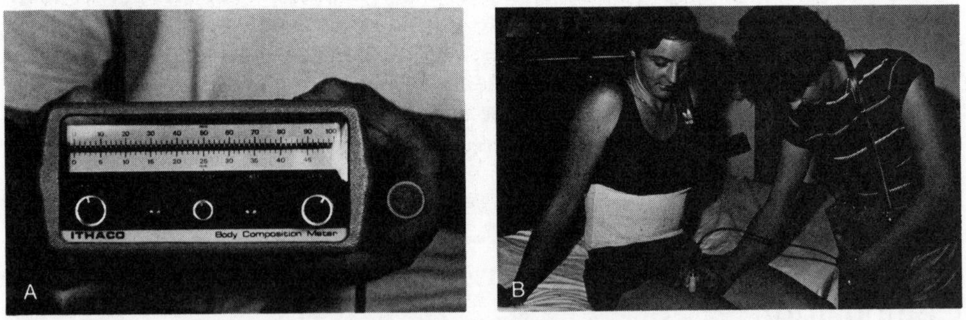
ITHACO
Body Composition Meter
A
B

Figure 5-5. *Ultrasound measurement. A. Portable body composition meter that includes a display scale on the meter to provide a direct readout of distance between skin-to-fat, fat-to-muscle, and muscle-to-bone. B. Measurement of upper leg fat and muscle thickness.*

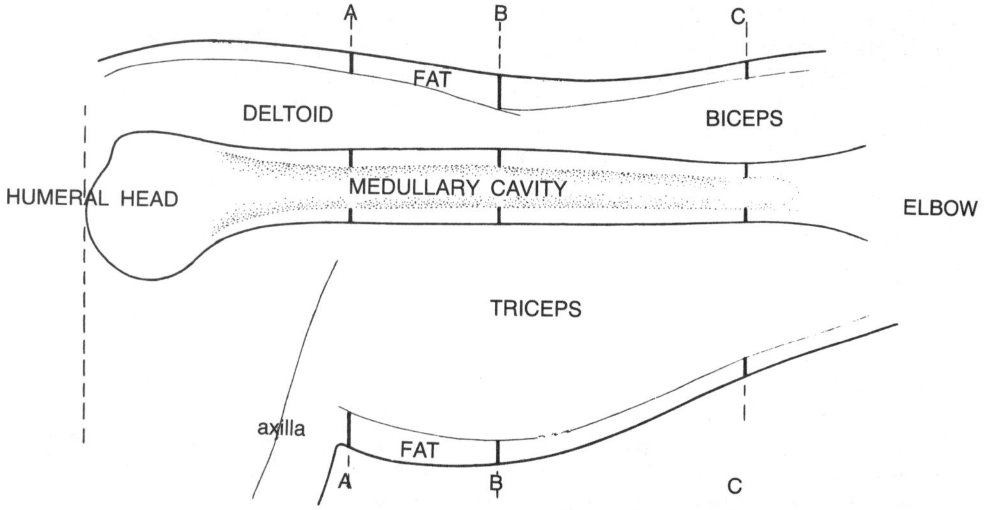
A
B
C
FAT
DELTOID
BICEPS
HUMERAL HEAD
MEDULLARY CAVITY
ELBOW
TRICEPS
axilla
FAT
A
B
C

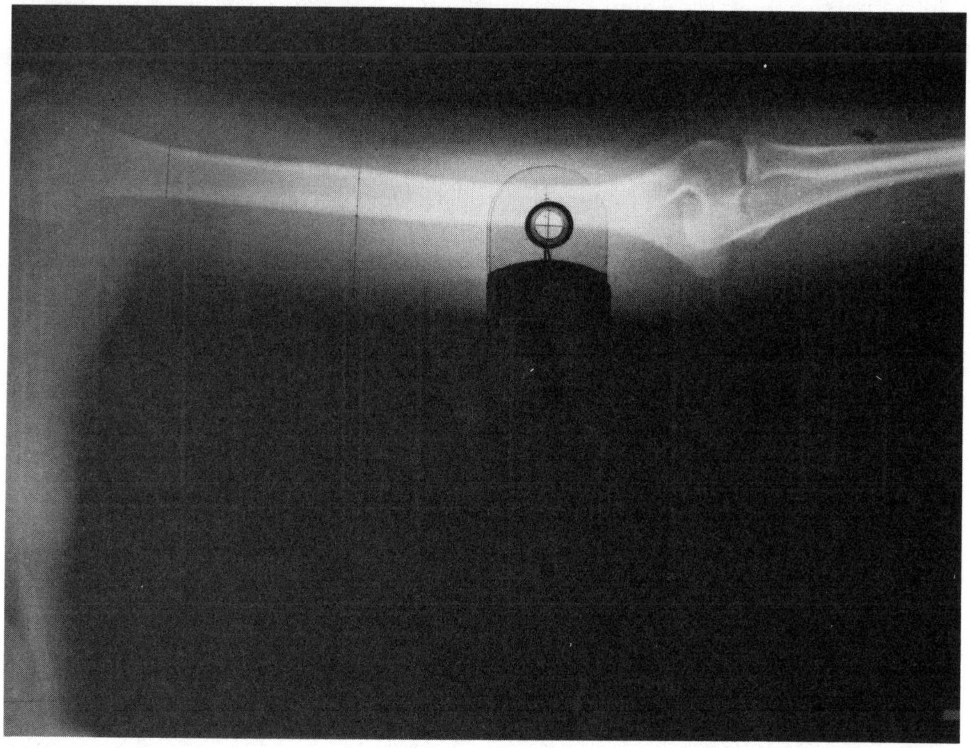

Figure 5-6. *Top. Schematic drawing of an arm x-ray of a 24-year-old female. The six fat widths are represented by the vertical lines drawn perpendicular to the long axis of the humerus at points A, B, and C. Bottom. There is a demarcation on the x-ray between fat, muscle, and bone that permits an accurate assessment of radiographic widths. Total body fat determined from this x-ray was 23.6%; by underwater weighing, body fat was 23.3%. The technician is using a digitizer to calculate fat width on the x-ray. The information from the digitizer is processed by a computer to a printer and graphics plotter.*

the fat layers at points A, B, and C are measured accurately with either a caliper or electronic measuring instrument interfaced with a sonic digitizer and computer graphics system. Muscle and bone (medullary and cortex) thickness can also be measured. Total radiation (10 millirems) is low; it is approximately one-half that of a chest x-ray film or about one-tenth the background radiation accumulated in 1 year living at sea level.

There is a high degree of association between percent body fat determined by hydrostatic weighing and fat thickness from the x-ray picture (correlation or r = .90). This remarkable relationship, in conjunction with a person's height and weight, permits the conversion of the fat thickness shown on x-ray film to total body fat. For a given individual, the conversion to percent body fat is accurate to within plus or minus 3% actual units for body fat determined by the hydrostatic weighing method. The technique is valid for Caucasian and Black young and older men and women, for young and older men and women classified as high or low in fitness status assessed by treadmill maximal oxygen consumption, and for males and females who reduced total body fat content by dietary restriction and increased exercise. The arm x-ray technique to assess body fat was only marginally effective in cardiac and pulmonary patients. Recent studies in one of our laboratories involved measurement of the fat, muscle, and bone cortex and medulla in the arms of postmenopausal women, half of whom had osteoporosis and half who did not. We related upper body muscular strength to upper arm muscle thickness from the x-ray, as well as the relation between upper body muscular strength and the ratio of upper arm bone cortex to medulla. Preliminary results were very encouraging and suggested that an objective measure of muscular strength may be as good a predictor of the degree of osteoporosis as is bone mineral content assessed by photon beam absorptiometry.

COMPUTED TOMOGRAPHY (CT)

The CT scanning procedure produces radiographic images at any section of the body. In the first studies to use CT for body composition evaluation, researchers were able to accurately differentiate fat accumulation in the abdominal area. By use of appropriate computer software, the scan provides pictorial and quantitative information for total tissue area, total fat area, and intra-abdominal fat area. Figure 5-7 shows a CT scan of both upper legs and a cross section at the mid-thigh region in a professional walker who completed an 11,200 mile walk through the 50 United States in 50 weeks. A comparison of CT scans prior to and after the walk showed a significant increase in the total cross section of muscle area and corresponding decrease in subcutaneous fat in the mid-thigh region. In the most recent studies using CT scans, scientists have been able to determine the relationship between the outer thickness of fat at the abdomen and the visceral fat within the abdominal cavity. Suprisingly, there was little relation in both males and females between the external and internal measure of fat! The CT scan procedure and the newer technology of magnetic resonance imaging can provide valuable information about the body's various tissue compartments following exercise training, nutritional supplementation and dietary regimens, as well as during growth and aging.

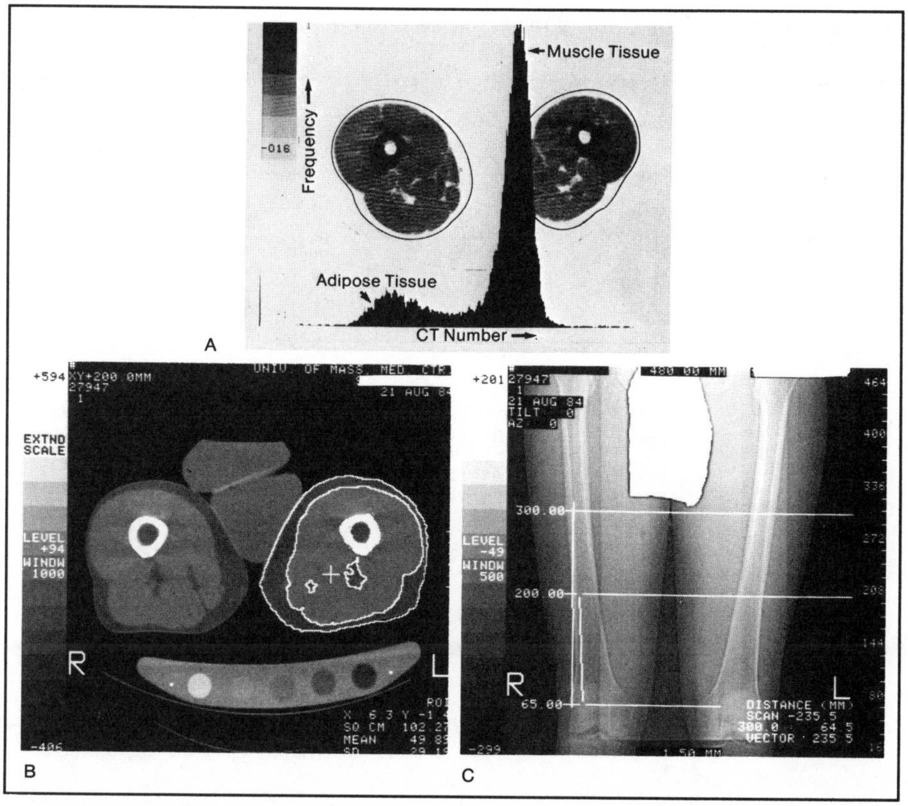
Muscle Tissue
Frequency
Adipose Tissue
CT Number
A
B
C

Figure 5-7. *CT scan. A, Plot of pixel elements that illustrates extent of adipose tissue and muscle tissue in the cross-section of the thigh. B, C, Anterior view of both upper legs and cross-section at mid thigh prior to an 11,200 mile walk around the United States. (A, courtesy of Dr. Steven Heymsfeld, M.D., Emory University School of Medicine. B, C, courtesy of the University of Massachusetts Medical School, Department of Radiology, Worcester, Mass.)*

Average Values for Body Composition

Values for body fat for a sample of men and women throughout the United States are presented in Table 5-1. In comparing your values for body fat with these results, keep in mind that these data represent average values. We have also included values that are plus and minus one standard deviation in the table to give some indication of the amount of variation or spread from the average. The column headed "68% variation limits" indicates the range of values for percent body fat that includes 1 standard deviation or about 68 of every 100 people measured. As an example, the average value for percent body fat for young men from the New York sample is 15.0%, and the 68% variation limits are from 8.9 to 21.1% body fat. Interpreting this statistically, it could be expected that for 68 of every 100 people measured, values for percent fat would range between 8.9 to 21.1%. Of the remaining 32 young men, 16 would possess more than 21% body fat, while for the other 16

Table 5-1. *Average values of percent body fat for younger and older women and men from selected studies.*

STUDY	AGE RANGE	HEIGHT cm	WEIGHT kg	PERCENT FAT[a]	68% VARIATION LIMITS
Younger Women					
North Carolina, 1962	17–25	165.0	55.5	22.9	17.5–28.5
New York, 1962	16–30	167.5	59.0	28.7	24.6–32.9
California, 1968	19–23	165.9	58.4	21.9	17.0–26.9
California, 1970	17–29	164.9	58.6	25.5	21.0–30.1
Air Force, 1972	17–22	164.1	55.8	28.7	22.3–35.3
New York, 1973	17–26	160.4	59.0	26.2	23.4–33.3
North Carolina, 1975		166.1	57.5	24.6	—
Texas, 1978	18–26	165.0	57.4	25.5	21.1–30.0
Massachusetts, 1987	17–31	165.2	57.7	21.9	16.7–27.7
Older Women					
Minnesota, 1953	31–45	163.3	60.7	28.9	25.1–32.8
	43–68	160.0	60.9	34.2	28.0–40.5
New York, 1963	30–40	164.9	59.6	28.6	22.1–35.3
	40–50	163.1	56.4	34.4	29.5–39.5
North Carolina, 1975	33–50	—	—	29.7	23.1–36.5
Massachusetts, 1987	31–52	165.3	58.8	25.2	19.2–31.3
Younger Men					
Minnesota, 1951	17–26	177.8	69.1	11.8	5.9–11.8
Colorado, 1956	17–25	172.4	68.3	13.5	8.3–18.8
Indiana, 1966	18–23	180.1	75.5	12.6	8.7–16.5
California, 1968	16–31	175.7	74.1	15.2	6.3–24.2
New York, 1973	17–26	176.4	71.4	15.0	8.9–21.1
Texas, 1977	18–24	179.9	74.6	13.4	7.4–19.4
Massachusetts, 1987	17–32	178.3	76.4	12.9	7.8–19.2
Older Men					
Indiana, 1966	24–38	179.0	76.6	17.8	11.3–24.3
	40–48	177.0	80.5	22.3	16.3–28.3
North Carolina, 1976	27–50	—	—	23.7	17.9–30.1
Texas, 1977	27–59	180.0	85.3	27.1	23.7–30.5
Massachusetts, 1987	31–52	177.1	77.4	19.9	13.2–29.5

[a]Percent body fat computed from body density measured by hydrostatic weighing, Percent fat = 495/Density − 450.

people, body fat would be less than 8.9%. Certainly a value within the 68% variation limits for body fat could be considered "normal." In the next chapter we will discuss what is considered abnormal or excessive fatness.

Although considerable data are available concerning the average body composition of many groups of men and women of different ages and fitness levels, there has been no systematic evaluation of the body composition of representative samples from the general population that would warrant setting up precise norms or desirable values of body composition. At this time, the best we can do is to present the average values from various studies of different age groups.

A general conclusion based on these data is that with increasing age, the percentage of body fat tends to increase in both men and women. This average change does not necessarily mean the trend should be interpreted as being desirable or "normal." Changes in body composition with age could in part occur because the aging skeleton becomes demineralized and porous. Such a process reduces body density because of the decrease in bone density. Another reason for the relative increase in body fat with age is the reduction in the level of daily physical activity. The adaptation to a more sedentary life style could increase the deposition of storage fat and reduce the quantity of muscle mass. This would occur even if the daily caloric consumption remained unchanged. The exact interaction of the aging process per se and the numerous ramifications of the sociology and psychology of aging on fitness and body composition in industrialized societies have not as yet been adequately evaluated.

DESIRABLE BODY WEIGHT

Although excess quantities of body fat are undesirable for good health and fitness, precise statements cannot be made as to an optimum level of body fat or body weight for a particular individual. More than likely, this optimum varies from person to person and is greatly influenced by a variety of genetic factors. Based on data from physically active young adults and competitive athletes, it would be desirable in our opinion to strive for a body fat content of 15% for men (certainly less than 20%), and about 25% body fat for women (certainly less than 30%). Some fitness enthusiasts have advocated that men should be no higher than 10% body fat and women no higher than 20%. We think these limits are an unreasonable standard that most people would find extremely difficult to achieve and maintain. An "optimal" or "desirable" body weight can be computed using a desired level of body fat as follows:

$$\text{Desirable body weight} = \frac{\text{Lean body weight}}{1.00 - \text{\% fat desired}}$$

Suppose a 200-pound man, who has 20% body fat, wishes to know the weight he should attain so that this new lower body weight would contain 15% body fat. The computations would be:

$$\text{Fat weight} = 200 \text{ lbs} \times .15 = 30 \text{ lbs}$$

$$\text{Lean body weight} = 200 \text{ lbs} - 30 \text{ lbs} = 170 \text{ lbs}$$

$$\text{Desirable body weight} = \frac{170 \text{ lbs}}{1.00 - .10}$$

$$= \frac{170 \text{ lb}}{.90}$$

$$= 188.9$$

Desirable fat loss = Present body weight − Desirable body weight

$$= 200 \text{ lb} - 188.9 \text{ lb}$$
$$= 11.1 \text{ lb}$$

If this man lost 11.1 lbs of body fat, his new body weight of 188.9 lbs would have a fat content equal to 15% of body weight. For practical purposes, it is prudent to recommend a *desirable weight range*, rather than an absolute value for the desirable weight. In this example, an appropriate weight range would be 187 to 197 lbs. *We believe that the notion of an upper and lower limit around the desired weight is the best procedure to use when prescribing optimal levels of body composition.*

In our opinion, the weight loss should always be accompanied by a planned, systematic program of increased physical activity. This will ensure that the lost weight is mostly fat and not the lean tissues.

6

Obesity

AMERICANS CONSUME more fat per capita than any other nation in the world. They also consume more than 90% of the foods high in saturated fats and processed sugars. The end result of this national preoccupation with food and effortless living is that an estimated 60 to 70 million adults and 10 to 12 million teenagers are "too fat" by a total of 2.3 billion pounds. In calories, this excess fat represents an energy equivalent of 5.7 trillion kcal, or the potential energy in 1.3 billion gallons of gasoline! This is sufficient energy to power 900,000 automobiles a year or provide the annual residential electrical requirements of Boston, Chicago, San Francisco, and Washington, D.C.

Until recently, it was commonly believed that the major cause of progressive weight gain (and resulting obesity) was simply a problem of overeating. However, if gluttony and overindulgence were the only factors associated with accumulation of excess fat, the easiest way to reduce body fat would simply be to decrease food intake. As we all know, it's much more complicated. If there were a simple method to help cure the overfat condition, obesity would surely be eliminated as a major health concern. There are obviously other factors that include genetic, environmental, psychological, and social influences. Research suggests that individual differences in specific factors such as eating patterns, body image, resting metabolic rate, basal body temperature, hypothalamic control, levels of cellular enzymes, and brown fat may predispose a person to excessive fat gain. It is also becoming increasingly clear that the lack of adequate energy expenditure in daily physical activity is an important predisposing factor to obesity.

We can state with certainty that excess fat is the end result of an imbalance between the number of calories consumed and the number of calories expended to sustain daily activities. It also is clear to us that treatment procedures devised so far, be they dietary, surgical, drug, or behavioral, either alone or in combination, have not been particularly successful in controlling obesity on a long-term basis. Although research has provided some information about the possible causes of the imbalance between calorie intake and energy output, as yet no unifying theory has emerged to explain exactly why some people become too fat, while others remain relatively thin despite an apparently large caloric intake.

This chapter deals with the development of obesity and examines the following topics: (1) the definition of obesity; (2) medical and health aspects of obesity; (3) methods of determining the size and number of fat cells and their comparison in normal and obese subjects before and after weight gain and reduction; (4) development of adipose cellularity in animals and humans; and (5) the influence of diet and exercise in modifying fat cell size and number.

What Is Obesity?

PERCENT BODY FAT AS A CRITERION

Obesity can be defined as an excessive enlargement of the body's total quantity of fat. The line of demarcation between normal levels of body fat and obesity is somewhat arbitrary. In the previous chapter we suggested that the normal range of body fat in adult men and women encompasses at least plus and minus one unit of variation from the average population value for body fat. The variation unit is approximately 5% body fat for men and women between the ages 17 to 50 years. Within this statistical boundary, overfatness would correspond to any value for percent body fat that exceeds the average value for fatness for a particular age and gender, plus 5%. For young men whose body weight averages 15% fat, the borderline for obesity is 20% body fat. For older men average fatness is approximately 25%. Consequently, overfatness for this group would be a body fat content in excess of 30%. For young women aged 17 to 27, obesity would correspond to a body fat content above 31%, while for older women aged 27 to 50, borderline obesity would be about 37% body fat. It should be emphasized that although the average population value for percent body fat increases with age, *this does NOT imply that men and women should be expected to get fatter as they grow older. To the contrary, the criterion for overfatness should probably be that established for younger men and women—above 20% for men and above 30% for women.*

It should also be pointed out that there is a gradation of obesity that progresses from the upper limit of normal—20% for men and 30% for women—to as high as 50 to 70% of body weight in those who are massively obese. Common terms for the gradation of obesity include pleasantly plump for those just above the cut off, to moderately obese, excessively obese, and massively obese. The latter category includes people who weigh in the range of 375 to about 600 pounds, and whose fat content is above 55% of body weight, and often 60 to 65% or higher! In this situation body fat exceeds the lean body weight and obesity may be a life threatening condition.

STANDARDS FOR OVERFATNESS
Men—above 20%
Women—above 30%

FAT CELL SIZE AND NUMBER AS CRITERIA

In addition to the total percent of body fat, the *size* and *number* of fat cells has been proposed as a means to identify and study what is normal and abnormal with regard to body fatness. The body increases its quantity of adipose tissue in two ways. The first is by enlarging or filling existing fat cells with more fat. We refer to this as fat cell *hypertrophy.* The second way is by increasing the total number of fat cells, or fat cell *hyperplasia.*

MEDICAL AND HEALTH ASPECTS OF OBESITY

Nearly 34 million Americans weight 20% or more above their desirable body weight (for example, a 204 pound person whose ideal weight is 170), and more than 11 million of these men and women are severely obese and at greater risk of developing a variety of diseases related to their obesity. Although it has been argued that a moderate excess in body fat is not in itself harmful, a 1986 report of a 14-member panel convened at the National Institutes of Health concluded that obesity should be viewed as a *disease.* This is because there are multiple biological hazards at surprisingly low levels of excess fat that represent only 5 to 10 pounds above desirable body weight. In fact, it is now argued rather convincingly that obesity is a powerful heart disease risk that may be equal to that of smoking, elevated blood fats, and hypertension.

It is well established in the medical literature that chronic disease is more prevalent in obese than individuals of normal body fat. While it is not clear the degree to which obesity causes specific medical problems, the plight of the obese person in terms of increased medical and health complications include the following: (1) hypertension (5.6 times higher) and increased risk of stroke, (2) renal disease, (3) gallbladder disease, (4) diabetes mellitus (3 times as frequent), (5) pulmonary diseases, (6) problems with anesthesia during surgery, (7) osteoarthritis and gout, (8) breast and endometrial cancer, (9) abnormal plasma lipid and lipoprotein concentrations, (10) impairment of cardiac function due to an increase in the heart's mechanical work, (11) menstrual irregularities and toxemia of pregnancy, (12) psychologic trauma, (13) flat feet and intertriginous dermatitis (infection in fatfolds), (14) organ compression by adipose tissue, and (15) impaired heat tolerance.

It also appears that the distribution of adipose tissue, independent of total body fat, alters the health risks of obesity. For example, possessing a high ratio of waist to hip circumference (ratio > 0.90) is associated with an increased risk for illness, while possessing a "pear shaped" figure of equivalent fatness may not be as risky. This may occur because fat in the abdominal area is more active metabolically than fat located in the hips and thighs.

Methods of Determining Fat Cell Size and Number

Researchers have used a variety of techniques to study adipose cellularity in humans and animals. The most accurate method was developed in the 1960s in the laboratory of Dr. Jules Hirsch at Rockefeller University, New York City. The technique involves sucking small fragments of subcutaneous tissue, usually from the buttocks and abdomen, into a syringe through a needle inserted directly into a fat depot. The adipose tissue is then treated chemically so that the fat cells can be separated and counted.

Once the number of cells is determined for a known weight of fat tissue, the average quantity of fat per cell is determined by dividing the quantity of fat in the sample by the total number of cells present in the sample. If total body fat is known, a reasonable estimate can be made of the total number of fat cells in the body. Let us assume that a subject weighs 70 kg and is 18% fat as determined by the underwater weighing method outlined in Chapter 5. The weight of fat for this person is computed as body weight × percent body fat and equals 12.6 kg of fat. By dividing this value for the weight of fat by the average content of fat per cell, the total number of fat cells in the body can be determined.

$$\text{Total number of fat cells} = \frac{\text{Weight of body fat}}{\text{Fat content per cell}}$$

In this example, if the average fat cell contains 0.53 micrograms (μg) of fat, then there are 23.8 billion fat cells contained in the 12.6 kg adipose tissue depot.

In one of our laboratories, the needle biopsy procedure coupled with photomicrographic techniques are used to extract and measure the average size of fat cells in the buttocks, abdomen, and upper back area. After the fat sample is extracted, it is treated chemically and then photographed for later projection on a large screen. Figure 6-1 shows the biopsy procedure from the buttocks region and a photomicrograph of the fat cells that are counted and measured for diameter and volume with a light emitting pen that interfaces with a computer. For the middle-aged professor whose total fat content prior to a successful marathon run was 14.4 kg (184 lbs or 83.4 kg body weight, 17.2% body fat) with 0.68 μg of lipid per cell, the total number of fat cells was estimated to be 21.2 billion (14.4 kg ÷ 0.68 μg).

Fat Cell Size and Number of Normal and Obese Adult Subjects

There have been several comparative studies of adipose cellularity in obese and nonobese human subjects. These studies show quite conclusively that the accumulation of excess calories as fat in the obese is brought about either by the storage of larger quantities of fat in existing adipose cells (hypertrophy), by the actual formation of new fat cells (hyperplasia), or by a combination of both hypertrophy and hyperplasia.

Figure 6-2 graphically compares the body weight, total fat content, cell size, and cell number in a group of 20 subjects clinically classified as obese and in 5 nonobese subjects.

The body weight of the obese subjects averaged more than twice that of the nonobese, while their total fat content was nearly triple that of the leaner group. The weight of body fat in the obese ranged from 92 pounds to 227 pounds, while the average weight of fat for the nonobese was about 40 pounds. Further analysis of fat composition indicated that the average amount of fat within each fat cell was

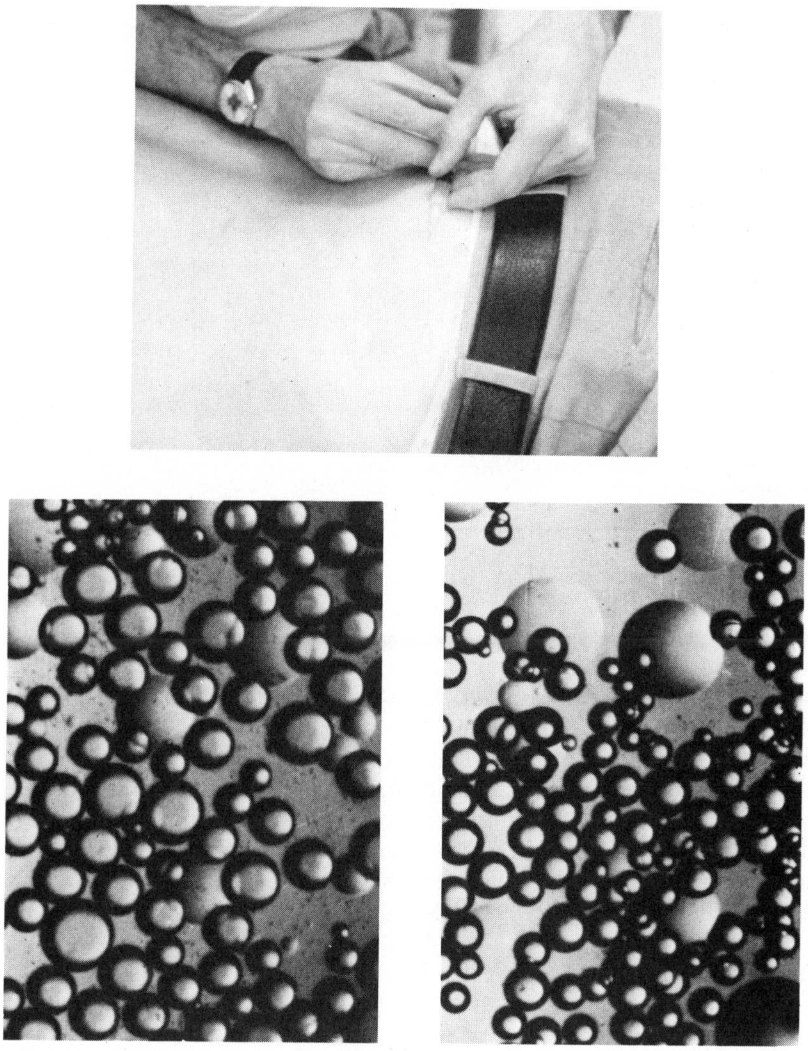

Figure 6-1. *Upper panel. Needle biopsy procedure for extraction of fat cells in the upper buttocks region. The biopsy needle is placed beneath the skin surface after the area is anesthetized. The syringe is used to collect the small tissue fragments after they are literally sucked from the site of the incision. Bottom panels. Photomicrograph of fat cells biopsied from the buttocks of the middle-aged, physically active professor. The large spherical structures in the background are lipid droplets. During a period of relative inactivity prior to 6 months of marathon training (5 day/ week, 10 to 16 miles/day), the average diameter of the buttocks fat cells was 8.6% larger than following the training regimen. The average volume of fat in each cell decreased by 18.2% compared to pretraining values.*

about 35% greater in the obese than in the nonobese. In addition, the total *number* of fat cells in the obese subjects was approximately 3 times greater than the number of fat cells in the nonobese—75 billion fat cells compared to 27 billion fat cells. This vividly illustrates that the major structural difference in adipose tissue mass between obese and nonobese people is in cell number.

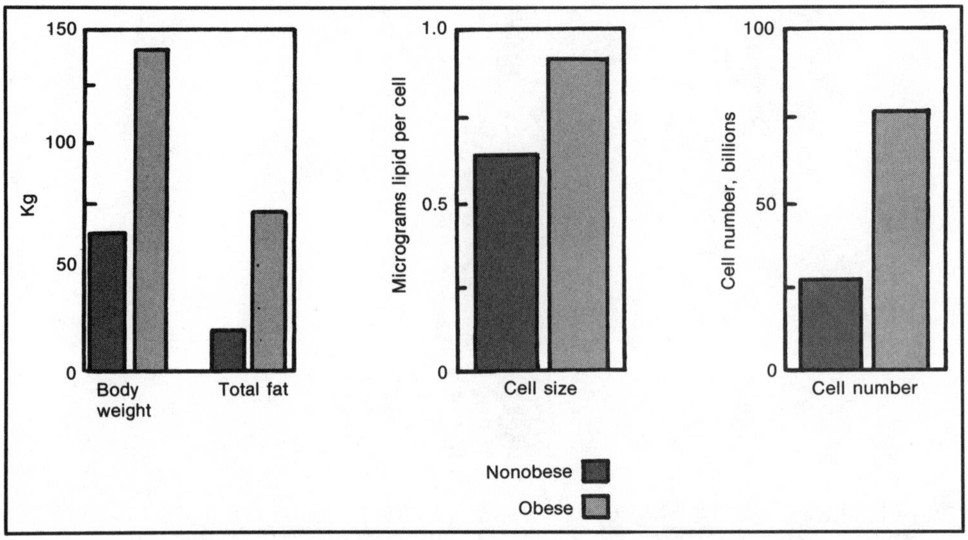
150
100
50
0
Kg
Body weight
Total fat
1.0
0.5
0
Micrograms lipid per cell
Cell size
100
50
0
Cell number, billions
Cell number
Nonobese
Obese

Figure 6-2. *Comparison of body weight, total body fat, cell size, and cell number in obese and non-obese subjects.*

We can illustrate the role of fat cell number in obesity further by relating total fat content to both cell size and cell number. The data in the left side of Figure 6-3 demonstrate the strong positive relationship between total weight of fat in the obese and the total number of fat cells. The obese person with the lowest fat content had the fewest number of fat cells, while the fattest subject had considerably more fat cells than the less fat subjects. On the other hand, the data displayed in the right panel of Figure 6-3 clearly show that there was little or no relationship between the total body fat of obese people and the average size of fat cells. This information suggests that there may be some biologic upper limit to how large fat cells can become. After this size is reached, cell number probably becomes the key factor in determining the extent of obesity. Even if the size of fat cells could double, their size would not account for the tremendous difference in the amount of fat in obese and nonobese people. The excessive quantity of adipose tissue in obesity, therefore, must occur by fat cell hyperplasia. As a frame of reference, an average nonobese person has about 25 to 30 billion fat cells. For the moderately obese the number of fat cells is about 60 to 100 billion, while for the massively obese, the number of fat cells may be as high as 300 billion or more.

Fat Cell Size and Number after Weight Reduction

Weight reduction in obese adults and children is accompanied by a decrease in the size of fat cells but no change in the number of cells. If a weight reduction program achieves normal body weight and fatness, then the individual fat cells will shrink and actually become smaller in size than the fat cells of people who have never been obese. The results of one study of weight reduction in obese adults are depicted in Figure 6-4.

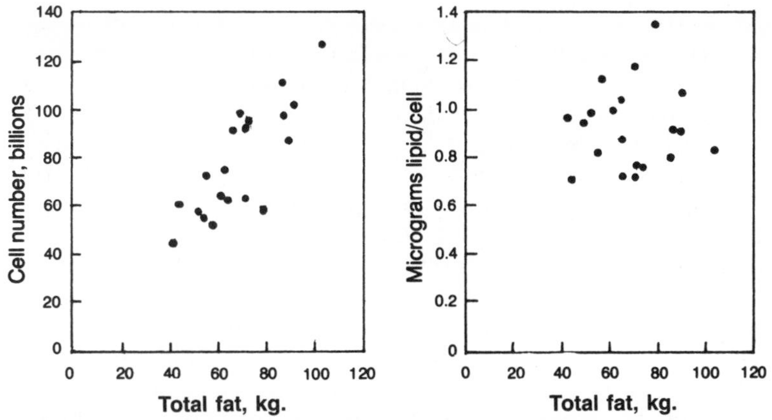
Cell number, billions
Total fat, kg.
Micrograms lipid/cell
Total fat, kg.

Figure 6-3. *Left panel: Adipose cell number related to the body's total weight of fat; right panel: Adipose cell size related to the body's total weight of fat.*

In this study 19 obese subjects who initially weighed 328 pounds reduced body weight by 101 pounds, weighing 227 pounds at the end of the first part of the experiment. Prior to weight reduction the average number of fat cells was approximately 75 billion. This number remained essentially unchanged after weight reduction. The average size of the fat cells, on the other hand, was reduced 33%, from 0.9 to 0.6 μg of fat per cell. When they lost 62 more pounds, the subjects attained a normal body weight. Cell number again remained unchanged, while cell size continued to shrink to about one-third the size of the fat cells of normal, nonobese subjects. Other experiments have confirmed these findings in adults and young children. *The major anatomic or structural change after weight reduction is a shrinkage in fat cell size with little or no change in cell number.*

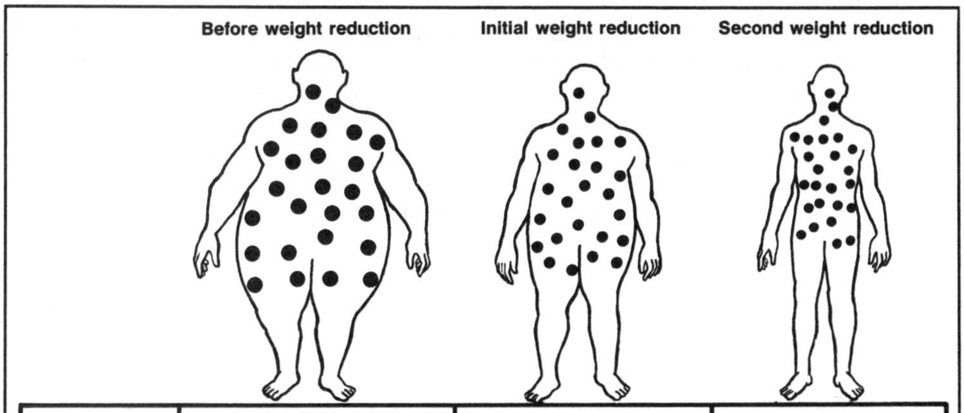
Before weight reduction
Initial weight reduction
Second weight reduction

	Before weight reduction	Initial weight reduction	Second weight reduction
Body weight	328 lb	227 lb	165 lb
Fat cell size	0.9 μg/cell	0.6 μg/cell	0.2 μg/cell
Fat cell number	75 billion	75 billion	75 billion

Figure 6-4. *Changes in adipose cellularity with weight reduction in obese subjects.*

These findings show that the formerly obese person who reduces body weight and even body fat to near average levels is still not "cured" of obesity, at least not in terms of the number of fat cells present. Clinical evidence reveals that such formerly obese patients have an extremely difficult time maintaining their new body size. It is tempting to suggest that this large number of relatively small fat cells in the reduced obese is somehow related to the appetite control center in the brain. When this appetite center is stimulated, the person craves food, overeats, and regains the lost weight. Some nutritionists have referred to the repetitive "yo-yo-like" cycle of weight loss and weight gain among the obese as the "plight of the starving fat cells."

Research indicates that using various dietary manipulations to help adult obese persons to reduce is not likely to alter their large number of fat cells, even if the dietary intervention is successful over a long period. This is a somewhat pessimistic outlook for the obese person who hopes to stay permanently reduced.

Fat Cell Size and Number after Weight Gain

An interesting series of studies dealing with the experimental development of obesity in humans was carried out by researchers at the College of Medicine, University of Vermont. Over a period of 40 weeks, adult male volunteers with an initial average body fat content of 15% deliberately tripled their caloric intake to about 7000 kcal per day. The subject shown in Figure 6-5 increased 25% in body weight, from 110 to 138 pounds. Body fat for this subject doubled from 14.6 to 28.2% of body weight. Consequently, of the 28 pounds gained during the period of overeating, 23 were caused by increased deposition of body fat.

In a similar experiment with a group of nonobese subjects with no previous personal or family history of obesity, body weight increased an average of 36 pounds from voluntary overeating. When the size and number of fat cells were compared before and after the 4-month experimental period, the average size of the fat cells had increased substantially, with no corresponding change in cell number. When the subjects were once again reduced to their normal weight by restricting caloric intake, body fat was reduced and the fat cells returned to their original size. These results indicate that the acquisition of excess fat produced in adults by overeating is caused by filling existing adipose cells with more fat rather than by increasing or proliferating new fat cells. There is also evidence that in mature-onset moderate to massive obesity, where the already fat adult becomes even fatter, new fat cells may be developed in addition to the expansion in size of the already existing cells.

Development of Adipose Cellularity

The development of adipose tissue during growth has been studied by several laboratories and can be categorized in terms of animal research and human research.

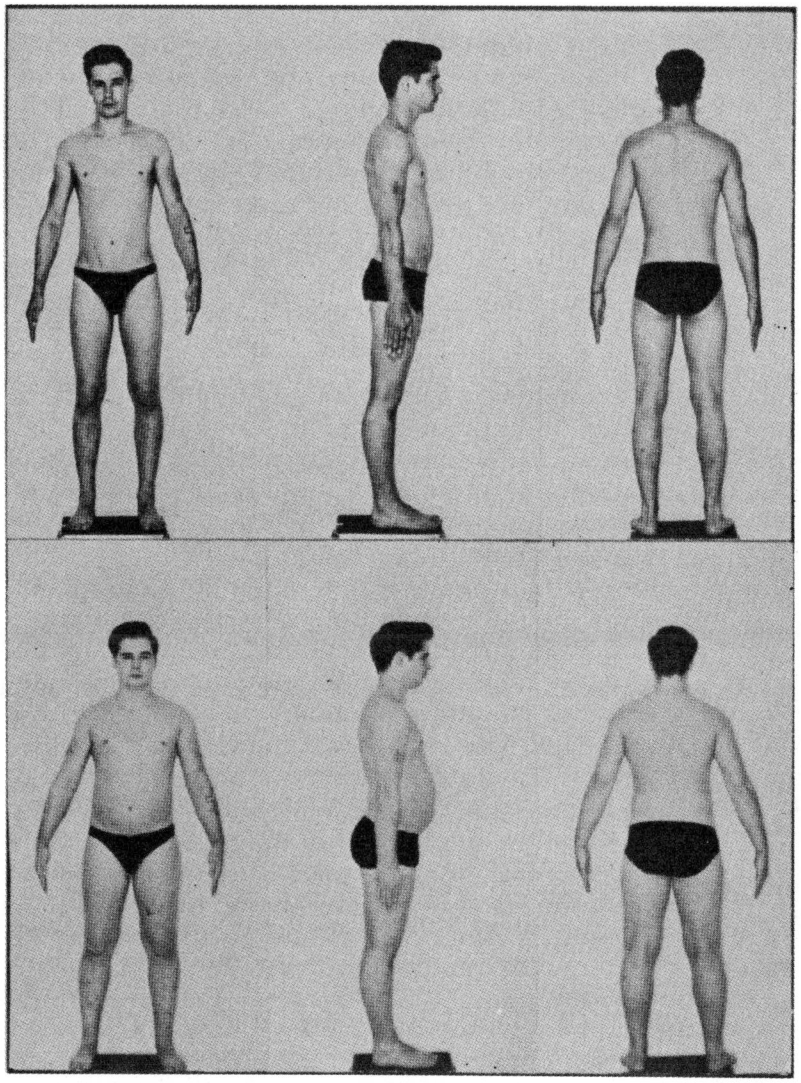

Figure 6-5. *Changes in body weight and percent body fat by deliberate overeating (top:14.6% body fat; bottom: 28.2% body fat). A 25% increase in body weight was accompanied by a 100% increase in body fat.*

ANIMAL STUDIES

Studies of fat cell development in different species of animals reveal two basic ways in which fat depots develop. The guinea pig, for example, expands its adipose tissue mass from 6 weeks to 1 year primarily by hyperplasia. The hamster and rat, on the other hand, increase adipose tissue mainly by fat cell hypertrophy, although hyperplasia also occurs. The most extensive studies of adipose cellularity have been conducted with rats because these mammals have a relatively short life span, and various diets and exercise regimens can be studied quite easily during the growth cycle. In establishing these growth curves, the experimenter determines adipose cellularity periodically from three main fat depots in the rat. What usually occurs is that the number and size of fat cells increases during weeks 6 through 16. Thereafter, as animals continue to gain in body weight and body fat, there is a corresponding increase only in the size of the fat cells. Thus, the additional increase in body fat occurs by filling existing cells rather than by developing new fat cells.

HUMAN STUDIES

In contrast to the many longitudinal studies of animals during their growth periods, few investigations are available on the time course of adipose tissue development in humans. In one human experiment, fat cell size and number were determined for 34 infants and children who ranged in age from a few days to age 13. Figure 6-6 plots some of these data to illustrate the relationship between fat cell size and age. The value for average cell size in normal adults is shown at the right of the figure.

These data suggest that the size of fat cells in newborn infants and children up to the age of 1 year is about one-fourth the size of adult fat cells. It is also evident from Figure 6-6 that fat cells triple in size during the first 6 years with little further increase in size to age 13. Data on adipose cell size during adolescence are scarce. We can assume, however, that cell size increases further during this growth period because in adulthood it is significantly larger than it was at age 13. Figure 6-7 illustrates data on fat cell number from birth to age 13.

During the *first year of life* cell number increases fairly rapidly. The total number of fat cells is about 3 times greater at 1 year than at birth. Scientists believe that most of the fat cells existing prior to birth are formed during the *last 3 months of pregnancy.* After the first year of life cell number increases more gradually up to the age of about 10. As was the case with cell size, the number of cells formed after age 13 continues to increase during the *growth spurt in adolescence* until adulthood; thereafter, there is little further increase in cell number. Thus, there appear to be three critical periods when the number of fat cells increases significantly. The first is during the last trimester of pregnancy, the second is during the first year of life, and the third occurs during the adolescent growth spurt. It is during adulthood

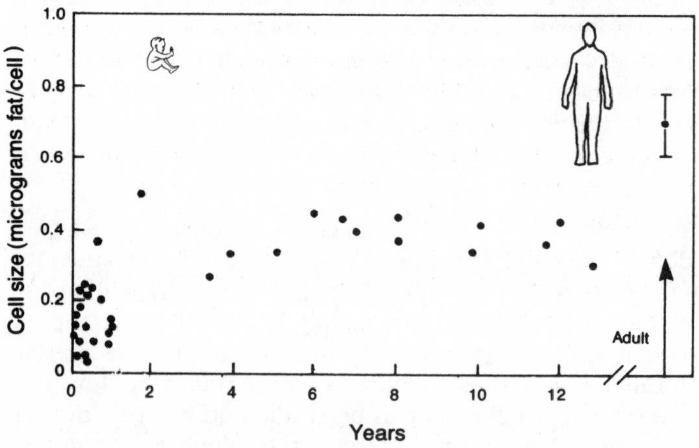
1.0
0.8
0.6
0.4
0.2
0
Cell size (micrograms fat/cell)
0
2
4
6
8
10
12
Adult
Years

Figure 6-6. *Changes in fat cell size from birth to adulthood.*

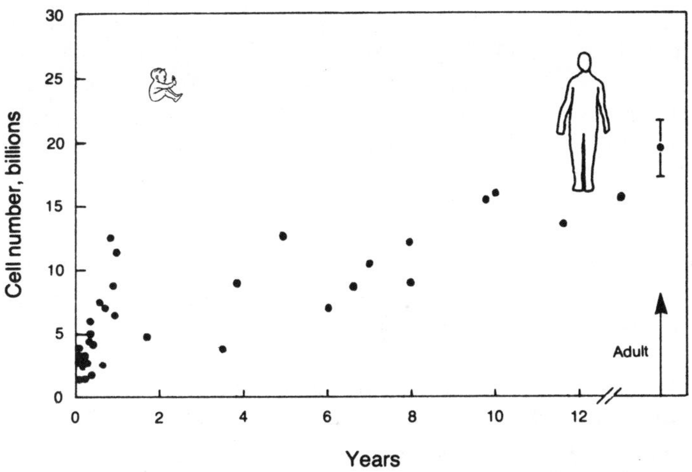
30
25
20
15
10
5
0
Cell number, billions
0
2
4
6
8
10
12
Years
Adult

Figure 6-7. *Changes in fat cell number from birth to adulthood.*

that the total number of fat cells probably cannot be altered to any significant degree; an exception is in the moderately or massively obese adult where further cell proliferation can occur. However, there are still no substantial data to indicate clearly if the final number of adult fat cells can be modified through some form of intervention at an earlier period of life. It is impossible to state with certainty whether the rate of fat cell development in humans can be reversed or at least slowed down. A fundamental question remains, "Can fat cell number be altered before adulthood, or is overfatness predetermined primarily by genetic code?"

Modification of Adipose Cellularity

Although the precise causes for fat cell development are poorly understood, it does appear that certain practices can affect body fat. In humans, for example, nutritional practices of the mother during pregnancy may modify the body composition of the developing fetus. A weight gain by the mother in excess of 40 lb was associated with a significantly larger fatfold thickness of the offspring than in women who followed a recommended weight gain during pregnancy. Bottle feeding and the early introduction of solid food may also be associated with the development of obesity. Conversely, breast feeding, allowing the infant to set the limits to food consumption, and a delayed introduction to solid food, may prevent overfeeding, the development of poor eating habits, and subsequent obesity.

Research in animals suggests that alterations in fat cell size and number can be achieved in two ways: (1) modification of early nutrition, and (2) exercise.

NUTRITIONAL INFLUENCES

Studies have demonstrated that *early nutritional practices* can influence the development of body fatness and adipose cellularity at a later time period in the animal's life. In one well-controlled study large numbers of rats were redistributed at birth, giving some mothers large litters of 22 animals and others smaller litters of 4 animals. After weaning at 21 days both groups were given unlimited access to food. At weaning and at each subsequent 5-week period to 20 weeks of age, both groups of rats differed significantly in body weight. Thus, the early (calorically deprived) nutritional deprivation produced by rearing animals in large litters for the first 21 days of life resulted in the permanent stunting of their growth, even though both groups of animals had free access to food after weaning. The underfed group reached a definite plateau in the number of fat cells by 15 weeks of age. In contrast, cell number continued to increase in the overfed, small-litter animals. In both groups cell size increased progressively during the 20-week experiment. These data certainly suggest there may be a critical time during the early growth period when permanent modifications in adipose tissue occur.

We would like to point out that it is difficult to extrapolate experimental results from rats to humans. However, some striking similarities appear in human and rat adipose tissue development. The excessive quantity of body fat of obese humans is associated primarily with a large increase in the number of fat cells, and to a lesser extent to increased size of individual fat cells. When obese adults lose a considerable amount of weight, the number of fat cells remains unchanged and total body fat is reduced almost exclusively by reducing fat cell size. Similar findings concerning fat cell number occur in studies with adult rats. When adult rats are calorically deprived by acute starvation or more prolonged semistarvation, the decrease in body weight is only temporary and is rapidly reinstated upon refeeding. The weight loss is due to a decrease in fat cell size with no corresponding change in cell number. When the starved animals again have normal access to food, the fat cells refill and attain the size they had prior to food deprivation. Except in already obese animals, overfeeding of adult animals produces an increase in total body fat, but as with humans, this increase is generally brought about by "stuffing" of cells with fat rather than by increases in cell number. Thus in both humans and rats, dietary manipulation does not appear to affect adipose cell number in adulthood; changes in the total quantity of body fat are brought about primarily by cellular enlargement. Furthermore, when the fat content of adult humans is reduced, cell size shrinks accordingly, only to expand again when the body's content of fat is restored.

Other studies have also shown that the early nutritional patterns in rats (controlled by weaning in small and large litters), can have a sustained effect on the total fat mass and total number of cells, but not necessarily the size of the cells. If the influence of early nutrition in the rat is paralleled by similar effects in man, then overfeeding during childhood may increase the tendency to adult obesity. It certainly seems prudent to encourage the parents of young children to avoid overfeeding their youngsters because this may temper their proclivity to obesity as adults. This may be especially true prior to age two.

EXERCISE INFLUENCES

Only a few experiments have evaluated the contribution of exercise to modifying adipose tissue cell size and number. Figure 6-8 summarizes the results of one such experiment on the effects of physical activity and food restriction on the growth of rats. In this study an exercise group with free access to food was subjected to a 14- to 16-week program of swimming early in the animals' growth period. The animals swam in plastic barrels 6 days a week. Initially the exercise

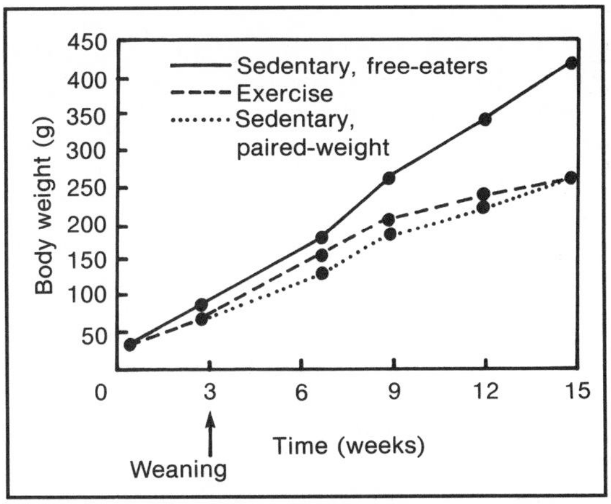
Sedentary, free-eaters
Exercise
Sedentary, paired-weight
Body weight (g)
450
400
350
300
250
200
150
100
50
0
3
6
9
12
15
Weaning
Time (weeks)

Figure 6-8. *Effects of exercise and food restriction on body weight of rats.*

sessions lasted 15 minutes; they lengthened gradually until the animals were swimming for 360 minutes at the end of 4 weeks. They continued to swim for 360 minutes until the end of the experimental period. They were then sacrificed and analyzed for fat content and adipose cellularity. During the experiment two adult groups of rats remained sedentary; one group had free access to food and water, while the other group was restricted in food intake to maintain their body weight at the same level as the exercise group.

The results were convincing; animals given unlimited food but forced to exercise for 15 weeks gained weight more slowly and had a lower final body weight than sedentary, freely eating rats. Because both groups consumed the *same* number of calories each day, the lower rate of weight gain in the exercisers could be attributed to the increased caloric requirements of the exercise. It was also shown that the total fat content of the nonexercise group was about 4 times higher than the fat content of the freely eating exercise group. The exercise intervention program during the growth period resulted in a significant reduction in total body fat due to a decrease in both cell size *and* number.

The total fat content of the sedentary, food-restricted group was lower than that of the sedentary animals who could eat freely. Reducing food intake resulted in a reduction in cell size and cell number. When the body fat of the food restricted and exercised animals was compared, the exercisers had fewer fat cells and less fat per cell, even though the final body weights of both groups were approximately equal. The results demonstrated that exercise performed *early* during the growth period depressed the growth of new fat cells. In a follow-up experiment, the fat-retarding effects of exercise or diet early in an animal's life were studied to determine whether either would reduce fat accumulation in adulthood.

Three groups of animals were used: an exercise group, a sedentary group with free access to food and water, and a sedentary group with restricted food intake. Exercise and food restriction were terminated after 28 weeks. Several animals from each group were then sacrificed and the group compared for growth, body fat, and adipose cell size and number. The remaining animals were subjected to 34 weeks of sedentary living without exercise and were allowed unlimited food and water. The animals were then sacrificed and the groups compared for body weight,

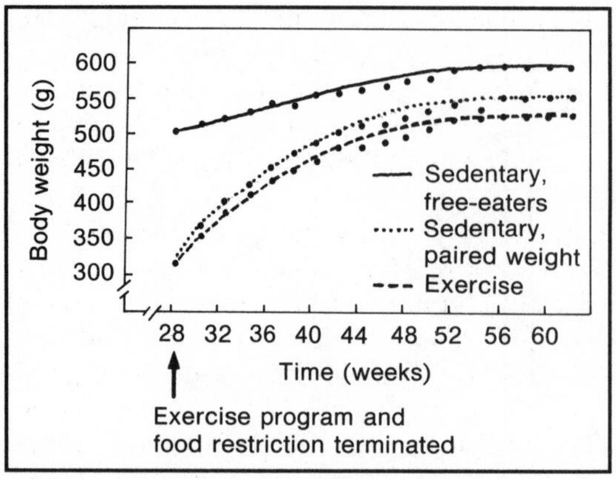
600
550
500
450
400
350
300
Body weight (g)
Sedentary, free-eaters
Sedentary, paired weight
Exercise
28 32 36 40 44 48 52 56 60
Time (weeks)
Exercise program and food restriction terminated

Figure 6-9. *Effects of 28 weeks of exercise and food restriction on body weight in rats followed by no exercise with unlimited access to foods.*

cell size, and cell number. The data in Figure 6-9 show that the exercised animals had lower body weights at 28 weeks of age than the other groups.

During the next 34 weeks of inactivity, the previously exercised animals continued to maintain a lower body weight than the sedentary animals. Thus, the 28-week exercise program performed earlier in life caused a reduction in body weight that was still evident at the end of the experiment. Comparing cell size and number at the end of the training period revealed that the exercised group had *fewer and smaller* fat cells than either sedentary group of animals. These results were in agreement with the previous experiment. The exercise group had a lower final body weight and reduced total body fat content than their sedentary counterparts, as well as significantly *fewer* fat cells in later life than animals in the other groups. Twenty-six weeks of exercise, begun early in life and then terminated, retarded the expansion and proliferation of fat cells during the growth period to adulthood, even though the exercise period was followed by 34 weeks of inactivity.

If these findings can be applied to humans, it is possible that the introduction of a diet and/or exercise program during the early stages of growth may aid in controlling the proliferation of new fat cells and the filling up of previously dormant ones. Programs of exercise and weight control begun later in life and maintained thereafter can be effective in lowering the body's total quantity of fat. As far as we know, only cell size can be reduced, not cell number. If exercise or dietary intervention is discontinued, then the existing adipose tissue mass is likely to increase again by expansion of the cellular volume. *Early prevention of obesity through exercise and diet, rather than correction of obesity once it is present, may be the most effective method to curb the grossly "overfat" condition so common in teenagers and adults.*

SPOT REDUCTION: A FUTILE EXERCISE TO SELECTIVELY REDUCE BODY FAT

There is widespread belief that by exercising one area of the body, more fat will be lost from that area in comparison to other body parts. It is also believed that disuse of a muscle group causes a disproportionate accumulation of local subcutaneous fat and, conversely, an increase in a muscle's activity facilitates a relatively large fat mobilization from the specific storage sites. While the notion of *"spot-reduction"* through selective exercise such as leg raises, sit ups, side bends, or twists is especially attractive from an aesthetic stand point (and monetarily to those who peddle special creams, shakers and rollers), the scientific evidence does not support such practices.

In an experiment to evaluate the spot reducing hypothesis, thirteen college men at the University of Massachusetts, Amherst, performed 5,004 sit-ups during a 27-day progressive sit-up exercise program. Sit-ups were performed with hands clasped behind the head and legs bent at a 90 degree angle at the knee. Cadence was maintained with a metronome. Table 6-1 outlines the regimen used to progressively increase the number of sit-ups. Detailed measurements of body composition were made before and following the experimental period. Total body fat was measured by hydrostatic weighing outlined in Chapter 5, as were selected fatfolds and girths. In addition, fat biopsies were taken from the abdominal, buttocks, and subscapular (base of shoulder blade) regions and the number of fat cells determined by the photomicrographic, computer-digitizing method discussed in a previous section.

If spot reducing worked due to the sit-up exercise, then the amount of fat in the abdominal fat cells should have reduced to a greater extent than the storage fat in the fat cells of the other areas. However, this did not occur. The reduction in cell diameter was the *same* for the three sites. While the amount of change in cell diameter was about 5% (equivalent to a 15 to 17% change in volume), there were no alterations in gross measures of body composition (body density, fatfolds, or girths) for the experimental subjects or control subjects that did not exercise. Under the conditions of this experiment, the notion of spot reducing was considered to be unattainable. Similar findings have been observed in comparisons of the circumferences and subcutaneous fat stores of the right and left forearms of elite tennis players. While the dominant or playing arm was significantly larger than the non-dominant arm, this was due entirely to a modest muscular hypertrophy, because there was no difference between the arms in terms of quantity of subcutaneous forearm fat. It seems clear that the mobilization of fat during selective exercise is not restricted to the underlying fatty area of the body part being exercised.

Table 6-1. *Progressive sit-up training program.*[a]

DAYS	BOUTS	TIME PER BOUT, SEC	SIT-UPS COMPLETED PER BOUT	TOTAL SIT-UPS
1–6	10 increase to 20	10	7	630
7–12	10 increase to 20	15	10	900
13–18	10 increase to 20	20	14	1260
19–24	10 increase to 20	25	15	1350
25–27	10 increase to 14	30	24	864
				5004

[a]A 10-sec rest interval remained constant between bouts on all training days.

From: Katch, F.I., Clarkson, P.M., Kroll, W., McBride, T., and A. Wilcox. Preferential effects of abdominal exercise training on regional adipose cell size. *Research Quarterly for Exercise and Sport. 55*:249, 1984.

Mobilization of fatty acids occurs from the fat depots throughout the body and the areas of greatest fat storage probably supply the greatest amount of energy, regardless of the muscle groups exercised.

Additional Reading

Ashwell, M. and C.J. Meade: Obesity: Can some fat cells enlarge while others are shrinking? *Lipids. 16:*475, 1981.

Berry, E.M. et al.: The role of dietary fat in human obesity. *International Journal of Obesity. 10:*123, 1986.

Björntorp, P.: Classification of obese patients and complications related to the distribution of surplus fat. *American Journal of Clinical Nutrition. 45:*1120, 1987.

Bray, G.A.: The energetics of obesity. *Medicine and Science in Sports and Exercise. 15:*32, 1983.

Bray, G.A., and J.E. Bethune, (Eds.): *Treatment and Management of Obesity.* New York, Harper & Row, 1974.

Bukowiecki, L. et al.: Mechanism of enhanced lipolysis in adipose tissue of exercise-trained rats. *American Journal of Physiology. 239:*422, 1980.

Chumlea, W.C. et al.: Adipocytes and adiposity in adults. *American Journal of Clinical Nutrition. 34:*1798, 1981.

Chumlea, W.C. et al.: Size and number of adipocytes and measures of body fat in boys and girls 10 to 18 years of age. *American Journal of Nutrition. 34:*1791, 1981.

Davies, P.S.W., Jones, P.R.M. and N.G. Norgan: The distribution of subcutaneous and internal fat in man. *Annals of Human Biology. 13:*189, 1986.

Drenick, E.J.: Risk of obesity and surgical indications. *International Journal of Obesity. 5:*387, 1980.

Duston, H.P.: Obesity and Hypertension. *Annals of Internal Medicine. 103:*1047, 1985.

Faust, I.M., P.R. Johnson, and J. Hirsch: Long-term effects of early nutritional experience on the development of obesity in the rat. *Journal of Nutrition. 110:*2027, 1980.

Frank, S., Colliver, J.A. and A. Frank: The electrocardiogram in obesity: Statistical analysis of 1,029 patients. *Journal of American College of Cardiology. 7:*295, 1986.

Garn, S.M. and P.E. Cole: Do the obese remain obese and the lean remain lean? *American Journal of Public Health. 70:*351, 1980.

Ginsberg-Fellner, F. et al.: Overweight and obesity in preschool children in New York City. *American Journal of Clinical Nutrition. 34:*2236, 1981.

Ginsberg-Fellner, F. and J.L. Knittle: Weight reduction in young obese children. 1. Effects on adipose tissue cellularity and metabolism. *Pediatric Research. 15:*1381, 1981.

Greenwood, M.R.C.: Adipose tissue: Cellular morphology and adipose tissue development. *Annals of Internal Medicine. 103:*996, 1985.

Hirsch, J., and P.W. Han: Cellularity of rat adipose tissue: Effects of growth, starvation and obesity. *Journal of Lipid Research. 10:*77, 1969.

Hirsch, J., and J. Knittle: Cellularity of obese and nonobese human adipose tissue. *Federation Proceedings. 28:*1516, 1970.

Iverius, P.H. and J.D. Brunzell: Obesity and common genetic metabolic disorders. *Annals of Internal Medicine. 103:*1050, 1985.

Johnson, F.E.: Health implications of childhood obesity. *Annals of Internal Medicine. 103:*1068, 1985.

Kasiske, B.L. and J.T. Crosson: Renal disease in patients with massive obesity. *Archives of Internal Medicine. 146:*1105, 1986.

Katch, F.I., et al.: Effects of situp exercise training on adipose cell size and adiposity. *Research Quarterly For Exercise and Sport, 55:*242, 1984.

Kissebah, A.H. et al.: Relation of body fat distribution to metabolic complications of obesity. *Journal of Clinical Endocrinology and Metabolism. 54:*254, 1982.

Knittle, J., and J. Hirsch: Effect of early nutrition on the development of rat epididymal fat pads: Cellularity and metabolism. *Journal of Clinical Investigation. 47:*2091, 1968.

Krotkiewski, M. et al.: Impact of obesity on metabolism in men and women—importance of regional adipocyte size in man. *Journal of Clinical Endocrinology and Metabolism. 72:*1150, 1983.

Larsson, B., Bjorntorp, P. and G. Tibblin: The health consequences of moderate obesity. *International Journal of Obesity. 5:*97, 1981.

Leibel, R. and J. Hirsch: Metabolic characterization of obesity. *Annals of Internal Medicine. 103:*1000, 1985.

National Institutes of Health. Health implications of obesity. National Institutes of Health Consensus Development Conference Statement. Vol. 5, No. 9. U.S. Government Printing Office, 1985.

Oscai, L., et al.: Effects of exercise and of food restriction on adipose tissue cellularity. *Journal of Lipid Research. 13:*588, 1972.

Oscai, L., et al.: Exercise or food restriction: Effect on adipose tissue cellularity. *American Journal of Physiology. 227:*901, 1974.

Rebuffé-Scrive, M. et al.: Regulation of human adipose tissue metabolism during the menstrual cycle, pregnancy, and lactation. *Journal of Clinical Investigation. 75:*1973, 1985.

Roche, A.F.: The adipocyte-number hypothesis. *Child Development. 52:*31, 1981.

Salans, L.B., et al.: Studies of human adipose tissue: Adipose cell size and number in non-obese and obese patients. *Journal of Clinical Investigation. 52:*929, 1973.

Schutz, Y. et al.: Diet-induced thermogenesis measured over a whole day in obese and non-obese women. *American Journal of Clinical Nutrition. 40:*542, 1984.

Sims, E.A.H., and E.S. Horton: Endocrine and metabolic adaptation to obesity and starvation. *American Journal of Clinical Nutrition. 21:*1455, 1968.

Snowden, D.A., Phillips, R.L. and W. Choi: Diet, obesity, and risk of fatal prostate cancer. *American Journal of Epidemiology. 120:*244, 1984.

Stern, J. and M.R.C. Greenwood: A review of development of adipose cellularity in man and animals. *Federation Proceedings. 33:*1952, 1974.

Thompson, J.K. et al.: Exercise and obesity: Etiology, physiology, and intervention. *Psychological Bulletin. 91:*55, 1982.

Ylitalo, V.: Treatment of obese school children. *Acta Paediactrica Scandinavica.* Suppl. 290, 1981.

7
Weight Control

IT IS TRULY REMARKABLE that the body weight of most adults fluctuates only slightly during the year, even though the annual intake of food averages between 1600 to 1900 pounds; this includes 280 eggs, 15.6 pounds of breakfast cereal, 184 pounds of meat, 200 pounds of fruit, 250 pounds of vegetables, 68 pounds of bread, and 429 soft drinks, 2 gallons of wine, 24 gallons of beer, and 2 gallons of liquor! This relative stability in body weight is rather impressive when you consider that a slight but prolonged increase in food intake can cause a substantial increase in body weight. Eating just an extra handful of peanuts each day would increase body weight by about 10 pounds in 1 year. However, because the body weight of most adults does not usually increase by this amount illustrates the body's exquisite regulatory control in balancing caloric intake with daily energy expenditure. *It is only when the number of calories ingested as food exceeds the daily energy requirements that the excess calories are stored as fat in adipose tissue.* To prevent an increase in body weight and body fat because of a caloric imbalance, an effective program of weight control must establish a balance between energy input and energy output.

Balancing Energy Input with Energy Output

The many popular books that advocate exotic diets or exercise plans to help reduce body weight have one thing in common: They all claim their plans are so easy and effortless to follow that results can be guaranteed! If this were the case, and a simple procedure could maintain the "perfect" body size permanently, then the estimated 60 to 70 million American adults and at least 10 to 12 million American teenagers who are overfat could be cured easily. Even when a particular diet plan gains widespread popularity as a result of an advertising blitz that "documents" examples of actual weight loss, these schemes often place a dieter's total health in jeopardy. Many professional organizations have voiced strong opposition to various dietary practices, in particular the *low-carbohydrate, high-fat,* and *high-protein* diets. The American Medical Association Council on Food and Nutrition severely criticized the popular Atkins high-fat diet as "bizarre" by stating it was without scientific merit, and lacked prior experimentation concerning the validity of the claims made. Advocates of this diet emphasize carbohydrate restriction while ignoring the total caloric content of the diet. It is argued that with minimal carbohydrate for energy the body must metabolize its fat stores. This supposedly generates sufficient ketones bodies (by-products of incomplete fat breakdown) to cause urinary loss of these unused calories to account for significant weight loss despite an allegedly high caloric intake. It is argued that this caloric loss will be so great that dieters can eat all they wish, as long as carbohydrates are restricted. At best, the calories lost by a urinary excretion of ketones would equal only 100 to 150 calories a day. This would account for only a small weight loss of approximately 1 pound a month—not very appealing when the major proportion of the daily calorie intake amounts to a fat intake that may be as high as 60 to 70% of the food consumed. Also, any initial weight loss on this diet may be due largely to dehydration brought about by an extra solute load on the kidneys that increases the excretion of urinary water. Such water loss is of no lasting significance in a program designed to reduce body fat. Low carbohydrate diets have the potential for causing the body to lose significant amounts of lean tissue. This is certainly an *undesirable* side effect for a diet designed to bring about fat loss.

High-fat, low-carbohydrate diets are also potentially hazardous in a number of ways. The diet can raise serum uric acid levels and lower potassium levels that facilitates undesirable cardiac arrhythmias, causes acidosis, aggravates kidney problems due to the extra solute burden placed on the renal system, elevates blood lipids thus increasing a primary heart disease risk factor, depletes glycogen reserves and contributes to a fatigued state, and causes a relative dehydration. The diet is definitely contraindicated during pregnancy because adequate carbohydrate metabolism is essential for proper fetal development.

A *starvation diet* or *therapeutic fast* may be recommended in cases of severe obesity where body fat exceeds 40 to 50% of body weight. Such diets are usually prescribed for up to 3 months, but only as a "last resort" prior to undertaking more extreme medical approaches that include various surgical treatments. The starvation approach to weight loss is predicated on the hope that abstinence from food will break established dietary habits and this, in turn, may improve the long term prospects for successful weight loss. This form of dieting must be closely supervised, usually in a hospital setting. There are ample examples of famous movie stars who advocate fasting as the ultimate method to "cleanse" the body of so-called "toxins". *We recommend strongly that such strategies be abandoned—not only can they be dangerous, but its basis is sheer poppycock and hokum.*

Other dietary plans, specifically the various modifications of a *high-protein* diet, can be potentially harmful. The high-protein diet has been extolled as the "last chance diet" for the obese as well as those who are less overweight. It is argued that protein diets cause suppression of appetite through the body's excessive reliance on fat mobilization. This effect has yet to be supported with careful research. It is also argued that the elevated calorie-burning thermic effect of dietary protein as well as its relatively low coefficient of digestibility ultimately reduce the net calories available from this food compared to a well-balanced meal of equal caloric value. This calorigenic effect of protein ingestion is believed to be due largely to digestive processes as well as the extra energy required by the liver to assimilate amino acids. Although this point may have some validity, many other factors must be considered in formulating a sound program for weight loss—not to mention the potentially harmful strain on kidney and liver function, and accompanying dehydration, electrolyte imbalance, and lean tissue loss resulting from diets excessively high in protein. When the protein is in liquid form, the "miracle liquid" is made palatable with artificial flavoring, and often includes a blend of ground-up animal hooves and horns, and pigskin mixed in a broth with enzymes and tenderizers to "predigest" it. In 1979, according to the Federal Drug Administration, this particular brand of protein elixir and others like it were associated with 58 deaths. Sixteen of the victims were obese women who lost an average of 83 pounds within 2 to 8 months. None had a previous history of heart disease; they all died suddenly while on the diet or shortly thereafter. Formal complaints were received from 165 people who reported a variety of side effects that included hair loss, nausea, headaches, constipation, neural disorders, bad breath, faintness, muscle weakness, decreased libido, and gastrointestinal disorders. Table 7-1 summarizes the principles and main advantages and disadvantages of some of the popular dietary approaches to weight loss.

While most diets produce a weight loss during the first several weeks, most of the weight lost is body water. Unless a person can maintain a reduced caloric intake for a considerable time, the weight will eventually be regained. The net result is a return to original body size, often at the expense of feelings of hunger and other psychologic stresses while the diet plan is actually followed. Anyone who has seriously tried to maintain a diet knows the difficulties encountered. While it is certainly possible to lose 15, 20, or even 30 or more pounds through diet, few people have enough self-control to stick with a diet plan long enough to change body size successfully and permanently.

A review of the scientific literature dealing with weight loss in obese subjects reveals that people who are initially successful in modifying their body composition are usually *unsuccessful* in permanently maintaining their desired body size and shape. This has been pointed out in numerous studies dealing with follow-up measurements of patients who have participated in weight reduction programs where caloric intake was carefully regulated and monitored. In one survey of the effectiveness of obesity clinics in weight control management during a 10-year period, it was observed that the dropout rate varied from 20 to 80%. Of those who remained in a program, no more than 25% lost as much as 20 pounds and only 5% lost 40 pounds or more. Such statistics are rather discouraging and indicate that the long-term maintenance of a particular low-calorie diet is extremely difficult; it is especially difficult in the relaxed atmosphere of a person's home, where access to food is relatively easy. Similarly, increasing energy expenditure through physical activity, while not unpleasant in itself, does require a personal commitment in terms of time and lifestyle that many people are not willing to make. *Reducing body size through diet and exercise is only half the battle; staying reduced requires a serious commitment to a new life style.*

WHEN IS IT TIME TO REDUCE?

In the previous chapter on evaluating body composition we described a simple tape measure technique for determining the body's fat content. By referring to the suggested guidelines for optimal fatness in Chapter 6, you can make a good esti-

Table 7-1. *Some popular weight loss methods.*

TYPE OF METHOD	PRINCIPLE	ADVANTAGES	DISADVANTAGES	COMMENTS
Surgical procedures	Alteration of the gastrointestinal tract changes capacity or amount of absorptive surface.	Caloric restriction is less necessary.	Risks of surgery and post-surgical complications include death.	Radical procedures include stapling of the stomach and removal of a section of the small intestine (a jejunoilieal bypass).
Fasting	No energy input assures negative energy balance.	Weight loss is rapid (which may be a disadvantage). Exposure to temptation is reduced.	Ketogenic. A large portion of weight lost is from lean body mass. Nutrients are lacking.	Medical supervision is mandatory and hospitalization is recommended.
Protein-sparing modified fast	Same as fasting except protein intake helps preserve lean body mass.	Same as above.	Ketogenic. Nutrients are lacking. Some unconfirmed deaths have been reported, possibly from potassium depletion.	Medical supervision is mandatory. Popular presentation was made in Linn's *The Last Chance Diet*.
One-food-centered diets	Low-caloric intake favors negative energy balance.	Being easy to follow has initial psychological appeal.	Being too restrictive means nutrients are probably lacking. Repetitious nature may cause boredom.	No food or food combination is known to "burn off" fat. Examples include the grapefruit diet and the egg diet.
Low-carbohydrate high-fat diets	Increased ketone excretion removes energy-containing substances from the body. Fat intake is often voluntarily decreased; a low caloric diet results.	Inclusion of rich foods may have psychological appeal. Initial rapid loss of water may be an incentive.	Ketogenic. High-fat intake is contraindicated for heart and diabetes patients. Nutrients are often lacking.	Popular versions have been offered by Taller and Atkins; some have been called the "Mayo," "Drinking Man's," and "Air Force" diets.
Low-carbohydrate/ high-protein diets	Low-caloric intake favors negative energy balance.		Expense and repetitious nature may make it difficult to sustain.	If meat is emphasized, the diet becomes one that is high in fat. The Pennington diet is an example.
High-carbohydrate/ low-fat diets	Low-caloric intake favors negative energy balance.	Wise food selections can make the diet nutritionally sound.	Initial water retention may be discouraging.	

mate of whether or not you are overfat for your age and gender. Consider the example of a 23-year-old female who weighs 175 pounds.

The three circumference measurements used to compute fatness from Appendix C are mid-abdomen = 36 inches, right thigh = 26.5 inches, and right forearm = 10.0 inches. By using the appropriate constants and substituting into the formula, percent body fat is computed as 40.6% of total body weight. This amounts to a total quantity of body fat of 71.1 pounds (175 pounds × 0.406), and 103.9 pounds of lean tissues (175 pounds body weight − 71.1 pounds fat). Knowing these values of body composition, you could ask, "How do these body composition measures compare to the average woman for this age range?" Refer to Table 5-1 to compare the obtained value for percent body fat and that of an average woman. The last two columns in this table show the average values for percent body fat as well as the acceptable limits for body fat. A value of 40.6% body fat is well above the average and even exceeds one variation unit that includes the normal range. When compared to the 1983 Massachusetts data, the value for fat is 18.7% units higher than the 21.9% average fat value for the Massachusetts women, and 6.3% units higher than the upper range of the 1967 data for young women in Colorado. Thus, this hypothetical 23-year-old woman possesses considerably more fat than the average woman reported in these studies.

Recall also that the average value plus or minus one variation unit gives a range for body fat that includes about 68 out of every 100 persons tested. The value of one variation unit is 5% body fat; thus two variation units above average would correspond to the average percent of fat plus an additional 10%. If you use the 1967 values of fatness for New York women, then 37% would represent the body fat value two variation units above the average. The observed value of 40.6% body fat is still above this limit; this woman is fatter than about 95 out of every 100 women measured. Admittedly, the diagnosis is not too cheerful, especially when her degree of fatness is related to what is known about fat cell size and fat cell number. Compared to the average young women who possesses about 25 to 30 billion fat cells, this woman could have anywhere from 60 to 300 billion fat cells. To complicate matters further, the average size of her fat cells is also much larger than that of the fat cells of normal people. The important question to ask in this situation is, "What can be done to reduce to normal body size?"

THE ENERGY BALANCE EQUATION

Before someone develops a plan for establishing normal body composition, the rationale underlying the *energy balance equation* must be considered. The equation states that *body weight will remain constant when caloric intake equals caloric expenditure.* Any imbalance in energy output or energy input will result in a change in body weight. Figure 7-1 shows the ideal situation in which energy input (calories in food) *exactly balances* energy output (calories expended in daily physical activities). As long as this equilibrium is maintained within narrow limits, there will be relatively little fluctuation in body weight. The middle part of the figure depicts what happens all too frequently when energy input *exceeds* energy output. Under such conditions the number of calories consumed in excess of daily requirements is stored as fat in the adipose tissue depots. As we will discuss shortly, *3500 "extra" kcal on either the input or output side of the equation equal approximately 1 pound of stored fat.* The body has a way of keeping track of the extra calories consumed above the requirement level. It simply does not forget about the

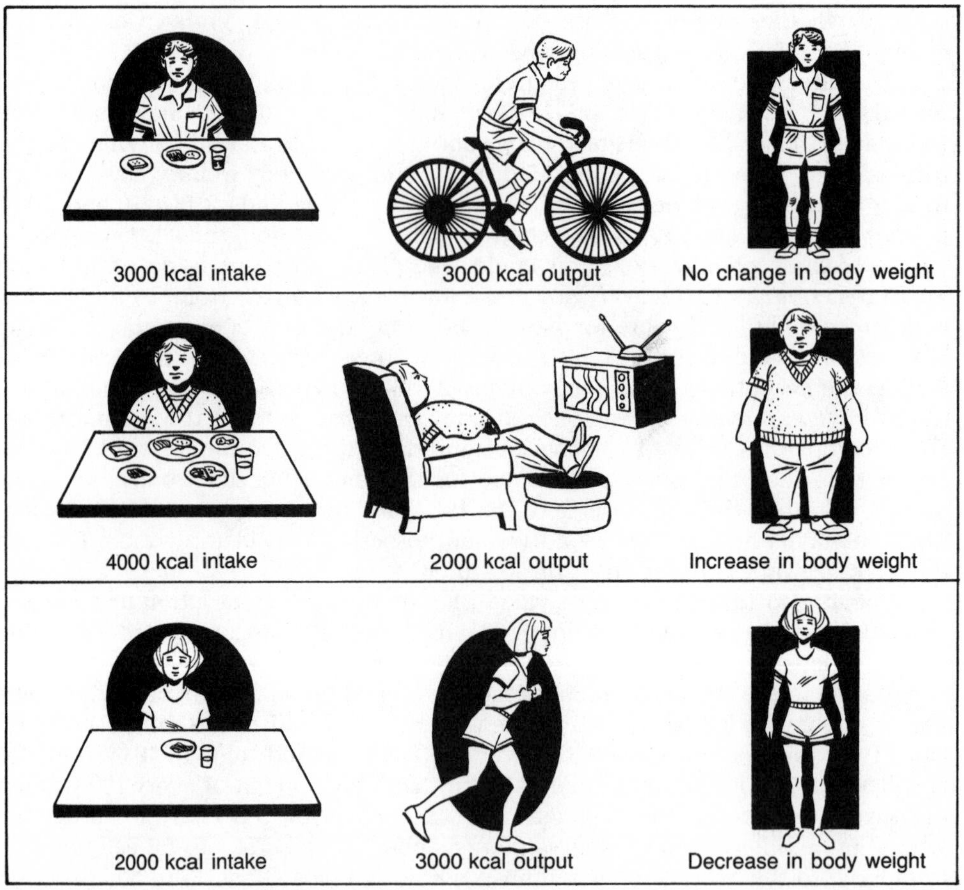
3000 kcal intake
3000 kcal output
No change in body weight
4000 kcal intake
2000 kcal output
Increase in body weight
2000 kcal intake
3000 kcal output
Decrease in body weight

Figure 7-1. *The energy balance equation.*

extra slice of cheese, cola, or additional helping of pizza or strawberry ice cream with chocolate jimmies on top. The bottom of the figure illustrates what occurs when energy intake is *less than* energy output. In this case, the body obtains the required calories from its energy stores and weight and fat become reduced.

There are three ways to "unbalance" the energy balance equation and cause a reduction in body weight: (1) reduce caloric intake *below* daily energy requirements, (2) maintain regular food intake and *increase* caloric output through additional physical activity *above* daily energy requirements, and (3) combine methods (1) and (2) by *decreasing* daily food intake and *increasing* daily energy expenditure.

To understand how sensitive the energy balance equation is in regulating overall energy balance, consider the situation where calorie intake exceeds calorie output by only a hundred kcal per day. This could be achieved by eating only one extra banana each day. On an annual basis, the surplus number of kcal consumed would be 365 days × 100 kcal or 36,500 kcal. Because 1 pound of body fat contains about 3500 kcal, the small daily increase in calories consumed would result in a gain of 10.4 pounds of fat in a year. If the same eating habits were maintained and energy output remained unchanged, then theoretically there would be a gain in fat weight of 52 pounds in 5 years! On the other hand, reducing food intake by only 100 kcal a day and increasing energy expenditure by 100 kcal by jogging a mile each day would reduce total body fat by 21 pounds in 1 year. There's simply no way of getting around the fact that when the total extra calories consumed add up to 3500, approximately 1 extra pound of fat is gained. This cannot be undone by magic potions, trick diets, or special formula foods.

We believe one of the major reasons that weight control is so difficult is because most Americans are not willing to display the discipline or initiative to curb their appetites and get their bodies moving. We are all mesmerized to varying degrees by modern technologies that provide convenience rather than rely on the body's own power for movement and exercise. In the next chapter, we will discuss practical ways to help 20th century man and woman fight the battle of the energy balance equation to avoid defeat by 21st century technologies.

Personal Assessment of Eating Behavior

We usually eat for two reasons. First, we consume food because we are truly hungry. This hunger enables us to maintain a food intake to supply the energy to power the body's vital processes and sustain life. Second, we eat food to satisfy our appetites, which in America are usually "programmed" to be stimulated 3 times each day. Even after finishing the most delicious and satisfying meal, few of us could not be coaxed into eating "just a bit more of a delicious piece of pie or home made cheesecake", even if we felt full. Such overeating, although quite common, apparently occurs more in obese than in lean people. It appears that human eating behavior is intimately tied to environmental cues as well as to internal biochemical cues that signal a real need for caloric intake. The external "food cues" include the sight of food, its packaging, display, and advertising, the time and physical environment in which the food is eaten, and the taste, smell, and size of the portions.

Several experiments have demonstrated how external factors can influence eating behavior. In one study, normal and obese subjects were deceived into believing they were participating in an elaborate psychologic experiment. In actuality the experimenters wished to determine whether or not the visual presence of food affects eating behavior. After missing lunch, normal and obese subjects were tested in their responses to meaningless psychophysic stimuli. They were then left in a room to complete a questionnaire supposedly concerned with the experiment. In the room subjects found either 1 or 3 roast beef sandwiches and soda. Subjects were told to eat as much as they wanted and to help themselves to more food from the refrigerator. When 3 sandwiches were left in the room, the obese subjects consumed an average of 2.3 sandwiches compared with 1.9 sandwiches eaten by the normal-sized subjects; when only 1 sandwich was in view, the obese subjects ate fewer sandwiches (1.5) then the nonobese subjects (2.0).

Another experiment concerned the effects of taste on eating behavior. Before the experiment, obese subjects normally consumed 3500 kcal per day while non-obese subjects consumed 2200 kcal per day. Then for 3 weeks subjects in both groups were offered a bland liquid diet; the nonobese subjects continued to consume 2200 kcal of this liquid meal each day, whereas the obese subjects decreased their daily caloric intake to only 500 kcal. These results demonstrated that obese subjects were influenced considerably more by the *taste of food* then by its caloric content. Results of this type illustrate how external environmental cues can significantly affect eating behavior, especially in the obese.

Daily events quite unrelated to food itself can also trigger the urge to eat. Depression, frustration, boredom, "uptight" or anxious feelings, guilt, sadness, or anger can all be linked to periods of excessive food intake. The importance of food cues in dieting is that the prospective dieter must learn to make an accurate appraisal of his or her eating behavior in terms of the quantity, frequency, and circumstances of eating. A first step in such a self-analysis is to become keenly aware of daily caloric intake. Once this is accomplished, "undesirable" food cues must be eliminated, and a new set of desirable eating responses must replace previously learned behaviors. In the following chapter we will discuss such a process that is referred to as *eating behavior modification.*

In addition to caloric restriction through diet coupled with attempts to modify eating behavior, we believe that the final component of a successful program of weight control is the adoption of a physically active life style. This does not mean that the dieter simply plays a token game of tennis twice a year, goes for a swim on weekends during the summer, or walks to the store when the car is being repaired. *Modifying personal exercise habits entails a serious commitment to changing the daily routine to include regular periods of relatively vigorous physical activity.*

HOW TO DETERMINE CALORIC INTAKE FROM FOODS

To determine the average total number of calories consumed each day, the dieter should keep a *daily log* of food intake for 7 consecutive days. Many experiments have shown that people who calculate caloric intake from accurate records of their daily food consumption are usually within 10% of the actual number of calories consumed. For example, suppose the caloric value of your daily food intake were directly measured in the bomb calorimeter and averaged 2130 kcal. If you kept a 7-day dietary history and estimated your daily caloric intake, the daily value would vary by about 10% from the actual value or from 1920 to 2350 kcal. As long as you maintained a careful record, the degree of accuracy for daily caloric determinations would be within acceptable limits.

Before beginning to record daily caloric intake for the 7-day period, you must become familiar with "honest" calorie counting. To do this you must first acquire 4 items for measuring food: a plastic ruler, a standard measuring cup, measuring spoons, and a small, inexpensive balance or weighing scale. You can purchase these items at most hardware stores. Second, familiarize yourself with the caloric value of foods. Consult Appendix D for this purpose that includes a listing for alcoholic beverages as well as the nutritive value of specialty and "fast-food" items sold at 12 popular take-out restaurants. You should obtain an inexpensive calorie-counting guide as a supplement. This is available at newsstands and bookstores and gives the average caloric values for most foods. Guides that list foods according to brand names are also helpful.

Measure or weigh each of the food items in your diet that are listed below. This is the only reliable way to get an accurate estimate of the size of a food portion. If you elect to use Appendix D to estimate kcal value, you need only to weigh each food item. If you use a supplementary calorie-counting guide, you may have to use the measuring cup, spoons, and ruler.

Food Categories

Meat and fish: Measure the portion of meat or fish by thickness, length, and width, or record weight on the scale.

Vegetables, mashed potatoes, rice, cereals, salads: Measure the portion in a measuring cup or record weight on the scale.

Cream or sugar added to coffee or tea: Measure the portion with the measuring spoons before adding to the drink or record weight on the scale.

Fluids and bottled drinks: Check the labels for volume or empty the container into the measuring cup. If you weigh the fluid, be sure to subtract the weight of the cup or glass. Sugar-free soft drinks usually have kcal values listed on their labels.

Cookies, cakes, pies: For cookies, measure the diameter and thickness with a ruler, or weigh on the scale. Evaluate frosting or sauces separately.

Fruits: Cut them in half before eating and measure the diameters, or weigh on the scale. For fruits that must be peeled or have rinds or cores, be sure the weight of the nonedible portion is subtracted from the total weight of the food. Do this for items such as oranges, apples, and bananas.

Jam, salad dressing, catsup, mayonnaise: Measure the condiment with the measuring spoon or weigh the portion on the scale.

If you eat a food item not listed in Appendix D or in the calorie guide, try to make an intelligent guess as to the ingredients and amount eaten. Sometimes this is impossible, however, and the only alternative is to use a somewhat arbitrary average value. If you are completely baffled, use 400 kcal for small portions, 600 kcal for medium to large portions, and 800 kcal for "giant" portions. It is better to overestimate the number of kcal consumed than to underestimate or to make no estimation at all. If you go to a restaurant for dinner, or to a friend's house where it may be inappropriate to take the measurements, then omit this day from the counting procedure and resume record-keeping the following day. Be sure to include a Friday, Saturday, and Sunday sequence as part of the 7-day record. Research has shown that caloric intake is significantly higher on the weekend than on weekdays. Because the purpose of keeping records for 7 days is to obtain an accurate appraisal of the average daily calorie intake, recordkeeping during the weekend is extremely important. Be sure to record everything you eat. If you are not completely "honest," you are wasting your time. Most people find it easier to keep accurate records if they record food items while preparing a meal or immediately afterwards when eating snack items. Table 7-2 presents an example of a daily dietary intake form for 1 of the 7 days. The caloric value for each food item consumed during the day was estimated from Appendix D.

COMPUTE DAILY CALORIC INTAKE FOR 7 DAYS

You should keep meticulous records of food intake for 7 consecutive days. At first it is normal to become preoccupied with the food you eat, so much so that you may unconsciously begin to diet by omitting foods you would usually eat. Be aware of this temptation and try not to limit normal food intake during the evaluation period. It is important at this point to obtain an accurate estimate of daily caloric intake. Many people like to believe they eat less than they actually do. An overfat person rarely takes delight in knowing that he or she consumes 5000 or 8000 calories per day. Initially, most people who need to restrict food intake will underestimate their true kcal intake, perhaps from fear of confirming what they already know. We have had experience with overfat people who actually believed they

Table 7-2. *Form used to record the caloric equivalent of food consumed on a daily basis.*

FOOD ITEM	AMOUNT	KCAL VALUE
Breakfast		
eggs, boiled	2	160
orange juice	6 oz	110
Cheerios	1¼ cup	111
skim milk	8 oz	90
Snack		
Taco Bell beef burrito	1	466
Pepsi Cola	12 oz	160
Lunch		
tuna fish, white	2 oz	113
white bread	2 pieces	140
mayonnaise	1 tbsp	100
skim milk	8 oz	90
plums	4	100
Snack		
ice cream, rocky road, sugar cone	2¼	204
Dinner		
Burger King chicken sandwich	2	1376
french fries	small	214
banana split, 3 scoops vanilla, topping, whipped cream	average	550
Snack		
Burger King vanilla shake	10 oz	320
	Total	4304

were consuming only 500 to 600 kcal each day. These people never seemed to lose weight and some even gained weight during a 16-week physical conditioning course. We kept a 7-day dietary record for one middle-aged woman who stated she was adhering strictly to a low-calorie diet; however, we determined that her total daily calorie intake was approximately 6 times higher than she had originally "guesstimated."

Once the number of calories consumed for 7 days is determined, compute the number of kcal consumed for a typical day by dividing the total by 7. For a quick but less reliable appraisal of caloric and nutrient intake, a 3-day recall could be used but is not recommended. Record keeping such as this accomplishes two things; (1) it provides the dieter with an objective list of the foods actually consumed (rather than a guess as to what had been eaten), and (2) it triggers an important aspect of the dietary process that must occur before any measure of success can really be achieved—self realization or awareness of current food habits and preferences. Most people who keep meticulous records are often "shocked" at not only how much they actually eat, but the wide range of foods they consume. For many people, the act of eating food has truly become an unconscious act, so much so that they have difficulty remembering what they ate, let alone the quantity of food consumed, the frequency of consumption, or the situations that trigger the urge to eat.

Unbalancing the Energy Balance Equation

The preceding means for estimating caloric intake provides useful information with regard to the energy balance equation. By knowing the average daily caloric input and whether or not body weight is increasing, decreasing, or remaining stable, it is relatively easy to determine if caloric intake is equal to, less than, or exceeds the average daily expenditure of energy. If body weight remains relatively stable from week to week, caloric input exactly matches the caloric requirements of daily living. Part of this food energy is needed to maintain the resting requirements and the remainder is used for physical activity. On the other hand, if the intake of calories *exceeds* that expended for rest plus other daily energy needs, then a positive caloric imbalance will result and body weight will increase. *It is simply not possible to consume more calories than are expended without increasing body weight.* If, however, the equilibrium is disturbed in favor of less input than output, body weight will decrease.

In a previous section we pointed out that 1 pound of adipose tissue contains approximately 3500 kcal of energy. It follows that consuming an additional 3500 kcal above that required to sustain the daily energy requirements will result in a weight gain equal to about 1 pound of body fat. Conversely, to decrease the body's fat content by 1 pound, it would be necessary to create a caloric deficit of 3500 kcal. If the goal is to reduce 2 pounds of fat, then the caloric deficit must be about 7000 kcal. For a 3-pound fat loss, the deficit would be 10,500 kcal; to lose 4 pounds, the necessary deficit would be 14,000 kcal, and so on.

Unbalancing the energy balance equation is the most important step in a weight loss program, and it puts theory into practice by creating a *disequilibrium* of the equation. Energy input must become less than energy output, or energy output must become *greater* than energy input. In either instance, weight reduction will occur.

DIETING TO TIP THE ENERGY BALANCE EQUATION

The approach to weight loss creates an imbalance in the energy balance equation by reducing energy intake, usually by about 500 to 1000 kcal a day below the daily energy expenditure. Let us assume that a hypothetical 23-year-old obese woman who consumes 2833 kcal per day and maintains body weight at 175 pounds wishes to lose 5 pounds. If her daily level of physical activity remains unchanged, her energy output of 2833 kcal would remain the same. Suppose the woman decreases her daily food intake to create a caloric deficit of 1000 kcal. Caloric restriction of greater than 1000 kcal per day is poorly tolerated over prolonged periods, and this form of semi-starvation greatly increases the chances for poor nourishment. Instead of consuming 2833 kcal each day, she reduces daily caloric intake to

1833 kcal. In 7 days, the caloric deficit would equal 7000 kcal (1000 kcal/day × 7 days). This would be accompanied by a corresponding loss of approximately 2 pounds of body fat. Actually, more than 2 pounds would be lost during the first week because the carbohydrate stores that contain fewer calories per pound than fat, and considerably more water, would be metabolized first. To reduce fat content by another 3 pounds the reduced daily caloric intake of 1833 kcal would have to be maintained for another 10.5 days. By adhering to the 1833 kcal diet, she would reduce body fat at the rate of 1 pound of fat every 3.5 days, provided that caloric output remained at 2833 kcal. If the dieter continued to maintain this energy deficit for a prolonged period, she would lose 10 pounds of fat after 35 days, 20 pounds after 70 days, and 30 pounds within 100 days. While the mathematics of weight loss through caloric restriction may seem rather straightforward, uncomplicated, and encouraging, several basic assumptions could, if violated, reduce the effectiveness of weight loss through diet or even cause the energy balance equation to become unbalanced in the opposite direction.

The *first assumption* is that energy expenditure remains relatively unchanged throughout the period of caloric restriction. This is somewhat difficult to control, however, as there can be considerable variation in someone's daily and weekly energy output. For some people, caloric restriction and its resulting depletion of the body's carbohydrate stores may cause lethargy and actually *decrease* the level of energy expenditure. In addition, as body weight is reduced the energy cost of moving the body is reduced proportionately. Again, the energy output side of the equation may become smaller. The *second assumption* is that a dieter can maintain reduced caloric intake until the desired body size is achieved. These two assumptions could probably be met quite adequately if humans functioned without individual variation. Because physiologic functioning is in continuous interaction with the internal and external environment and subject to its many and varied fluctuations, we cannot expect "perfect" results with regard to weight loss with a low-calorie diet. If weight loss was indeed proportional to caloric restriction, a progressive decrease in body weight would depend directly on the extent of the caloric deprivation. However, changes take place during caloric restriction that can affect the rate at which weight loss occurs. One such change is in the resting metabolic rate.

SETPOINT THEORY: A CASE AGAINST DIETING

When reviewing the scientific literature on the success of weight loss through dieting, one is forced to conclude that, on a long-term basis, dieting just does not work. Surely, one can crash off large amounts of body weight in a relatively short time period by simply not eating. However, this success is short-lived and eventually the urge to eat wins out and weight is regained. The reason for this failure lies in "setpoints" that differ from what the dieter would like to have. The proponents of a *setpoint theory* argue that the body has an internal control mechanism, a setpoint, probably located deep within the brain's *hypothalamus*, that drives the body to maintain a particular level of *body fat*. In a practical sense, this would be the body weight you would tend to achieve when you are not counting calories. The problem is that we all have different setpoints, and various factors such as the drugs amphetamine and nicotine, as well as exercise, lower the particular setting—while dieting has no effect. Each time we manage to reduce our fat level below our "natural" setpoint by dieting, the body makes internal adjustments to resist this change and conserve body fat. One well-documented occurrence is the dramatic reduction in resting metabolic rate. In fact, the decrease in resting metabolism is often greater than the decrease attributable to the weight loss. For example, severe caloric restriction depresses resting metabolism by as much as 45%! This calorie-sparing effect may even become more apparent with repeated bouts of dieting so the depression of resting metabolism is enhanced with each subsequent attempt to reduce caloric intake. This greatly conserves energy and causes dieting to become progressively less effective. As a result, a plateau in weight loss is reached and further decreases in weight are considerably less than predicted from the mathematics of the restricted food intake. When the rewards of one's efforts are no longer apparent, the dieter usually quits and reverts to the previous eating behaviors. Figure 7-2 displays the results from one study of 6 obese men in which body weight, resting oxygen consumption (minimal energy requirements), and caloric intake were carefully monitored for 31 consecutive days. The subjects consumed 3500 kcal per day for the first 7 days of the experiment. For the remaining 24 days the daily caloric intake was reduced markedly to 450 kcal.

During the prediet period, body weight and resting oxygen consumption remained stable. For this group, 3500 kcal a day was just adequate to equal the daily

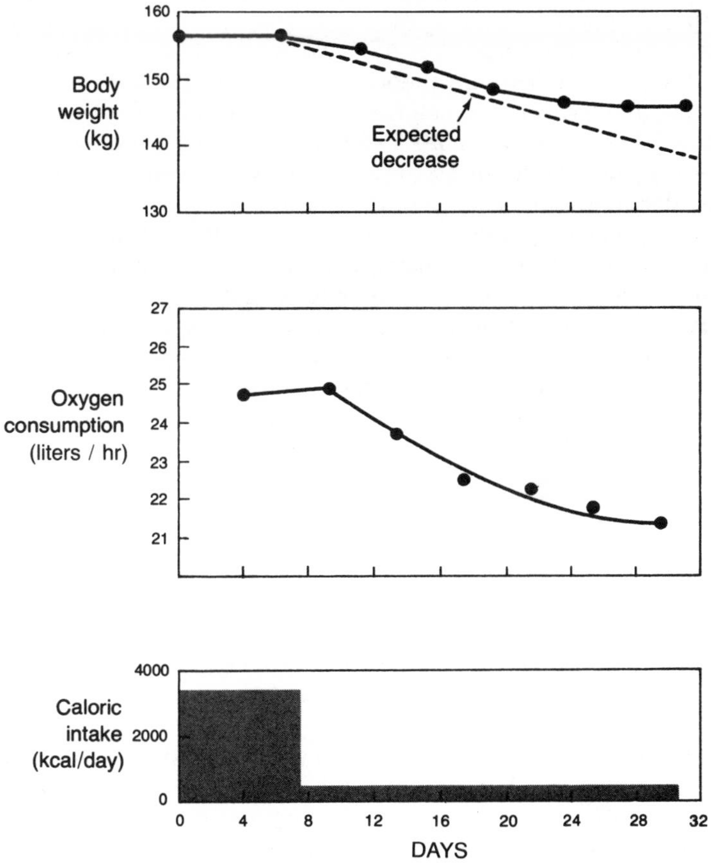
160
150
140
130
Body
weight
(kg)
Expected
decrease
27
26
25
24
23
22
21
Oxygen
consumption
(liters / hr)
4000
2000
0
Caloric
intake
(kcal/day)
0
4
8
12
16
20
24
28
32
DAYS

Figure 7-2. *Effects of two levels of caloric intake on changes in body weight and resting oxygen consumption.*

energy expenditure. However, when the subjects switched to the low-calorie semistarvation diet, both body weight and resting metabolism declined. Interestingly, the percentage decline in resting energy expenditure was greater than the decrease in body weight. The dashed line represents the expected weight loss for this 450-kcal diet. The decline in resting energy metabolism actually conserved energy and caused the diet to be less effective. More than half the 22.6-pound total weight loss occurred within the first 8 days of the 24-day diet, with the remaining weight loss occurring during the final 16 days. This slowing up of the theoretical weight loss curve often leaves the dieter frustrated and discouraged. Dieters are anxious for weight loss to occur rapidly and progress steadily according to an expected schedule.

Classic starvation studies in the 1940s to help the military plan the repatriation of war prisoners showed that even when an extreme diet ends and food intake is increased above the daily energy output, the dieter usually remains preoccupied with food. In fact, binge eating and psychologic distress continued until the original weight and fat level were attained. The fact that the body itself demands a certain amount of adipose tissue, as proposed by the setpoint theory, was further substantiated by a series of experiments in 1960 in which sedentary prisoners gained weight by increasing their food intake. As body weight and fat increased, concurrently the resting metabolic rate increased so it took an astounding 7000 kcal per day for weight gain to continue!

What then can safely affect the setpoint and lower it toward a more desirable level? One factor put forth by the setpoint theorists is *sustained, vigorous exercise.* Americans now eat about 10% fewer calories than they did 20 years ago, yet they weigh an average of 4 or 5 pounds more. Certainly, if dieting were effective, this reduction in caloric intake should bring the national body weight to a lower, not higher level. Notwithstanding the renewed interest in exercise, the American population has become increasingly sedentary, *not* increasingly gluttonous. Most fat people eat normal quantities of food and sometimes even less than thin people eat. The main difference between fat and lean people is often the level of daily physical activity—lean people move around much more and consequently expend more calories than their obese counterparts. For overweight men and women who exercise regularly, food intake tends to drop initially, despite the increase in caloric output, and body fat decreases. Eventually, as an active lifestyle is maintained, caloric intake balances the daily energy requirements so body weight is stabilized at a *lower* level.

HOW TO SELECT A DIET PLAN

The most difficult aspect of dieting is to decide on exactly what foods to include as part of the daily menu. There are literally hundreds of diet plans to choose from. There are water diets, drinking man's diets, fruit diets, egg diets, meat diets, fast food diets, ice cream diets, eating to win diets, name of city diets like New York City and Beverly Hills diets, and vegetable diets, not to mention the potentially dangerous varieties of the high-fat, low-carbohydrate and protein diets. Some authors have even preached that it's not total calories that contribute to weight loss, but the order in which foods are eaten! One popular diet book states that eating a grapefruit every morning counteracts the effects of consuming foods high in calories, and another that drinking extra water dilutes the number of calories in the foods ingested. *Of course, such claims are erroneous and misleading, but for those desperate to shed excess weight, such plans establish or reinforce negative eating behaviors.* A vicious cycle of failures is repeated. Someone who wants to reduce a given amount of weight tries a particular diet plan that, for whatever reason, is not accompanied by the expected weight loss. The dieter, who may have lost a few pounds, is easily discouraged and quickly regains the lost weight. After a pep talk or some counseling by friends, another attempt is made, this time with a diet "guaranteed" to work! The cycle continues, usually with the same results—the dieter has not changed appreciably in appearance and is still overfat.

As a general rule, it is unwise to follow some prescribed or packaged exotic diet plan in a commercially popular book or magazine. Instead, dieters should eat well-balanced meals but in smaller quantities. A calorie counting approach to weight loss should provide a well-balanced diet that contains all of the essential nutrients. The general recommendation is that low-calorie diets be composed of the appropriate RDA for protein, 20 to 30% fat (with reduced saturated fats), and the remainder consisting predominantly of unrefined, fiber-rich complex carbohydrates. The dietary fiber may add to a feeling of fullness and speed the transit of food through the digestive tract so that fewer calories are absorbed. *Calories do count;* the trick is to keep within the specified daily limits as determined by the amount and rate of fat loss desired. Recall from the previous section that the daily energy requirement is determined by two factors: (1) the minimal resting energy requirements, and (2) energy expenditure accounted for by daily physical activities. As long as the diet is nutritionally sound, it really is not important *what* is eaten, but rather *how many calories* are consumed. If a true caloric deficit exists and calorie input is less than calorie output, weight loss must occur quite independently of the diet's composition. When caloric intake is below the daily energy requirement, the initial decrease in body weight occurs primarily from water loss and a corresponding depletion of the body's carbohydrate reserves. With further weight loss, a larger proportion of body fat is metabolized to supply the caloric deficit created by restricting food intake or increasing physical activity.

There is simply no compelling evidence to support the contention that the popular "fad" diets have any advantage over a calorically-restricted, well-balanced diet. Weight loss occurs with reduced caloric intake regardless of the diet's composition of carbohydrate, protein, and fat. When obese patients consumed either a high-fat or high-carbohydrate 800 kcal diet, weight loss on each diet was nearly identical, as was the percentage of fat tissue lost during a 10-day period. These findings illustrated an important principle of dieting and weight control; *there is no magic metabolic mixture to assure a more effective weight loss than a well-balanced, low-calorie diet,* even though a low-calorie diet high in fat content may seem more filling and perhaps produce less hunger. A professional with competence and expertise in nutrition, exercise, and the energetics of weight control should be consulted in planning a dietary modification that deviates from the recommended low-calorie but well-balanced meal plan.

USING THE COMPUTERIZED MEAL PLAN AND EXERCISE APPROACH

The computerized meal and exercise plan discussed in Chapter 2 and illustrated in Appendix A is an alternative method to combine dietary control with exercise. The weight loss curve provides a picture of the progress likely to be made if one follows the nutrition *and* exercise prescription. As will be pointed out in Chapter 8, it is crucial to modify both eating and exercise behaviors if positive and permanent changes are to occur in body size and shape. The weight loss curve on the computer printout is not a straight line, but rather is curvilinear to account for *changes* that occur in metabolism and body composition as one progresses through the program of exercise and reduced food consumption.

There are three major advantages of utilizing a computer in the dietary and exercise prescription.

1. Because the meal plans are based on the dietary exchange method, foods of one's preference can easily be substituted within a given meal to offer tremendous variety in planning the daily menus. Such flexibility still maintains the integrity of the nutritional adequacy of the meals, and assures a constancy to the recommended level of caloric intake.
2. The major difference between the computer meal plan for dieting and the myriad of typical "diets" is that with the former, there is direct participation in the creation of well-balanced meals without having to follow a preset selection of foods chosen by someone else, often some self-appointed "expert." People who become actively involved in planning their daily meals are much more likely to remain with the program than if nutritional choices are unavailable. If a person selects to eat a particular food, then he or she probably will; having to eat disliked foods as part of a particular diet regimen is negative reinforcement and usually leads to failure (rejection of the diet) before achieving a particular goal (i.e., 15 pound weight loss). The same is true for exercise. If the plan calls for jogging, and jogging is despised with a passion, what are the chances of sticking with it? Slim of course. We all know men and women who refuse to exercise regularly because they've been led to believe that long-distance running is the only beneficial exercise. With a choice of activities, as well as an appropriate starting level, however, the chances are excellent for rapid progress. To this end the computer stands ready with its variety of *choices.*
3. The computerized exercise prescription allows a person to interchange between activities and still expend about the same number of calories. For example, if it rains one day and jogging is not preferred, then the computer allows alternative activities like swimming, cycling or racquetball to be performed at about the same caloric expenditure. The example in Appendix A shows the equivalency in gross caloric output between walking, swimming, cycling, and nine sport activities. Without a computer, such calculations would literally require hundreds of hours, particularly because the exercise output is matched to the dietary plan, and both are individualized to the needs of the particular person desiring a particular weight loss.

EXERCISE TO TIP THE ENERGY BALANCE EQUATION

Exercise can play an important role in helping to unbalance the energy balance equation and produce a caloric deficit. Too frequently, however, the importance of exercise in weight control has been played down. One reason is the common belief that participation in additional exercise *always* causes an increase in appetite and food intake. Also, it is often believed that the amount of energy expended during physical activity is so *small* that a dieter would have to spend an inordinate amount of time exercising before achieving a substantial caloric deficit. In the following section we will explore the basis for these two misconceptions.

Misconception One. Exercise Effects on Appetite. It appears that physical activity is necessary for the normal functioning of the brain's feeding control mechanisms. A fine balance between energy expenditure and food intake is not maintained in sedentary people. For them, the daily caloric intake generally exceeds energy requirement. The lack of precision in regulating food intake at the low end of the physical activity spectrum may account for the "creeping obesity" commonly observed in highly mechanized and technically advanced societies. On the other hand, for individuals who exercise on a regular basis, appetite control is in a "reactive zone" where it is simpler to match food intake with the daily level of energy expenditure. In considering the effects of exercise on appetite and food consumption, we must make a distinction between the type and duration of the exercise. There is no question that lumberjacks, farm laborers, and certain athletes who regularly perform hard, physical labor, often consume about twice the daily calories (4000 to 7000 kcal) than do more sedentary people (2000 to 3000 kcal).

In a study of 32 Scandinavian woodcutters who spent 4 days in national competition splitting and cutting lumber, the daily kcal intake ranged from 4120 to 7210 kcal, with an average intake of 5460 kcal. Other studies of Swedish lumbermen also revealed similar high daily caloric intakes. In one study the average caloric ingestion was 5700 kcal per day, while another study reported a 6200-kcal daily food consumption. This latter value is similar to 6425 kcal consumed each day by loggers in the Pacific Northwest and lower than the value of 8083 kcal estimated for lumberjacks working the forests of Maine. Because these workers are usually quite lean, such high caloric intakes are necessarily required to balance the extremely high caloric expenditure during lumberjacking and logging.

The same situation exists for many athletes who devote considerable time to strenuous physical training. Table 7-3 lists the estimated daily caloric intake of

Table 7-3. *Estimated daily caloric intake for athletes in various sport activities.*

SPORT	AVERAGE BODY WEIGHT KILOGRAMS	ESTIMATED DAILY KCAL INTAKE
Cross-country skiing	67.5	6105
Bicycle racing	68.0	5995
Canoe racing	75.0	5995
Marathon racing	68.0	5940
Soccer	74.0	5885
Field hockey (men)	75.0	5720
Handball (European)	75.0	5610
Basketball	75.0	5610
Ice hockey	68.0	5390
Gymnastics (men)	67.0	5000
Sailing	74.0	5170
Fencing	73.0	5000
Sprinting (track)	69.0	4675
Boxing (middle and welter weight)	63.5	4675
Diving	61.0	4620
Pole vault	73.0	4620

Reprinted with permission of Macmillan Publishing Co., Inc., from Encyclopedia of Sport Sciences and Medicine by the American College of Sports Medicine. Copyright © 1971 by Macmillan Publishing Co., Inc.

various international-caliber athletes. It should be emphasized that athletes of this status devote as much as 8 hours a day to training. Notice that endurance athletes like marathon runners, cross-country skiers, and cyclists consume about 6000 kcal each day. Yet some of these athletes are the leanest in the world! Obviously, this extreme caloric intake is required just to meet the energy requirements of their training.

When an evaluation of dietary intake is made for people who train for relatively short periods of time, the appetite-stimulating effect of exercise is *not* readily apparent. This was demonstrated for college women in an experiment that evaluated daily calorie intake before and after a season of competitive swimming and tennis. The physical conditioning programs for the two groups of women differed both in duration and intensity. Swimming workouts were conducted each day for 2 hours from January to May. Daily swimming distance ranged from between 2000 and 4000 meters during January and March to 1000 to 2000 meters in April and May. The tennis players practiced daily for 1 hour. The workouts consisted of 10 minutes of rope-skipping, 45 minutes of organized practice and games, followed by a half-mile jog. Rope-skipping and jogging were discontinued after January. Average daily caloric intake was assessed for each woman before and after the 5-month training and competitive season by use of the 7-day dietary inventory discussed previously.

Inspection of Table 7-4 shows that the average caloric intake of the swimmers remained about 15% higher than that of the tennis players. Within each group, however, there were only small increases in caloric intake during the season compared with values before and after the experiment. This was also true for proportions of proteins, fats, and carbohydrates consumed. During the 5-month evaluation there was no change in body weight, percent body fat, and lean body weight for both groups of athletes. Average body weight remained constant at 132 pounds for the swimmers and 129 pounds for the tennis players.

Many other studies provide supporting evidence that vigorous exercise of moderate duration does not markedly increase appetite and food intake. In one study, obese young men participated in a 3-phase, 18-week physical conditioning program. For the first 8 weeks (phase 1), subjects exercised 1 hour each day by running, swimming, performing calisthenics, and playing handball. For the next 5 weeks (phase 2) the daily exercise was terminated and subjects resumed their sedentary life style. Then the daily exercise program was resumed for another 5 weeks (phase 3). Daily caloric intake was assessed before and during the experiment. Before the program of physical activity, daily caloric intake averaged 2003

Table 7-4. *Average kcal intakes of swimmers and tennis players before and after a five-month training and competitive season.*

GROUP	CALORIES		PROTEINS		FATS		CARBOHYDRATES	
	BEFORE	AFTER	BEFORE	AFTER	BEFORE	AFTER	BEFORE	AFTER
Swimmers	2091	2065	80.8	71.8	92.3	90.0	247.9	240.6
Tennis players	1811	1797	78.1	74.2	78.9	78.8	192.6	195.2

Values for proteins, fats, and carbohydrates are expressed in grams.

Source: F.I. Katch et al.: Effects of physical training on the body composition and diet of females, *Research Quarterly, 40*:99–104, 1969.

kcal. During the first 8 weeks of exercise, caloric intake increased only slightly to 2148 kcal. During the next 5-week period of sedentary living, daily caloric intake increased only slightly. These data are in agreement with the pattern of caloric intake of the swimmers and tennis players reported in Table 7-4.

In summary, vigorous exercise of relatively short duration does not necessarily stimulate appetite and cause increased food intake. While there were no changes in body composition for the female swimmers and tennis players who were already within the normal range, exercise produced significant reductions in body weight and body fat for the obese men. Compared to their initial values before the exercise program, there was a 12.3% decrease in body weight, a 17% decrease in total pounds of fat, a 5.2% increase in lean body weight, and an 80% reduction in the sum of 8 skinfold measures. These modifications in body size can be attributed to the calorigenic effects of the exercise per se, since caloric intake remained essentially *unchanged.*

Misconception Two. Exercise Effects on Energy Expenditure. The second misconception concerns the number of calories that can be expended through regular exercise. Some authors argue that a person must perform an inordinate amount of exercise just to lose 1 pound of body fat. Usually cited is the fact that one must chop wood for 10 hours, golf for 20 hours, perform mild calisthenic exercises for 22 hours, or play Ping-Pong for 28 hours or volleyball for 32 hours or run 35 miles just to reduce body fat by 1 pound. Understandably, such a commitment is overwhelming and discouraging to the overweight person who plans to lose up to 20 or 30 pounds or more. From a different perspective, however, if golf was played only 2 hours (about 350 kcal per day), 2 days per week (700 kcal), it would take about 5 weeks or 10 golfing days to lose 1 pound of fat (3500 kcal). Assuming you could play golf year round, playing golf 2 days a week would result in a 10-pound loss of fat during the year, provided the food intake remained fairly constant. While most of us would probably not play golf this frequently (nor are we likely to play golf for 20 consecutive hours), the point is that the calorie expending effects of exercise are cumulative; *a caloric deficit of 3500 kcal is equivalent to a 1-pound loss of fat, whether the deficit occurs rapidly or systematically over a long time.*

In calculating the caloric cost of various physical activities, we must assume that the energy cost for people of a particular body size maintains a certain constancy. Recall that in Chapter 4 we pointed out that the values of energy expenditure determined for most physical activities were only averages based on few observations. Consequently a wide range of values may be possible because of individual differences in performance style and technique, and because of environmental factors such as terrain, temperature, and wind resistance, as well as the intensity of participation.

Two "average" golfers playing a typical course for 4 hours might expend considerably different amounts of energy. For that matter, the same golfer playing 2 or 3 consecutive days would never duplicate the same energy expenditure. This would also be true for most sport activities; however, under relatively constant exercise conditions, the energy requirements will remain fairly stable and can be estimated with considerable accuracy.

The values of energy expenditure for physical activities presented in Appendix B should not be considered absolute. These are "average" values, applicable under "average" conditions when applied to the "average" person of a given body weight. However, these values do provide a good approximation of energy expenditure and are quite useful in establishing the appropriate caloric cost of an exercise program.

DIET PLUS EXERCISE: THE IDEAL COMBINATION

A negative caloric balance produced either by dietary restriction or by exercise can result in a desirable modification in body composition; that is, a decrease in body weight and percent body fat. Certainly, combinations of exercise and diet offer considerably more flexibility for achieving a negative caloric balance and accompanying fat loss than either exercise alone or diet alone. The question remains, however, is exercise combined with a reduced caloric intake more effective in fat loss and weight control than either dietary restriction alone or exercise alone? To provide insight into this complex question, many factors must be considered.

If weight reduction is attempted by simply reducing food intake, then one must consider how many calories to consume. While there are no hard and fast rules, considerable experimental data as well as clinical observations have shown that adverse changes in psychologic behavior can occur if caloric intake is reduced too much over an extended period of time. In addition, prolonged dieting greatly increases the chances of developing a variety of nutritional deficiencies. The obvious alternative to achieving a negative caloric balance through dieting is to blend diet with exercise to establish a caloric deficit. To create a daily caloric deficit of 1000 kcal, for example, a combination of diet and exercise would seem an easier method than either diet alone or exercise alone.

Most nutrition experts agree that a loss in body fat of up to *2 pounds each week* is within acceptable medical limits. This guideline is partially based on the observation that people who have been successful in achieving and maintaining a desirable body weight lost no more than 1 to 2 pounds per week during the period of caloric deficit. A more conservative approach would establish a target loss of only 1 pound per week. Then even under the best circumstances the dieter would require 20 weeks to lose the 20 pounds of fat.

Suppose the target time selected to achieve a 20-pound fat loss is 20 weeks. The average weekly deficit must therefore be 3500 kcal; the daily caloric deficit is then 500 kcal (3500 ÷ 7). To achieve a daily deficit of 500 kcal by dieting, caloric intake must be reduced from 2100 to 1600 kcal per day. Remember, this level of "semistarvation" needs to be maintained for 5 months to achieve the desired pound-per-week or total 20-pound fat loss. However, if the dieter performed a half hour of moderate exercise equivalent to 350 "extra" kcal 3 days a week, then the weekly caloric output would increase by 1050 kcal (3 days per week × 350 kcal per exercise session). With additional exercise, the weekly caloric restriction necessary to lose the 1 pound of fat each week would now only have to reach 2450 kcal instead of 3500 kcal. The additional 1050 are "burned" during the weekly exercise. Instead of excluding 500 kcal from the daily diet, the caloric intake need only be restricted by 350 kcal, because the caloric contribution of the exercise averages 150 kcal a day (1050 kcal per week ÷ 7). If the same exercise were undertaken 5 days a week, the daily intake of food could be increased by an additional 100 calories and the pound-per-week fat loss would still be attained. If the *duration* of the 5 day-per-week workouts was extended from 30 minutes to 1 hour, then no reduction in food intake would be necessary to lose weight, because the required 3500 kcal caloric imbalance or deficit would have been created entirely through exercise.

If the *intensity* of the 1-hour exercise performed 5 days a week was then increased by only 10% (cycling at 22 miles per hour instead of 20 miles per hour; running a mile in 9 minutes instead of 10 minutes; swimming 50 yards in 54 seconds instead of 60 seconds), the number of calories burned each week through exercise would increase an additional 350 kcal (3500 kcal/week × 10%). This new weekly deficit of 3850 kcal or 550 kcal per day would actually permit the dieter to *increase* the daily food intake by 50 calories and still lose a pound of fat each week!

Clearly, physical activity can be used effectively by itself or in combination with mild dietary restriction to bring about an effective loss of body fat. Perhaps equally important, the feelings of intense hunger and other psychologic stressors may be minimal compared with a similar program of weight loss that relies exclusively on caloric restriction. Furthermore, exercise in a weight reduction program provides protection against the significant loss in lean tissue usually observed when weight loss is achieved by diet alone. The preservation of the lean tissue mass is partly due to aerobic exercise training that enhances the mobilization and breakdown of fat from the body's adipose depots. In addition, vigorous exercise tends to increase the rate of protein build up in skeletal muscle, while at the same time retarding its rate of breakdown. This protein-sparing effect causes a greater portion of the caloric deficit to be made up by the breakdown of *fat.*

Optimal Duration of Exercise Plus Diet Program

During the first few days of food restriction, when caloric intake is below the daily energy requirement, the observed decrease in body weight occurs primarily from a depletion of the body's carbohydrate stores and a corresponding loss in body water. As weight loss continues, a larger proportion of body fat is metabolized for energy to supply the caloric deficit created by food restriction.

Figure 7-3 shows the percentage composition of the average daily weight loss for water, protein, and fat that occurred during 24 days of a low-calorie diet consisting of 1000 kcal of carbohydrates per day. In addition to caloric restriction all subjects were exercised daily for 2½ hours in a prescribed activity program. Dur-

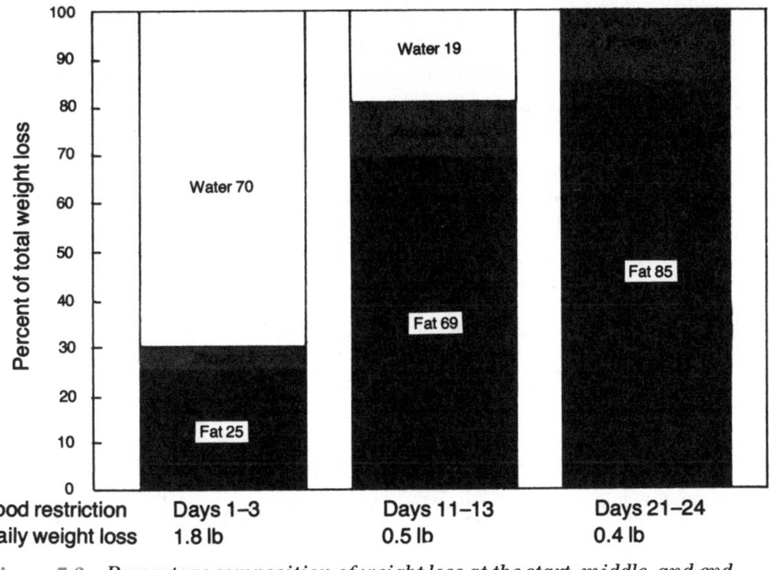
Percent of total weight loss
0
10
20
30
40
50
60
70
80
90
100
Water 70
Fat 25
Water 19
Fat 69
Fat 85
Food restriction
Days 1–3
Days 11–13
Days 21–24
Daily weight loss
1.8 lb
0.5 lb
0.4 lb

Figure 7-3. *Percentage composition of weight loss at the start, middle, and end of 24 days of food restriction (1000 kcal per day) plus enforced exercise of 2.5 hours per day.*

ing the first 3 days of the program, water loss represented 70% of the weight loss. The reduction of body water became progressively less as weight loss continued, and during days 11 to 13 water loss represented only 19% of the weight lost. In addition, the proportion of fat loss increased from 25 to 69% during this period. From day 21 to day 24, 85% of the weight loss occurred by reduction in body fat without a corresponding increase in water loss. The percentage of weight loss from protein increased from 5% initially to 12% during days 11 to 13 and to 15% by the end of the period of caloric restriction.

A relationship also exists between the proportion of water, protein, and fat lost and the amount of water consumed during the first few days of caloric restriction. Carefully conducted experiments have demonstrated that restricting water intake during the first 3 days of a diet significantly *increases* the proportion of water loss through dehydration and *decreases* the proportion of fat loss. The total quantity of fat lost was essentially the same regardless of the *quantity* of fluid ingested. It is therefore important to provide adequate hydration during the period of caloric restriction as *water restriction in no way facilitates fat loss.*

Figure 7-4 graphically displays the results of 6 experiments in terms of the caloric equivalent of each kilogram of weight loss. As shown in the figure, the caloric equivalent of each kilogram of weight loss increases substantially as the duration of caloric restriction increases. *This is the major reason why it is so important to maintain a caloric deficit for extended periods of time; shorter*

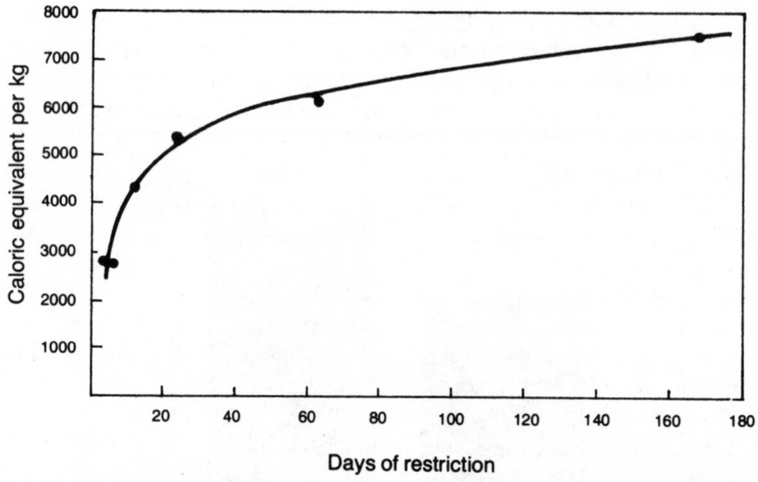
Caloric equivalent per kg
8000
7000
6000
5000
4000
3000
2000
1000
20
40
60
80
100
120
140
160
180
Days of restriction

Experiment	Number of subjects	Duration (days)	Average weight loss (kg)	Total calorie deficit	Caloric equivalent
1	1	4	2.85	8,107	2,845
2	6	5	5.50	15,590	2,835
3	6	12	5.90	25,368	4,300
4	13	24	7.60	40,480	5,326
5	12	63	14.10	87,000	6,170
6	32	168	16.82	126,420	7,516

Figure 7-4. *Caloric equivalent of weight loss in relation to the duration of calorie restriction. Each data point represents an experiment as summarized in the accompanying legend.*

periods of caloric restriction result in a larger percentage of water and carbohydrate loss per unit of weight reduction with only a minimal decrease in body fat. While the caloric equivalent of 1 kg of weight approaches only 3000 kcal during the first 4 or 5 days on a reduced caloric intake, the caloric equivalent more than doubles after 2 months of maintaining a caloric deficit.

The major findings of studies that evaluate the efficacy of various approaches to establishing a caloric imbalance are as follows:

1. Exercise combined with dietary restriction appears to be a more effective approach for achieving a negative caloric balance compared with exercise or diet alone.
2. During the first few days of weight reduction, the rapid weight loss is due primarily to a loss in body water and carbohydrates; at least 2 months of weight reduction is associated with a substantially greater loss of fat per unit of weight loss.
3. Water intake should not be restricted when beginning a weight reduction program because this can precipitate dehydration but no additional fat loss.
4. Undesirable psychologic and medically related problems may occur with prolonged caloric restriction maintained below minimal energy requirements.
5. Weight loss by diet alone causes a significant loss of muscle mass. Exercise appears to protect against lean tissue losses; thus, more of the weight loss is fat loss.

Additional Reading

American Medical Association Council on Food and Nutrition: *Journal of the American Medical Association. 224:*1418, 1973.

American College of Sports Medicine: Position statement on proper and improper weight loss programs. *Medicine and Science in Sports and Exercise. 15*(1):1X, 1983.

Baron, J.A. et al.: A randomized controlled trial of low carbohydrate and low fat/high fiber diets for weight loss. *American Journal of Public Health. 76:*1293, 1986.

Bennett, W. and J. Gurin: The Dieter's Dilemma. New York, Basic Books, Inc., 1982.

Bjorntorp, P., et al.: Effect of an energy reduced dietary regimen in relation to adipose tissue cellularity in obese women. *American Journal of Clinical Nutrition. 28:*445, 1975.

Brownell, K.D. and F.S. Kaye: A school-based behavior modification, nutrition education, and physical activity program for obese children. *American Journal of Clinical Nutrition. 35:*277, 1982.

Craighead, L.W., et al.: Behavior therapy and pharmacotherapy for obesity. *Archives of General Psychiatry. 38:*763, 1981.

Frank, A., et al.: Fatalities on the liquid-protein diet: An analysis of possible causes. *International Journal of Obesity. 5:*243, 1981.

Grande, F.: Nutrition and energy balance in body composition studies. In: Techniques for Measuring Body Composition. Washington, D.C., National Academy of Sciences-National Research Council, 1961.

Isner, J.M. et al.: Sudden unexpected death in avid dieters using the liquid-protein-modified fast. *Circulation. 60:*1401, 1979.

Karvonen, M.J., et al.: Consumption and selection of food in competitive lumber work. *Journal of Applied Physiology. 6:*603, 1954.

Katch, F.I., et al.: Effects of physical training on the body composition and diet of females. *Research Quarterly. 40:*99, 1969.

McArdle, W.D., and M.M. Toner.: Application of exercise for weight control: The exercise prescription. In: *Eating Disorders Handbook: Complete Guide to Understanding and Treatment.* Edited by R. Frankle and M.-U. Yang. Maryland, Aspen Publications. (In Press)

McArdle, W.D., and Magel, J.R.: Weight management: diet and exercise. In: *The Medical Aspects of Clinical Nutrition.* Edited by J. Bland, and N. Shealy. New Canaan, CT, Keats, 1983.

Mirkin, G.B. and R.N. Shore: The Beverly Hills diet: dangers of the newest weight loss fad. *Journal of the American Medical Association. 246:*2235, 1981.

Newmark, S.R. and B. Williamson: Survey of very-low-calorie weight reduction diets. I. Novelty diets. *Archives of Internal Medicine. 143:*1195, 1983.

Newmark, S.R. and B. Williamson: Survey of very-low-calorie weight reduction diets. II. Total fasting, protein-sparing modified fasts, chemically defined diets. *Archives of Internal Medicine. 143:*1423, 1983.

Nisbett, R.E.: Eating behavior and obesity in men and animals. *Advances in Psychosomatic Medicine. 7:*173, 1972.

Schachter, S.: Obesity and eating: Internal and external cues differentially affect the eating behavior of obese and normal subjects. *Science. 161:*751, 1968.

Schachter, S.: Some extraordinary facts about obese humans and rats. *American Psychologist. 26:*129, 1971.

Snook, J.T., Delany, J.P. and V.M. Vivian: Effect of moderate to very low fat defined formula diets on serum lipids in healthy subjects. *Lipids. 20:*808, 1985.

Sours, H.E., et al.: Sudden death associated with very low caloric weight reduction regimens. *American Journal of Clinical Nutrition. 34:*453, 1981.

Stricker, E.M.: Biological bases of hunger and satiety: Therapeutic implications. *Nutrition Reviews. 42:*333, 1984.

Stunkard, A.J., and M. McLaren-Hume: The results of treatment for obesity. *Archives of Internal Medicine. 103:*79, 1959.

Weissman, C. et al.: Semistarvation and exercise. *Journal of Applied Physiology. 60:*2035, 1986.

8

Modification of Eating and Exercise Behaviors

THE HUMAN ORGANISM is remarkably adaptable. People can modify existing food and exercise behavior patterns as long as they establish a clear-cut need for change and they have a good possibility of success. One of the techniques used to alter behavior is referred to by psychologists as *behavior therapy* or *behavior modification*. This approach helps the person to identify, control, and modify undesirable behaviors so they become desirable.

An excellent example of the application of behavior modification is the treatment of *anorexia nervosa*, a condition where the person actually stops eating. As a result, body weight is reduced considerably, in some instances by as much as 50%. This disorder occurs mostly in young women and is associated with severe psychologic problems.

In one study women patients hospitalized for treatment of anorexia nervosa walked considerable distances around the hospital (averaging 6.8 miles per day) compared to an average distance of 4.9 miles walked each day by women of normal body weight living at home. This degree of hyperactivity was used as the behavioral modifier to induce patients to eat and subsequently gain weight. The patients were permitted to walk only if they made a daily gain in body weight. Any time the patient's body weight was at least a half pound above the weight of the previous day, she was allowed 6 hours of unrestricted activity outside the hospital. Within 1 week, the patients' body weights increased significantly. On the average, body weight increased 4 pounds per week during the 6 weeks of hospitalization. Case studies of this type illustrate that a behavioral disorder (refusal to eat) can be altered by providing positive reinforcement (opportunity to engage in physical activity) once a permanent feature of the disorder is uncovered (hyperactivity).

Another application of *eating behavior modification* involved the treatment of a 17-year-old woman who weighed 50 pounds. The search for a potential positive reinforcer was unsuccessful until the young woman began to complain about the sedative effects of a particular drug that was administered as part of her treatment. The doctors used this aspect of her behavior (complaint) as the reinforcer. Following each day in which there was a further loss or no change in body weight, they administered a large dose of the sedative drug. On the other hand, a quarter-pound weight gain resulted in a smaller drug dose; for a half-pound weight gain, an even smaller dose was given, and if 1 pound was gained no drug was administered. The decrease in drug dosage served as the positive reinforcer; the young woman eventually gained an average of 6 pounds each week. Ultimately, normal dietary patterns were established and a systematic weight gain occurred.

In the following sections we will present some basic principles of behavior modification, with special application to weight reduction by means of dietary modification and increased energy expenditure through physical activity. We use four basic steps in applying the principles of behavior modification to eating and exercise. These are: (1) description of the behavior to be modified, (2) replacement of established patterns of behavior with more desirable behaviors, (3) development of techniques to control behaviors, and (4) positive reinforcement or reward for controlling, altering, or modifying the undesirable behaviors.

Modification of Eating Behavior

While numerous treatment approaches have been used to rehabilitate obese people, none has been particularly successful in achieving long-term results. In fact, one doctor well known for his work in the treatment of obesity stated that "most obese patients won't even come for treatment. Those who do come often drop out, and the ones that don't drop out don't lose much weight. Finally, those who do lose weight usually regain it." The results of many studies provide ample support for this statement, especially with regard to long-term weight loss. The success record for weight loss in obese people is less than encouraging, and underscores the difficulties encountered with most traditional weight control programs in achieving either short-term or long-term results.

An apparent breakthrough was made in the treatment of obesity in 1967 when a behavioral psychologist reported the results of a 1-year treatment program for obesity using behavior modification techniques. Treatment sessions were conducted for 30 minutes, 3 times a week over a 4- to 5-week period. Subsequent sessions were conducted at 2-week intervals for 12 weeks; thereafter sessions were held only once a month or as needed. The total number of sessions attended by each person varied from 16 to 41 during the year. Of the 8 obese women 3 lost more than 40 pounds and 5 lost more than 26 pounds. The magnitude of these changes was the highest ever reported for the treatment of obesity in a group of subjects not confined to a hospital or clinic environment. Figure 8-1 shows the results for the 8 women in the study. These results were impressive because normally no more than 1 of 4 obese subjects who seek treatment loses more than 20 pounds, and no more than 1 of 20 loses more than 40 pounds.

The following sections summarize the basic principles of eating behavior modification as applied to programs of weight control.

DESCRIPTION OF THE BEHAVIOR TO BE MODIFIED

The first step is to describe the various eating behaviors and habits of the dieter and *not* immediately to change the diet. The subject is asked to keep meticu-

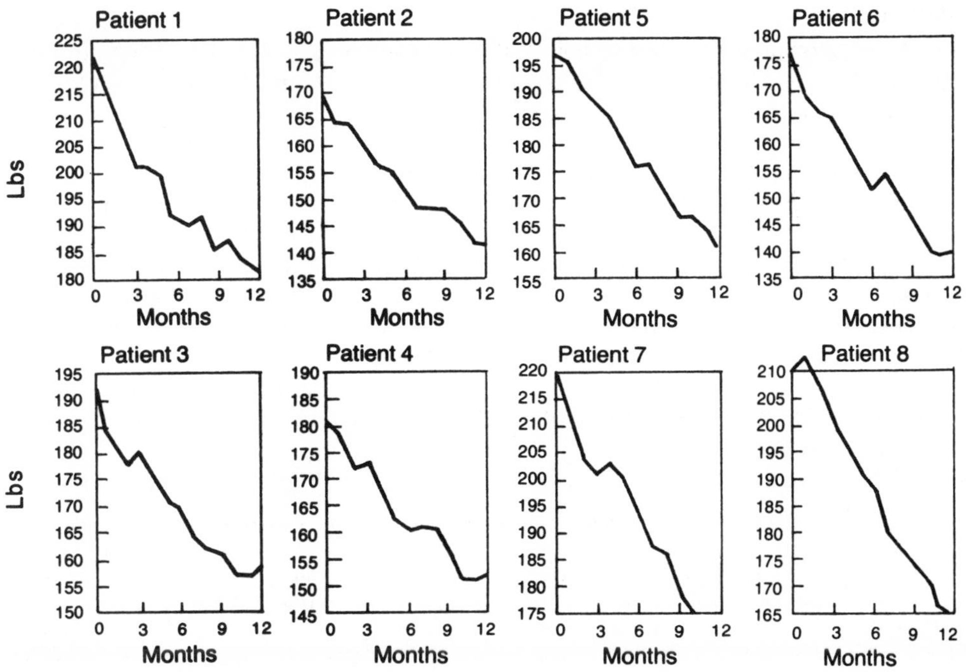
Patient 1
Patient 2
Patient 5
Patient 6
Patient 3
Patient 4
Patient 7
Patient 8
Lbs
Months

Figure 8-1. *Weight profile of 8 women undergoing behavior therapy for overeating. (From R.B. Stuart, "Behavioral Control of Overeating,"* Behavior Research and Therapy, 5:*364, Fig. 1, 1967.)*

lous records to provide answers to the following questions:

1. Where are meals eaten?
2. When are meals eaten?
3. What is the mood, feeling, or psychologic state during the meal?
4. How much time was spent at the meal?
5. What activities were engaged in during the meal (watching television, driving a car, sewing)?
6. Who was present during the meal?
7. What and how much food was eaten?

This time-consuming and often annoying record-keeping provides the dieter with objective information concerning personal eating behaviors. A careful examination of such records will reveal certain recurring patterns of behavior associated with eating. For example, the dieter may discover that feelings of depression are usually followed by eating candy; that he or she eats snacks while watching television, gets hungry at a particular time of day, goes on an ice-cream binge after an argument, or never eats breakfast or lunch at the kitchen table. Once an analysis is made of eating behaviors, the next step is to substitute alternate behaviors for the ones where a clear pattern has been established. Because circumstances intimately related to established eating patterns apparently signal the eating response, the objective is to eliminate or substitute these undesirable signals.

SUBSTITUTING ALTERNATIVE BEHAVIORS

Many alternate acceptable behaviors can replace a particular set of environmental cues associated with eating. Below is a list of some examples of existing behaviors associated with eating, as well as possible substitute behaviors.

Established behavior patterns	**Replacement behavior**
1. Eating candy while driving	1. Singing along with the radio while driving
2. Eating snacks while watching television	2. Sewing, painting, or writing letters while watching television
3. Feeling hungry at 4:00 p.m.	3. Going for a walk at 4:00 p.m.
4. Eating ice cream after an argument	4. Doing 10 repetitions of an exercise after an argument
5. Never eating breakfast or lunch at the kitchen table	5. Eating breakfast and lunch only at the kitchen table
6. Visiting the kitchen during TV commercials	6. Jogging in place; doing sit-ups

While we can give numerous other examples, the major aim of this approach is clear: *to create new associations to replace the old established patterns of behavior.*

DEVELOPMENT OF TECHNIQUES TO CONTROL THE ACT OF EATING

There are many useful techniques to gain control over eating habits once undesirable environmental cues have been identified and replaced or eliminated. Examples include the following:

1. Make the act of eating foods a ritual; limit eating to one place in the house and no matter what foods you eat, follow a set routine. Use a place mat, set the table with silverware, and use the same dishes at each meal. Do this for main meals as well as for snacks. One dieter who continually snacked between meals curbed this habit by dressing up in a tuxedo and eating by candlelight for each meal and snack. Snacking between meals soon stopped. To discourage bread eating, take only one slice of bread at a time and toast it before eating. For each slice get up from the table, unwrap the loaf of bread from its package, take out a slice, rewrap the loaf and replace it in the cupboard, toast the slice, and return to the table to eat it. Following an inconvenient routine to obtain some special food item often suppresses the desire for such food.
2. Use smaller dishes; the impetus to finish the meal may not be the food per se, but the desire to view an empty plate or glass.
3. Eat slowly; fight the urge to eat quickly by taking more time at meals. You can do this by cutting food into smaller pieces and chewing each piece 10 to 15 times before swallowing. Another technique is to place the knife, spoon, or fork back on the table after each 2 or 3 bites, and allow for a 1- or 2-minute rest pause between mouthfuls.

PROVIDE POSITIVE REINFORCEMENT OR REWARDS

The ultimate long-term rewards of achieving the desired outcomes of a positive weight control program are 3-fold: (1) improvement in personal appearance,

(2) subtle but observable changes in psychologic behaviors, and perhaps (3) better overall health because of physiologic changes. Dieters can set up short-term goals to provide interim rewards. After you maintain a given amount of weight loss for several months (say, 5 pounds), buy a new article of clothing; after the next substantial weight loss (10 pounds), go on a trip. Continue to provide rewards until you reach the eventual goal. Another useful technique is to maintain a weight chart and plot changes in body weight. Keep separate charts for recording daily caloric intake from food and caloric expenditure due to exercise, as well as recording changes in various body dimensions such as the abdomen, buttocks, and thighs.

The positive and negative reinforcing power of money can also be used as an incentive. This may work better in a group situation, however. For example, a given amount of money is given to the group leader at the start of the program. A portion of the deposit is returned to the group members depending on the amount specified for a given weight loss (for example, $10 per pound). If a member quits the program or fails to maintain the weight loss for at least 1 week, the deposit is forfeited and divided equally among the remaining participants at the end of a specified time period. Many variations of such procedures are possible. Remember, though, that merely providing information about the techniques of eating behavior modification will not in itself ensure their continued use. *Encouragement* and *positive reinforcement* must be built-in features of the weight control program. They must continue until subjects establish mastery over eating behaviors and achieve a proper balance between energy input and energy output so that body size can hopefully stay permanently reduced.

Modification of Exercise Behavior

In the past, it was generally accepted that the obese condition was the result of excessive food intake. Clearly, then, the effective approach to weight control would be some form of caloric restriction through dieting. However, research studies concerned with eating patterns and exercise behaviors of the obese show consistently that a low caloric output due to a lack of physical activity, rather than an inordinately high caloric (food) intake, is a prime factor associated with overfatness. *In fact, one is hard pressed for evidence that groups of overweight individuals actually eat more on the average than people of normal weight.* In the early 1940s, psychologists pointed out that only a small percentage of obese people participated in physical activities within the range usually observed for non-obese people of the same age and gender. This characteristic sedentary behavior pattern of the obese has been demonstrated in 6 of 9 studies conducted between 1953 and 1981. The surprising finding was that in all of the experiments, the food intake of the obese was *no greater* than for people of normal body size. Recent research conducted at Tufts University and Harvard Medical School indicated that in teenagers and younger children, the greater the hours of TV watching the fatter the child. More specifically, the prevalence of adolescent obesity increases 2% for each hour of television viewed daily. Also, the earlier in life TV watching begins the greater the obesity and the more profound the problem becomes in teenage years. In addition, the excess weight gain throughout life closely parallels reduced physical activity rather than increased caloric intake. For example, obese infants do not characteristically consume more calories than either the recommended dietary standards of counterparts of normal weight. Also, infant offspring of obese parents display less spontaneous movements than infants of normal weight parents. This suggests that such subdued movement patterns are abnormal and may reflect inherited characteristics.

It is of interest to point out that similar results of the relation between energy output and food consumption have been observed in genetically obese strains of mice and rats. Those strains of animals that fatten easily display significantly lower levels of motor activity than their relatively lean counterparts. Thus, in both obese humans and animals, physical inactivity appears to be a characteristic feature of their daily living habits.

Table 8-1 shows the results for one of the human experiments that compared the extent of participation in daily physical activities as well as average daily caloric intake of 28 obese and 28 normal high school girls. While time-in-motion analysis revealed that there was *little difference* between the two groups in the amount of time spent sitting, standing, grooming, baby-sitting, driving a car, or doing housework, a considerable difference was demonstrated in the extent of participation in active sports and other strenuous activities. "Extra" physical activity was engaged in for 4 hours a day on the average by the obese, while the nonobese girls consumed 27% *fewer* calories each day than the nonobese girls; only 3 of 28 obese girls consumed more than 2500 kcal each day.

In a similar study conducted several years later with young boys, almost identical findings were observed; obese boys consumed fewer calories each day than a group of nonobese boys. Daily food intake averaged 3011 kcal for the obese and 3476 kcal for the nonobese boys during the school year, and 3430 kcal and 4628 kcal for the obese and lean boys, respectively, during an 8-week summer camp. Researchers observed little difference between the groups in the amount of time they participated in light and moderate exercise; however, the degree of participa-

Table 8-1. *Physical activity and calorie intake of obese and nonobese adolescent girls.*

WEEKLY PHYSICAL ACTIVITY (HOURS)

GROUP	SLEEP, LYING STILL AWAKE	SITTING	STANDING	GROOMING	BABY-SITTING	PLAYING PIANO, DRIVING CAR	HOUSE-WORK	ACTIVE SPORTS AND OTHER VIGOROUS ACTIVITY
Obese	61	81	1	7	1	1.4	3.6	4
Nonobese	63	75	3	10	1	1.2	3.3	11

DAILY CALORIE INTAKE (KCAL/DAY)

GROUP	2500	2500–2000	2000	AVERAGE
Obese	3	6	19	1,965
Nonobese	15	10	3	2,706

Source: M.L. Johnson et al., "Relative importance of inactivity and overeating in the energy balance of obese high school girls," *American Journal of Clinical Nutrition,* 4:37–44, 1956.

tion by the obese boys in more strenuous activities was generally less than for the nonobese.

This observation that fat people often eat the same or even less than thinner ones is also true for adults as they become less active and slowly begin to add weight. In one experiment, the physical activity levels were compared for a group of obese and nonobese men and women who were matched for age, occupation, and socioeconomic background. Physical activity expressed in miles walked each day was assessed by means of *pedometers*. These small instruments are usually hooked from a belt worn around the waist. The pedometer is calibrated to the person's stride length and is operated by an internal pendulum that registers each stride. Total mileage walked was recorded daily for 1 week by the women and for 2 weeks by the men.

The results for the women were unequivocal; the average distance walked by the obese women was about 41% shorter than that walked by the nonobese women. Total miles walked each day averaged 2.0 miles for the obese and 4.9 miles for the nonobese. A comparison of the data for the men showed a similar pattern with regard to distance walked; the obese men walked an average of 39% less than their nonobese counterparts.

The data from the above studies illustrate clearly that inactivity is a major behavioral characteristic that distinguishes overfat from nonobese people. *Individuals who maintain physically active lifestyles or who become involved in appropriate exercise programs generally maintain a desirable level of body composition.* Consequently the obese must not only relearn or modify existing eating behaviors, but also reverse the existing syndrome of insufficient caloric output due to a sedentary life style. Learning how to replace daily periods of relative inactivity (low caloric output) with more strenuous activity requiring a greater energy expenditure may seem a difficult task. Experiencing *enjoyment* and *success* in a given activity is the most important aspect of this relearning process. Only a few people will continue to participate in exercise that is so taxing from a physiologic standpoint that little or no enjoyment is possible. A good example is running. It is not much fun to run for a minute or two when the end result is shortness of breath, wobbly legs, and a "stitch" in the side. All the personal motivation you can muster cannot overcome the genuine discomfort you feel when you pursue unrealistic goals. Even jogging for 5 minutes at a relatively slow pace is not easy, especially for people who have previously been sedentary. If there is little chance for enjoyment and success, then most people will become discouraged and discontinue participation. In psychologic behavior terms, they have received negative reinforcement from the activity participation. However, walking and walking/jogging as well as other programs of physical activities *can be enjoyable* if the probability of *success* is maximized. This necessitates a carefully planned, systematic approach with long-term rather than short-term goals. If the long-term goal is to jog continuously for 30 minutes each day, then the beginning jogger should plan to achieve this goal over a period of weeks or months, rather than trying to run this distance on the first or second day.

DESCRIPTION OF THE BEHAVIOR TO BE MODIFIED

The first step is to determine the daily pattern of physical activity, including such minimal daily requirements as sleeping, eating, going to the bathroom, and bathing. An activity profile can be constructed by keeping a daily record of the actual time allotted for the various activities for 7 consecutive days. The activity profile for a physically active college professor during a typical day of summer vacation is presented in Table 8-2. This record includes a description of the activity, its duration, and its classification into one of three broad categories of energy expenditure: light exercise (under 150 kcal per hour), moderate exercise (150 to 250 kcal per hour), and heavy exercise (over 250 kcal per hour). The actual caloric values of energy expenditure for various physical activities are included in Appendix B.

The results present a fairly detailed picture of the variations in caloric output during a work day. For the professor, the following results are clear: an average of 1350 minutes each day were spent in relatively sedentary activities, and 90 minutes per day were for activities requiring a relatively high energy output. If it were not for the hour and a half devoted to strenuous activities, the energy output level for this person would be classified as sedentary.

Any hope of changing the pattern and quantity of daily physical activity is predicated on an accurate appraisal of the energy cost of the activities that make up a person's life style. Once this has been determined, the next step in exercise behavior modification is to substitute more strenuous activities for those that rate low on energy expenditure.

SUBSTITUTING ALTERNATE BEHAVIORS

Moderate to strenuous physical activity can easily replace the more sedentary activities only when the dieter is willing to become more physically active. This substitution process should begin after an analysis is made of the amount of time devoted to the various daily activities.

There are many ways to increase energy expenditure within the time allotted to daily routines. The important considerations are to determine *when* and *how* to make changes. For example:

1. When driving to work, park a half mile away and walk the remaining distance. Brisk walking to and from the car each day, 5 days a week, will burn up the caloric equivalent of about 7 pounds of fat in 1 year.
2. When taking public transportation, get off 8 to 10 stops early and walk the remaining distance.
3. When traveling relatively short distances, walk instead of taking a cab or bus.
4. Don't go to a restaurant for lunch; participate in some form of physical activity, such as walking, that you can continue for 30 to 45 minutes.
5. Wake up an hour early and take a brisk walk, cycle, row, or swim before breakfast.
6. Replace the cocktail hour with 20 minutes of exercise.
7. Replace coffee breaks with exercise breaks.
8. Walk up and down several flights of stairs after each hour of work.
9. Sweep the sidewalks in front of your house or apartment. One of our dear colleagues, a world-renowned 85-year-old scientist, used to sweep the perimeter of a 4-square-block park in San Francisco, 2½ hours a day, 5 to 6 days a week! He did this not only as a public service, but to augment his generally

Table 8-2. *Detailed record of physical activity for 1 day.*

ACTIVITY	BEGIN ACTIVITY	END ACTIVITY	TOTAL TIME, MINUTES	CLASSIFICATION
1. Wake up	6:45 A.M.			
2. Use bathroom	6:45	6:53 A.M.	8	Light
3. Go back to bed	6:53	7:30	37	Light
4. Eat breakfast	7:30	7:50	20	Light
5. Use bathroom	7:50	8:00	10	Light
6. Dress	8:00	8:06	6	Light
7. Drive to school	8:06	8:17	11	Light
8. Walk to office	8:17	8:25	8	Light
9. Work in office	8:25	10:00	95	Light
10. Pick up mail—walk up and down stairs	10:00	10:10	10	Light
11. Work in office and lab	10:10	12:10 P.M.	120	Light
12. Go to locker room—get dressed	12:10 P.M.	12:16	6	Light
13. Walk to track	12:16	12:20	4	Light
14. Wait for friend	12:20	12:30	10	Light
15. Run to park and back	12:30	2:00	90	Strenuous
16. Walk to locker room	2:00	2:04	4	Light
17. Shower and dress	2:04	2:20	16	Light
18. Walk to office	2:20	2:24	4	Light
19. Have student conference (eat lunch)	2:24	3:00	36	Light
20. Work in office	3:00	5:05	125	Light
21. Walk to library	5:05	5:12	7	Light
22. Work in library	5:12	6:05	53	Light
23. Walk to dean's office	6:05	6:10	5	Light
24. Meet with dean	6:10	6:35	25	Light
25. Walk to office	6:35	6:43	8	Light
26. Walk to car	6:43	6:51	8	Light
27. Drive home	6:51	7:03	12	Light
28. Change clothes	7:03	7:07	4	Light
29. Wash up	7:07	7:11	4	Light
30. Play with baby	7:11	8:00	49	Light
31. Watch TV	8:00	8:30	30	Light
32. Eat dinner	8:30	9:00	30	Light
33. Mail letter	9:00	9:05	5	Light
34. Listen to stereo	9:05	9:30	25	Light
35. Watch TV	9:30	10:30	60	Light
36. Wash up	10:30	10:38	8	Light
37. Read in bed	10:38	11:15	37	Light
38. Turn off lights	11:15	6:45 A.M.	450	Light
		Total	Light	1350
			Moderate	0
			Strenuous	90

sedentary life style with physically demanding tasks to maintain his arm and leg strength. When he was 84 years old and no longer able to work in the park, he substituted what he termed "arm aerobics" as his exercise. He carried two, 3 pound dumbbells around his apartment several times a day.

10. When going on a family outing, allow time for exercise: (a) Get out of the car before reaching your destination; let your family drive the rest of the way while you walk or jog. (b) Instead of eating at half-time or intermission at sport events, walk around the stadium or arena. Climb up and down stairs instead of using elevators or escalators.

11. Replace the hired help and undertake some of these tasks yourself:
    a. Gardening
    b. Mowing the lawn
    c. Painting
    d. Washing and waxing the car
    e. Walking the dog
    f. Plowing the driveway

12. During television commercials, run in place, jump rope, jog up and down stairs, or perform vigorous calisthenics.

13. Replace power tools and appliances with manually operated devices:
    a. Lawn care equipment
    b. Automatic household appliances such as vacuum cleaners, eggbeaters, ice cream maker, juicers.
    c. Saws
    d. Drills
    e. Snow shovelers
    f. Garage doors

14. Play golf without a golf cart or caddy.

15. Walk or jog up and down the beach in addition to sun bathing.

The most difficult task in rearranging a daily routine is to replace conveniences with tasks that require more effort. Identifying possible areas for activity modification is easy because twentieth-century men and women have become accustomed to an automated, labor-saving society. Humans are slaves to machines; we have learned to live the "easy life." Learned behaviors, however, *can* be changed or modified; the major requirement is a willingness to commit yourself to a new life style that incorporates more vigorous activities within the fabric of the daily routine. Unless a person makes this commitment they will be unable to modify a sedentary life style. Unfortunately, most of us are too "locked into" daily routines even to try to modify existing behaviors. There may be a few things we are willing to do, such as use a hand lawnmower now and then or go for a brisk walk at lunchtime. However, it takes a real commitment to sweep the streets, jog around the block, bicycle to and from work, or walk up and down stairs without feeling embarrassed or self-conscious. People must overcome social pressures and constraints to attain permanent changes in life style.

DEVELOPMENT OF TECHNIQUES TO MAXIMIZE EXERCISE SUCCESS

Several techniques can be used to maximize the "fun" potential of exercise. These techniques may not apply to team or individual sports in which skill or competition are the key elements (tennis, badminton, basketball, golf, racquetball, squash), but to activities such as jogging, bicycling, swimming, and calisthenic exercises.

1. Progress slowly: People who have not exercised for a long time should progress slowly and not try to accomplish too much in the first few weeks. Instead of running 1 mile initially, run or even walk 1 block; instead of trying to cycle 10 miles, cycle 3 miles; instead of trying to do 100 sit-ups, do 5 to 10.
2. Include variety: Rather than perform the same exercise over and over again within a given time period, alternate exercises as well as the number of repetitions. For example, instead of jogging continuously around the track, intersperse other forms of exercise: Jog for 2 minutes—skip for 1 minute—hop on the right foot 20 times—hop on the left foot 20 times—jump up and down 20 minutes—skip 1 minute—jog 3 minutes—and so on, until you reach the desired end-point.
3. Become goal oriented: There are three ways to exercise using goal-oriented behavior: (1) Exercise for a certain amount of time; (2) continue to exercise until you reach a predetermined number of repetitions or distance; (3) combine both of the preceding approaches. Select one of these three methods depending on your personal preference. If a track is available, then total distance run becomes a convenient guide. One limitation with this approach, however, is the tedium of running the same route, over and over again, with little or no change in scenery. An alternative is to mark off a given distance (your house to the store, the store to the playground, the playground to the house), and then run this route.

   If exercise for a specific time is the goal, then run a predetermined route such as around a track or through the neighborhood. The latter alternative has the advantage of changing sceneries. For the novice jogger who may only run continuously for a minute or two between rest intervals, the goal should be to cover a given distance, such as running from a big tree to the fence post, the fence post to the red car, and the red car to the stop sign. Mastery of preset goals provides immediate positive reinforcement and minimizes chances of failure. At the same time the fun aspect of the activity is maximized because of the feeling of personal achievement.
4. Be systematic: Set aside certain times during the day to exercise. Don't permit outside factors such as watching television, shopping, and doing housework to interfere with *your* daily activity.
5. Wear clothes conducive to exercise: You need not be concerned with what clothes to wear while swimming or skiing, as the choices are limited and obvious. Many activities have no established patterns of dress, and people should follow their personal preferences. On hot and humid days, wear light clothing to permit rapid heat loss.

PROVIDE POSITIVE REINFORCEMENT OR REWARD

Positive reinforcement should be intimately tied to exercise, especially for the beginner.

1. Keep charts to record progress. Fill in the chart as soon as you achieve the preset goal. Such charts provide immediate feedback and serve the important purpose of helping to maintain motivation and interest.

2. Exercise with a "buddy" or in small groups. Exercising may be more enjoyable when performed in small groups of two or three people. Having to make commitments with others can be a subtle form of motivation, and can help to ensure exercise on a regular schedule.

3. Provide rewards. Self-made competition can be an effective means for achieving preset goals. This is especially true for people who are just beginning an exercise program and need some incentive. We have found that a simple game is effective in helping many people maintain a high degree of self-motivation. The game can be played by as many persons as desired. The object is to perform a given amount of exercise, and a painted button is awarded when the exercise goal is achieved. A predetermined reward is given for accumulating 10 buttons. To start, obtain 16 white shirt buttons. Then paint 10 of them a favorite color. Each of the remaining white buttons is equal to a given number of minutes of exercise. We make a 5-minute exercise period equal to 1 white button. When a person accumulates 6 white buttons (equal to 30 minutes of exercise), they are traded in for a painted button. When the person secures 10 painted buttons, he or she has won the game and receives a reward. The reward is chosen in advance, and can be anything the participant wants. We suggest that the painted buttons be stored in a prominent place in the house, where family members can keep track of progress and provide encouragement and support. For people just beginning an exercise program, the goal is to achieve 5 painted buttons each week. The exercise equivalent for each button can be increased as exercise capacity improves. For purposes of illustration, suppose 30 minutes of exercise is made to equal 1 painted button. For the person who weighs 200 pounds and accumulates 5 painted buttons each week by walking briskly, the "extra" caloric expenditure due to walking would be equal to approximately 1200 kcal per week, 4800 kcal per month, *or the equivalent of 16.5 pounds of fat per year.* It should be obvious that if the reducer achieved a corresponding decrease in calorie intake, the rate and quantity of fat loss would double!

While this particular game may at first seem inappropriate for both younger and older adults, its underlying principle provides for ample positive feedback and reinforcement. As long as the player places value on the reward, the process of striving to achieve it takes on new meaning and offers at least a fighting chance for success.

Additional Reading

Bjorvell, H. and S. Rossner: Long term treatment of severe obesity: four year follow-up of results of combined behavioural modification programme. *British Medical Journal. 291:*379, 1985.

Brownell, K.D.: Behavioral, psychological, and environmental predictors of obesity and success at weight reduction. *International Journal of Obesity. 8:*543, 1984.

Brownell, K.D. and F.S. Kaye: A school-based behavior modification, nutrition education, and physical activity program for obese children. *The American Journal of Clinical Nutrition. 35:*277, 1982.

Epstein, L.H. et al.: A comparison of lifestyle exercise, aerobic exercise, and calisthenics on weight loss in obese children. *Behavior Therapy. 16:*345, 1985.

Foreyt, J.P., and W.A. Kennedy: Treatment of overweight by aversion therapy. *Behaviour Research and Therapy. 9:*29, 1971.

Garner, D.M., Olmstead, M.P. and J. Polivy: Development and validation of a multidimensional eating disorder inventory for anorexia nervosa and bulimia. *International Journal of Eating Disorders. 2:*15, 1983.

Graham, L.E. et al.: Five-year follow-up to a behavioural weight-loss program. *Journal of Consulting Clinical Psychology. 51:*322, 1983.

James, W.P.T., et al.: Dietary recommendations after weight loss: how to avoid relapse of obesity. *American Journal of Clinical Nutrition. 45:*1135, 1987.

Jeffery, R.W. et al.: Behavioral treatment of obesity with monetary contracting: two year follow up. *Addictive Behaviors. 9:*311, 1984.

Johnson, M.L., et al.: Relative importance of inactivity and overeating in the energy balance of obese high school girls. *American Journal of Clinical Nutrition. 4:*37, 1956.

Jordan, H.A., and L.S. Levitz: Behavior modification in a self-help group. *Journal of the American Dietetic Association. 62:*27, 1973.

Leon, G.R.: The behavior modification approach to weight reduction. *Contemporary Nutrition. 4*(8): 1979.

Palgi, A. et al.: Multidisciplinary treatment of obesity with a protein-sparing modified fast: Results in 668 outpatients. *American Journal of Public Health. 75:*1190, 1985.

Penick, S.B., et al.: Behaviour modification in the treatment of obesity. *Psychosomatic Medicine. 33:*49, 1971.

Perri, M.G. et al.: Maintenance strategies for the treatment of obesity: an evaluation of relapse prevention training and post-treatment contact by mail and telephone. *Journal of Consulting Clinical Psychology. 52:*404, 1985.

Stuart, R.B., and B. Davis: Slim Chance in a Fat World: Behavioral Control of Obesity, Champaign, Ill., Research Press, 1971.

Stunkard, A.J.: Environment and obesity: Recent advances in our understanding of regulation of food intake in man. *Federation Proceedings.* 1367, 1968.

Stunkard, A.J., et al.: The management of obesity: Patient self help and medical treatment. *Archives of Internal Medicine. 125:*1067, 1970.

Stunkard, A.J.: New therapies for the eating disorders: Behavior modification of obesity and anorexia nervosa. *Archives of General Psychiatry. 26:*391, 1972.

Stunkard, A.J.: Behavioural treatment of obesity: the current status. *International Journal of Obesity. 2:*237, 1978.

Stunkard, A.J.: Conservative treatments for obesity. *American Journal of Clinical Nutrition. 45:*1142, 1987.

Stunkard, A.J. and S.B. Penick: Behavior modification in the treatment of obesity: The problem of maintaining weight loss. *Archives of General Psychiatry. 36:*801, 1979.

Wadden, T.A. et al.: Treatment of obesity by very-low calorie diet and behavior therapy. *Journal of Consulting and Clinical Psychology. 52:*692, 1984.

Wadden, T.A. and A.J. Stunkard: Social and psychological consequences of obesity. *Annals of Internal Medicine. 103:*1062, 1985.

Wilson, G.T., et al.: Behavior therapy for obesity: Including family members in the treatment process. *Behavior Therapy. 9:*943, 1978.

Wilson, G.T. and K.D. Brownell. Behavior therapy for obesity: An evaluation of treatment outcome. *Advances in Behavior Research and Therapy. 3:*49, 1980.

Wollersheim, J.P.: The effectiveness of group therapy based upon learning principles in the treatment of overweight women. *Journal of Abnormal Psychology. 76:*462, 1970.

Zuckerman, D.M. et al.: The prevalence of bulimia among college students. *American Journal of Public Health. 76:*1135, 1986.

PART III
Physiologic Conditioning for Total Fitness

The Concept of Total Fitness

PHYSICAL FITNESS to some reflects the trim legs and waist of the model or starlet who demonstrates stretching exercises in the popular glamour magazines or video tapes. To others, fitness means superior strength with its accompanying large muscular development. In the past, the popularity of health clubs, spas, and other exercise facilities has flourished in this image. At the other extreme the fit individual is exemplified by the lean, rather frail-looking competitive marathoner who runs at a 5-minute per mile pace for 26 miles.

The housewife, business executive, or college student may take a more moderate view and consider themselves physically fit by successfully completing a set of tennis, a round of golf, a game of racquetball, or climbing several flights of stairs without fatigue. This perspective places fitness on a continuum, with the necessary level of fitness being determined by the physical requirements of one's daily life. While this may be a practical view, medical evidence suggests that our bodies need *regular, vigorous aerobic exercise,* especially if our jobs are sedentary and our life styles inactive.

While it is difficult to formulate a precise definition of fitness, it is appropriate to view *total fitness* as a state of physical well-being that incorporates a balance between several well-developed fitness components. More specifically, total fitness requires adequate muscular strength and endurance, reasonable joint flexibility, an efficient cardiovascular system with a good level of aerobic fitness, and favorable body composition with acceptable control of body weight. Within this framework, exercise programs must be formulated on an individual basis using research-proven training principles and techniques with regular adjustments made to keep pace with the participant's changing level of fitness. *The approach to*

physiologic conditioning for men is basically the same as the approach to physiologic conditioning for women.

General Principles of Physiologic Conditioning

The term *physiologic conditioning* refers to a planned program of exercise directed toward improving the functional capacity of a particular bodily system. This improvement does not occur haphazardly; one must incorporate a basic training principle into an exercise program for physiologic adaptations to occur. This principle is *overload.*

OVERLOAD PRINCIPLE

Although programs of exercise differ considerably depending on a person's specific goals and expectations, any effective exercise program must be based on the proper application of physiologic stress or *overload.* By exercising a system of the body at a level above that at which it normally operates, that system will adapt and function more efficiently. The method and extent of the overload will directly affect the conditioning of the particular system involved. Overload can be accomplished in several ways:

1. Increase the *frequency* of exercise.
2. Increase the *intensity* of exercise within a given time period.
3. Increase the *duration* of exercise at a specified intensity.

Consider the following example of a sedentary woman who wishes to use jogging to train her cardiovascular system to improve her aerobic exercise capacity. If this woman jogged one block twice a week at a slow pace for 1 year, there is no doubt there would be some increase in exercise capacity. However, the improvement would be minimal. To more effectively use exercise for improving cardiovascular capacity above some minimal level, a person must select one of the preceding three methods of implementing the overload. The jogger could elect to speed up her running pace, thereby increasing the intensity of exercise. Other alternatives for overload would be periodically to increase the distance run or to increase the frequency of exercise to 5 days a week. The relative importance of frequency, duration, and intensity in physiologic conditioning will be developed more fully in the sections that follow. *The important point is that to ensure continued improvement in physiologic capacity during training, the relative degree of overload must keep pace with the adaptive changes that occur both in physiology and performance.* This concept of individualized and progressive overload applies to the athlete, the sedentary person, and even the cardiac patient.

A good example of the positive results of progressive overload is the cardiac patient who completely recovered from a heart attack and through a planned training program was able to run a 26-mile marathon in 4 hours. This extraordinary capability in exercise capacity did not occur within a few months. At first, walking for just a few minutes was strenuous. Soon, functional capacity improved and the patient could walk longer distances. In a short time the patient reached a plateau where further improvements in cardiovascular capacity and performance did not take place until additional overload was applied. Walking was replaced by slow jogging, that in turn was replaced by jogging at faster speeds. Simultaneously, distance gradually and systematically increased from a few yards to several blocks, to miles, and finally to a point that was personally rewarding. Of course, this can be carried to spectacular extremes: The world record for continuous swimming is 168 hours; the record for walking nonstop is 47 hours and 42 minutes (215 miles, 1670 yards); for running nonstop, the record is 22 hours and 27 minutes (121 miles, 440 yards); to cover 1000 miles it took 11 days, 9 hours and 41 seconds; for hiking, the record is 32 miles a day for 81 consecutive weeks over a distance of 18,500 miles.

SPECIFICITY PRINCIPLE

The important principle of *training specificity* will be expanded in the following two chapters. In a general sense, training specificity refers to adaptations in the *metabolic* and *physiologic* systems depending on the type of overload imposed. Exercise that develops one aspect of fitness generally contributes little to other fitness components. It is known that a specific exercise stress such as strength-power training induces specific strength-power adaptations. However, such strengthening exercises per se offer little stimulus for increasing the flow of blood through the body and provide only a minimal effect in terms of calories expended.

Research has indicated there is also a high degree of specificity in terms of improving a particular physiologic capacity. Evidence from these studies suggests strongly that a person should perform the training exercises in a manner as close as possible to the way he or she wishes to use this improved capacity. Developing the cardiovascular system for swimming, skiing, bicycling, or rowing, for example, can be achieved more readily when the exerciser works with the specific muscles involved in the particular activity. Consequently, fitness for bicycling is best achieved through cycling exercise, those desiring fitness for swimming should swim, while the runner is best conditioned through specific programs of run training. The same is true for improving the muscular system; performing an exercise with the arms in one pattern of movement, as in lifting a weight with two hands from the waist to a position above the head, does not necessarily mean that improvement in this specific type of lifting strength "transfers" to another arm movement such as the shot-put, even though both movements may use the *same* muscles. *Specific exercise elicits specific adaptations creating specific training effects.*

INDIVIDUAL DIFFERENCES PRINCIPLE

Many factors contribute to individual variation in training response. Of considerable importance is the person's relative fitness level at the start of training. It is unrealistic to expect different people to be in the same "state" of training at the same time. Consequently, it is counterproductive to insist that all individuals train the same way or at the same work rate. It is also unrealistic to expect all individuals to respond to a given training dosage in precisely the same manner. *Training benefits are optimized when programs are planned to meet the individual needs and capacities of the participants.*

PRINCIPLE OF REVERSIBILITY

Another important principle of physiologic conditioning is *reversibility.* The functional capacity of a bodily system is determined by the current level of overload. Once a person reaches a certain level of conditioning, a regular program of activity must be maintained to prevent deconditioning or a loss in functional capacity. When the normal level of exercise can no longer be applied, as occurs when an arm or leg is placed in a cast or when someone adopts a sedentary life style, the current level of physiologic capacity will regress to a lower level. For this reason the muscles of a limb immobilized in a cast will atrophy to a size smaller than the weight-bearing or opposite limb.

Some researchers estimate that once a conditioning program is discontinued, the improvements gained during the conditioning program are lost in 5 to 10 weeks. This is one reason why athletes in various sports begin a reconditioning program a month or two prior to the start of the competitive season. Many ex-athletes are in poorer physiologic condition several years after they retire from active participation than the 50-year-old business executive who has played handball 1 hour a day, 3 days a week, since college days.

An optimal state of functional capacity can be developed and maintained through activities such as tennis, handball, swimming, bicycling, volleyball, vigorous dancing, or backpacking, as well as through organized programs of jogging and calisthenics. In fact, the simple and practical activity of skipping rope or exercising to music can be easily adapted to formulate a program of aerobic conditioning. Many programs will work; the important point is to select a group of activities that blend with your personality and life style.

A Word of Caution Before You Begin

Before beginning a program a *medical checkup* is recommended. A sudden burst of vigorous exercise could be dangerous to some people. For example, intense physical activity coupled with certain environmental conditions may aggravate an existing asthmatic condition. People with a tendency toward high blood pressure should refrain from heavy lifting or straining exercises that may cause temporary yet rapid increases in heart rate and blood pressure above a safe level. Those over the age of 35 and certain "coronary-prone" younger people who possess a cluster of risk factors such as obesity, hypertension, diabetes, sedentary life style, cigarette smoking, and a family history of early heart disease are urged to obtain an electrocardiogram, preferably one administered during increasing levels of exercise.

There is no evidence that participation in intense physical exercise will damage a normal heart. In fact, the circulatory system adapts to exercise by an increase in its performance capacity. The exercise or *stress electrocardiogram*, may pick up subtle changes in the heart muscle that indicate the early development of coronary heart disease. Apparently healthy people may seriously harm themselves if after years of sedentary living, they decide suddenly to become active by running a mile, climbing a mountain, or shoveling the snow from the front walk. This does not mean that the coronary-prone or those with existing coronary heart disease should avoid exercise. On the contrary, with objective medical advice, exercise can properly be prescribed to improve capacity for exercise. Such programs may also have a positive effect in retarding the progression of the cardiovascular degenerative process. For this reason exercise "cardiac clubs" are flourishing throughout the country. Such groups engage in regular *aerobic exercise* at the proper intensity for the purpose of improving overall fitness and possibly reducing the risks of a heart attack.

9

Conditioning for Muscular Strength

IN TRAINING for muscular strength the overload principle is applied by the use of weights (dumbbells or barbells), immovable bars, straps, pulleys, or springs, or water, air, and oil hydraulic devices. There is nothing unique in the use of a barbell or spring, or any heavy object to improve muscular strength. In each case the muscle responds to the *intensity* of the overload rather than to a preference for the actual method of overload.

In general, the muscular overload is created by either increasing the load or *resistance*, increasing the number of times or *repetitions* the exercise is performed, increasing the *speed* of muscular contraction, or by various combinations of these.

Three exercise systems are commonly used for developing muscular strength: (1) *weight training*, (2) *isometric training*, and (3) *isokinetic training*.

Types of Strength Training

WEIGHT TRAINING

This is a popular system of strength training that involves the use of weight plates, barbells and dumbbells, or a variety of exercise machines in which the muscles exert tension to overcome a fixed or variable resistance during muscular contraction. There are three basic types of muscular contractions: *eccentric*, *concentric*, and *isometric*.

1. Eccentric contraction: This occurs when a muscle *lengthens* at a controlled rate as it contracts under tension. Figure 9-1A illustrates an eccentric muscular contraction. The weight is lowered but at a speed that acts against the force of gravity. The muscles of the upper arm increase in length as they contract eccentrically in an attempt to prevent the weight from crashing to the floor.

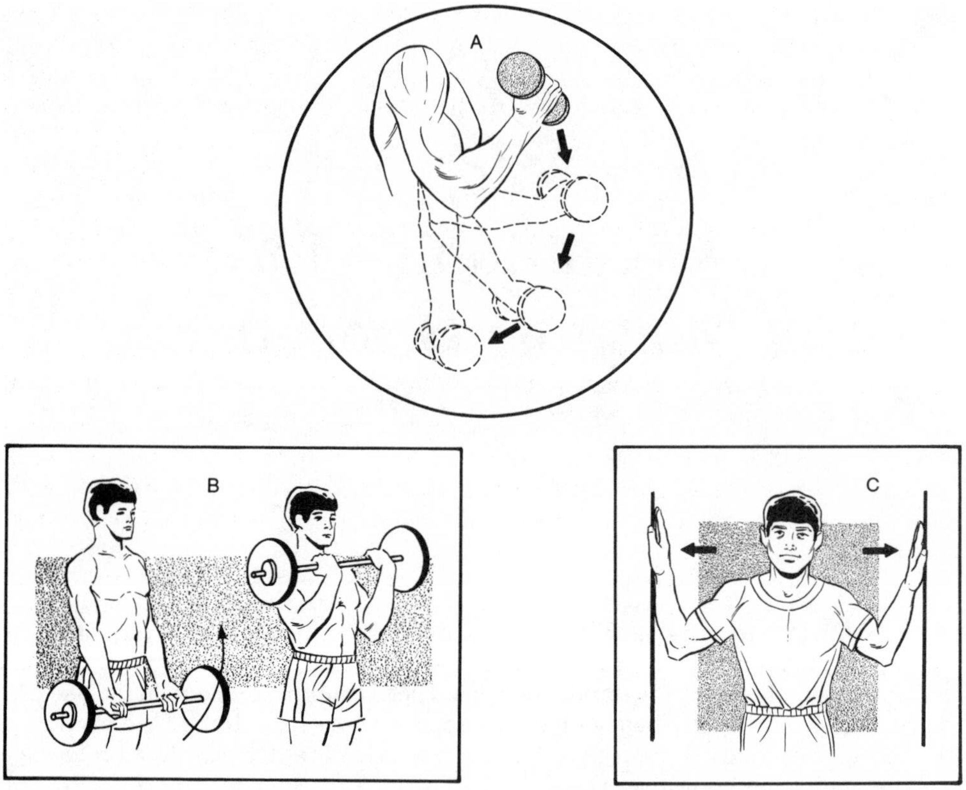
A
B
C

Figure 9-1. *A. Eccentric contraction; B. Concentric contraction; C. Isometric contraction.*

2. Concentric contraction: This is the most common type of muscular contraction and occurs in rhythmical activities where the muscle *shortens* as it develops tension. The muscles contract concentrically in most sport activities. Figure 9-1B illustrates a concentric muscular contraction during the raising of a dumbbell from the extended to the flexed position. It is possible to perform double concentric contractions (flexion and extension) with exercise equipment specifically designed for this purpose. Examples include Hydra Fitness hydraulic resistance machines (Hydra-Fitness Industries, Belton, TX) and Keiser Cam resistance machines (Keiser, Fresno, CA). With both systems, the flexion and extension movements are performed in rapid succession, and can be done "all out" to attempt to create maximum tension output throughout the range of movement at a particular contractile velocity of movement. The machines can be preset so movement occurs at either a pre-set speed that remains constant or a pre-set speed initially that then varies during movement depending on the exerciser's level of strength.

   In the latter situation, consider two people who both start an exercise at the same pre-set speed on the machine. If the first person is stronger, the exercise will be done at a faster contractile velocity (with a higher tension and power output) than the other person who is not as strong. In the case of hydraulic resistance exercise performed with Hydra-Fitness equipment, for example, the number of reps done in 20 seconds of "all-out" exercise at resistance setting 5 for arm curl/arm extension exercise by a strong person is 12 reps; for a weak subject, only 8 reps can be completed in 20 seconds. Both people pull and push as hard as they can, but the stronger person can sustain a higher power output during the double concentric exercise than the weaker person, and thus actually works at a faster rate of movement.

This form of exercise, where there is both a change in force output and a change in contractile velocity during the motion is referred to as *omnikinetic.* When the right and left limbs contract simultaneously, the contraction is *unidirectional;* when one limb can flex while the opposing limb extends, the contraction is called *bi-directional reciprocal.* If multiple contractions are performed by both limbs, the appropriate terminology would be *bi-directional, reciprocal alternating double concentric!* As you can see from this example, many movements are possible and the combinations are as difficult to keep track of for the scientist as for the exercisor!

3. Isometric contraction: This occurs when a muscle attempts to shorten but is unable to overcome the resistance. Considerable muscular force may be generated during an isometric contraction with *no noticeable shortening* of the muscle. Figure 9-1C illustrates an isometric muscular contraction.

   Both eccentric and concentric contractions are commonly referred to as *isotonic* because in both cases movement occurs. With such contractions, muscular force is developed either to overcome or to control the resistance during movement. The term isotonic is derived from the Greek word *isotonos* (*iso,* the same or equal; *tonos,* tension or strain). Actually, the use of this term is imprecise when applied to most muscular actions that involve movement because muscular tension varies as the joint angle changes—it does not remain constant.

ISOMETRIC TRAINING

This system of strength training was popular in the decade from 1955 to 1965. Research in Germany during this time showed that an increase in isometric strength of about 5% a week could be achieved by performing a single, maximum contraction of only 1 second's duration each day! Repeating this contraction between 5 and 10 times daily produced even greater increases in isometric strength. Although isometric training can provide a quick and convenient method for overloading and strengthening the muscular system, certain limitations make this means of strength training less than desirable, especially for most sport activities.

One major drawback of the isometric method is the difficulty of obtaining knowledge or results concerning the effectiveness of the program. Because there is almost no muscular movement, it is difficult to determine if the person's strength is actually improving, or if an overload force is being exerted. The measurement of isometric force requires specialized laboratory equipment not available at most exercise facilities. Another basic limitation is that isometric strength development is specific to the angle at which the isometric force is applied and developed. In other words, pushing against an immovable object as illustrated in Figure 9-1C will develop isometric strength at the particular joint angle at which the force is applied. The greatest increases in isometric strength will then occur when the strength is measured in nearly the exact position at which isometric training took place. There is little if any transfer of isometric strength developed at one joint angle to other body positions, even when the same muscles are involved! Thus, the muscle trained isometrically is stronger when measured isometrically, and particularly when measured at the specific joint angle at which the isometric overload was applied.

Isometric exercise can be effective for developing the "total" strength of a particular muscle or group of muscles if the isometric force is applied at four or five angles in the joint range of motion. This can be time-consuming, especially if conventional isotonic methods are available. Isometric training may be desirable and beneficial for special orthopedic applications that require accurate strength assessment and specific rehabilitation. With isometric training, the exact area of muscle weakness can be isolated and strengthening exercises administered at the proper joint angle.

ISOKINETIC TRAINING

Isokinetic exercise training is quite different from both the conventional isotonic and isometric systems. Recall that isotonic training occurs against an external load that generally remains constant throughout the movement, while isometric or static training is performed against an immovable load. In contrast, isokinetic exercise works against a resistance that permits movement at a preset, fixed speed, and enables the muscle to mobilize its maximum tension-generating capacity throughout the full range of movement *while shortening.* This is done with the aid of a mechanical device that contains a speed-controlling mechanism that accelerates to a preset speed when force is applied. Once a constant speed is attained, the isokinetic loading mechanism accommodates to provide a counterforce equal to the force generated by the muscle.

A distinction can be made between a muscle loaded isotonically and one loaded isokinetically. In isotonic or weightlifting exercises the inertia or initial resistance of the load must be first overcome; then the execution of the movement progresses. The weight of the resistance can be no heavier than the maximum strength of the weakest muscle acting in the particular movement. Otherwise the movement would not be completed. Consequently, the amount of force generated by the muscles during an isotonic contraction does not attain maximum levels throughout *all* phases of the movement. In an isokinetically loaded muscle the desired speed of movement occurs almost immediately, and the muscle is able to generate a peak power output at a specific but controlled speed of contraction.

The application of the isokinetic principle for overloading muscles to achieve their maximum power outputs has been used widely in sports medicine and athletic training. Many rehabilitation programs utilize isokinetic training to recondition injured limbs in their full range of motion.

Muscular Adaptations with Strength Training

The gross structural and microscopic changes that occur within muscle tissue as a result of overload training are fairly well documented. Considerable attention has also focused on the role of psychologic and learning factors in determining and modifying the expression of muscular strength.

PSYCHOLOGIC FACTORS

A unique series of experiments conducted in 1961 illustrated clearly the importance of psychologic factors in the acquisition of muscular strength. The strength of the arm muscles was determined for 17 male and 8 female subjects prior to various psychologic treatments. The strength scores served as the baseline for all subsequent comparisons. In one series of experiments, the researchers measured arm strength while intermittent gunshots were fired behind the subjects just before their exertions. At another time they instructed the subjects to shout or scream loudly at the moment force was exerted. Following the "shoot and shout" experiments, the experimenters measured subjects' strength under the influence of two disinhibitory drugs, alcohol and amphetamines or "pep pills." They also measured strength while subjects were in a posthypnotic state and were told their strength would be greater than ever before and they should have no fear of injury. In almost all of the "psychologic" conditions, arm strength was significantly greater than under normal conditions. The greatest strength increases were observed under hypnosis, the most "mental" of all the treatments. To explain these observations the researchers suggested that physical factors such as the size and type of muscle fibers and the anatomic lever arrangement of bone and muscle ultimately determine a person's capacity for muscular strength. They took the position that psychologic or mental factors within the central nervous system exert neural influences that prevent most people from achieving this strength capacity. *Inhibitions* within the central nervous system might be the result of social conditioning, unpleasant past experiences with physical activity, or an overprotective home environment. When performing under intense emotional conditions, such as athletic competition, an emergency situation, or posthypnotic suggestion, the inhibitory neural mechanisms may be reduced so much that the person is often capable of a "super performance" that more closely matches the physiologically determined capacity.

Observations such as these help to explain the apparent beneficial effects of "psyching" or the almost self-induced hypnosis of athletes before competition. Excellent examples of such *disinhibition* can be observed in weightlifters, high-jumpers and other track and field competitors, and self-defense experts who perform nontraditional skills such as smashing cement bricks with their hands and feet. The great feats of strength observed during emotionally laden emergency situations also fit nicely into this explanation. In addition, the rapid improvements in muscular strength made during the first few weeks of a strength training program may largely be due to a learning phenomenon as well as to the lessening of fear and psychologic inhibition as the person becomes more accustomed to performing in the strength activity.

MUSCULAR FACTORS

Although psychologic inhibitions as well as learning factors greatly modify ability to express muscular strength, the ultimate limit of strength development is determined by anatomic and physiologic factors within the muscle. These factors are not immutable and can be modified with strength training. The gross structural and microscopic changes in muscles that occur as a result of strength training are usually accompanied by substantial increases in muscular strength.

The large size of the skeletal muscles of weightlifters results from hypertrophy of individual muscle cells. Hypertrophy is due to an increase in the size of the already existing small muscle fibers in relation to the cross-sectional size of the larger fibers. The growth that occurs in the fast twitch fibers, results from an increase in the cellular materials within the muscle cell; there is an increase in the contractile proteins, actin and myosin, as well as an increase in enzymes and nutrients. There is no definitive evidence to indicate that muscular overload significantly stimulates the development of new muscle fibers. In addition to enlarging the existing muscle fibers, muscular overload thickens and strengthens the connective tissue that surrounds the muscle, the tendons that attach the muscle to the bone, and the ligaments that attach bones to bones.

Muscular Strength of Men and Women

When strength is compared on an *absolute* basis (that is total force applied or weight lifted), women generally possess about 70% of the force generating capacity of men. This difference is magnified in comparisons of upper body strength where the female is about 50% weaker than the male. Certainly there are exceptions to this generalization, especially for women involved in muscle strengthening and conditioning programs. When body size and body composition are considered, the large absolute strength differences between genders is reduced considerably. For example, when muscular strength is expressed in relation to force capacity per unit of lean body weight (body weight minus body fat), the strength differences are reduced considerably between men and women. These observations provide a strong argument that few gender differences exist in muscle quality; per unit of muscle size, men and women have similar strength. From a practical standpoint, however, because men generally develop a larger muscle mass than women, their absolute strength is proportionately greater. Also, because women usually have more body fat than men they are in a sense, loaded down with more "dead weight" than male counterparts of the same body weight. Consequently, their strength per unit of body weight is also usually lower.

Strength Training for Women

One of the more vivid and positive illustrations of the redefinition of women's roles in society has been their present attitude toward and participation in a wide range of competitive sport and physical activity experiences. Some women are still concerned, however, about the expected "masculinizing" effects of some activities, particularly strength development by use of resistance training procedures. Although muscular strength appears to be a major factor in achieving optimum performance in many sport activities, many women have shied away from strength training exercises for fear of developing the enlarged or bulging muscles that are so commonly observed for men. This is unfortunate because the failure of many women to learn the basic skills and improve in activities such as tennis, golf, dance, and gymnastics can be directly attributed to a lack of sufficient muscular strength, especially upper-body strength. A proper program of strength training can usually improve such muscular weakness.

Women who participate in resistance training programs are capable of making strength improvements similar to men's *generally without* the accompanying excessive muscular hypertrophy. In one series of studies, changes in the size and strength of 47 untrained college-aged women and 26 untrained college-aged men were evaluated during a 10-week weight training program. Before training, the men's strength was about 28 and 26% greater than that of the women for muscle groups of the upper and lower body, respectively. Much of these strength differences were due to the larger body size of the men because when strength was expressed in relation to body weight (strength per pound of body weight), no gender differences in strength appeared. After completing 10 weeks of weight training, both men and women showed significant and almost equal improvement in muscular strength, with improvements of approximately 30% in some areas of the body. It should be noted that the differences in muscular strength between genders observed at the beginning of the program still existed. However, after training the strength of the women was greater than that of the men as measured at the start of the program! While the muscles of the men became significantly enlarged with training, there was no increase in muscle size for the women. The authors suggested that hormonal differences between the genders, especially in the male hormone *testosterone*, account in part for the differences in muscular enlargement during strength training. Women can significantly increase their present level of muscular strength with conventional resistance training procedures with little fear of developing bulging or "overdeveloped" muscles.

Metabolic Stress of Resistance Training

Numerous claims have been advertised concerning the physical benefits to be derived from various strength training programs. These include the promise of improved "organic vigor," reduced body fat, and improved cardiovascular functioning. A properly planned program of resistance training can provide an effective means for developing and maintaining muscular strength.

Energy Cost of Weight Lifting. In a series of experiments in one of our laboratories, we studied the immediate effects of isometric and weight lifting exercises on overall cardiovascular functioning. The weightlifting exercises were performed with a weight that enabled the students to complete eight repetitions of a particular movement. A 6-second isometric contraction was performed against a bar placed in a position halfway through the range of motion of the corresponding weightlifting exercise. In this experiment we studied the two-arm curl, two-arm press, bench press, and squat.

The results we obtained for heart rate and oxygen consumption indicated that both isometric and weightlifting exercises would be classified as *light to moderate* in terms of energy expenditure, even though considerable stress is placed on the involved muscle groups. The rate of oxygen consumed during weight training was equivalent to walking at a pace of 4 miles per hour, gardening, or swimming at a slow speed. Although a person may perform 15 or 20 different exercises during a 1-hour weight training session, the amount of time devoted to the exercise per se is short, usually no longer than 6 or 7 minutes. This short activity period that produces only mild metabolic stress indicates that traditional isometric and weightlifting programs would not be effective for improving circulatory capacity for activities like running or swimming. Furthermore, they would not be effective as major activities in weight-reducing programs because the caloric expenditure during an exercise session is relatively low.

Energy Cost of Circuit Weight Training. By modifying the approach to standard strength training methods so that heavy muscle overload is deemphasized, it is possible to increase the caloric cost of exercise and bring about improvements in more than one aspect of fitness. Current research has focused on the energy cost and cardiorespiratory effect of *circuit weight training.* In this form of training, different resistance exercises are performed in a preestablished exercise-rest sequence. In most programs, the circuit consists of 8 to 12 exercise stations with a prescribed number of repetitions, usually 15 to 20, performed for each exercise. Exercise is usually performed at an intensity that requires between 40 and 50% of maximum force generating capacity.

In one experiment, the energy expended during circuit weight training was determined for 20 men and 20 women. They performed three exercise circuits (10 stations per circuit utilizing weight machines); there was a 15-second rest interval between exercises. The total time to perform the three circuits was 22.5 minutes. The net amount of energy expended, that excluded the resting metabolism, was 129 kcal for the men and 95 kcal for the women for the total exercise period. At this level of energy expenditure, the heart rate averaged 142 (72% maximum heart rate) and 158 beats per minute (82% max heart rate) for the men and women, respectively. This corresponded to an exercise intensity of about 41% of maximum oxygen uptake capacity for the men and 45% of maximum for the women. Because the rate of energy expenditure for this weight training circuit was related to an individual's body weight, the results in Table 9-1 for net energy expenditure are presented in terms of body weight. On the average, the level of energy expended for circuit weight training was approximately the equivalent of a slow jog (11 minutes:30 seconds per mile or 5.2 mph pace), hiking in the hills at a moderate pace, or playing

Table 9-1. *Net energy expenditure of circuit weight training in men and women.*

	KCAL EXPENDED PER MINUTE[a]											
BODY WEIGHT, POUNDS	100	110	120	130	140	150	160	170	180	190	200	210
Men			4.1	4.4	4.8	5.1	5.4	5.7	6.0	6.4	6.7	7.0
Women	3.4	3.6	3.7	3.9	4.1	4.3	4.4	4.6	4.8			

[a] Calculated from the data of Wilmore, J.H. and others. Energy cost of circuit weight training. *Medicine and Science in Sports 10:75,* 1978. To determine the total number of calories expended during workouts (over and above rest), multiply the value in the column that corresponds to your body weight by the duration of the circuit. For example, a 160-pound male who exercises on the circuit for 43 minutes would expend 232 kcal (5.4 kcal/min × 43 min).

in a basketball game, a tennis match, or leisurely swimming the crawl stroke. At this energy output, for example, a 130-pound woman working for 22 minutes per workout would expend an additional 1000 kcal a month if she performed the total circuit 3 times a week. At this rate, providing food intake and other physical activities remained unchanged, it would require about 14 weeks to reduce body weight the equivalent of 1 pound of fat. Her 170-pound male counterpart would burn 1500 extra kcal per month or the equivalent of 1 pound of fat every 9 to 10 weeks.

In terms of improving the cardiovascular system, there are conflicting reports concerning the improvements to be expected. While one experiment concluded that circuit weight training that made use of weight machines had a negligible effect on improving cardiovascular function and did little to improve flexibility, other studies report more positive results for both aerobic fitness and body composition. Clearly, more research is needed in this area, particularly for comparisons of different ways of measuring improvements and the various types of exercise circuits and equipment such as free weights, pulley and cam devices, hydraulic cylinders, isotonic-type machines, and especially the new generation of computer controlled, force and power resistive equipment.

Energy Cost of Hydraulic Resistance Exercise

Recent experiments in one of our laboratories have focused on the cardiovascular and metabolic response to omnikinetic* exercise (performed on hydraulic resistance equipment).

Experiment 1. *Pulse rate response during a 13-week circuit-type training program.* Pulse rate response was measured during and immediately following 11 different exercises that were performed in circuit fashion utilizing a 20-second exercise and 30-second rest period between exercises. Two circuits (22 exercises) were performed; the first at what would be classified as moderate resistance while the second was relatively hard exercise. Pulse rate was monitored daily in 15 college men and 13 women who participated in the 13-week, thrice weekly training program. In addition to higher pulse counts for men compared to women on all exercises at both resistive settings, the average pulse for both groups throughout the training period, including the rest pauses, exceeded 70% of maximum pulse. For exercise on some machines, notably the squat, the pulse averaged 85% of maximum for men and 84% of maximum for women.

Experiment 2: *Heart rate and metabolic response to shoulder, chest, and leg omnikinetic exercise.* Twenty college males exercised on two separate days; there were three sets of leg exercise (LE), chest exercise (CE), and shoulder exercise (SE). The duration of exercise was 20 seconds with a 20-second rest interval and 5-minute rest pause between each exercise mode. The average oxygen consumption based on the average of three sets for each exercise mode was 2.1 (LE), 1.9 (CE), and 1.7 (SE) liters/minute. In relation to the maximal aerobic capacity, the oxygen consumption was 57.4% (LE), 51.9% (CE), and 49.2% (SE) of the maximum

* Omnikinetic refers to concentric contractions that permit *variable* speed of movement and variable muscle power output, depending on the initial "strength" of the person. The hydraulic nature of the cylinders in the exercise machine permit such contractions to take place. These are in contrast to fixed, weight plates, cam devices, or other systems that permit movement at a *controlled* speed of movement that is set on the device manually, or by computer control.

response. In terms of caloric expenditure, it averaged 9.0 kcal a minute. The average heart rate response in relation to the maximum heart rate for LE was 85.4%, 85.2% for CE, and 83.1% for SE. These findings demonstrate that leg, chest, and shoulder omnikinetic exercise significantly augmented energy expenditure and heart rate response above the minimum threshold level recommended to promote improvements in cardiorespiratory function. As a frame of comparison in terms of calorie expenditure, the hydraulic exercises were approximately 35% higher than exercise with free weights, 29.4% greater than the average caloric expenditure based on two studies using Nautilus, and 11.5% higher caloric output than circuit exercise with Universal equipment. Walking at a normal pace on the level for a 150 pound man would require 5.4 calories a minute.

Experiment 3. *Physiological response and energy cost of submaximal and maximal rowing exercise in men and women.* Ten men and 10 women performed 2 submaximal and 2 maximal "all-out" tests on a hydraulic rower (Pro-Row 2000, Hydra-Fitness, Belton, TX), and treadmill (TM) $\dot{V}O_2$ max test. The first 4 stages of the max row tests were done at 30 cycles a minute and force output was set at 50% of maximal arm rowing force at the specified resistance settings. After stage 4, subjects performed "all out" to exhaustion. The Max 1 row test was 17 minutes in duration performed at 6 resistance settings (1 = easy, 6 = hard) for 5,5,3,2,1 and 1 minutes, respectively. The Max 2 row test was identical to Max 1 through stage 4, resistance was then reduced to setting 2 for the rest of the test. Caloric cost (open circuit spirometry) was also measured during two, 30 minute row tests (30 cycles a minute at resistance setting 3, and steady state $\dot{V}O_2$ and heart rate was calculated from minutes 15 to 30.

Oxygen Consumption (ml/kg · min)

	TM	MAX 1 ROW	MAX 2 ROW	STEADY STATE ROW
Men	56.6	39.5	46.6	31.6
Women	51.3	35.6	43.8	29.6

For the steady state rows, energy cost per minute was 11.6 kcal for men and 9.0 kcal for women; this was equivalent to level running on a treadmill at 6.0 mph for men and 4.7 mph for women. The Max 2 row was more effective than Max 1 row for eliciting near maximal cardiovascular responses (80–83% TM max and 85% TM max HR). Rowing for 30 minutes at 30 cycles a minute at 50% of maximal arm force capacity met the American College of Sports Medicine guidelines for exercise intensity to improve cardiovascular function. When the data for rowing with the hydraulic rower are compared to other forms of "large muscle" exercise, it turns out the *rowing exercise burns considerable calories,* and can certainly be classified as intense or unduly heavy exercise in terms of energy expenditure.

Specificity of Strength

The correct application of force in relatively complex, learned movements such as the tennis serve or the shot-put depends on a series of coordinated neuromuscular patterns and not *just* the strength of the muscle groups recruited during the movement. The complex interaction between the nervous and muscular systems provides some explanation for the observation that the leg muscles, when strengthened in an activity like squats or deep knee bends, do not usually show improved force capability when used in another leg movement such as jumping. In fact, a group of muscles strengthened with weights does not generate an equal improvement in force when measured isometrically. Consequently strengthening muscles for use in a specific activity such as golf, rowing, swimming, or football requires more than just identifying and overloading muscles involved in the movement. It requires that training be *specific* with regard to the exact movements involved. Training the muscles of the arms to become stronger by weightlifting does not necessarily mean that the performance of all subsequent arm movements will be improved. Generally, there will be little transfer of newly acquired strength to other types of movements, even though the same muscles are involved. *To improve a specific performance by the strengthened musculature, one must train the muscles with movements as close as possible to those used in the desired movement or actual skill.*

An intelligent application of the principle of specificity of strength training is used by football linemen who develop specific leg "strengths" by pushing weighted blocking sleds in a position and movement pattern similar to the act of blocking during a football game. Some swimmers apply specific overload to their back and shoulder muscles by using isokinetic-type "swimming machines" that enable them to train their muscles in a manner reasonably similar to the muscular action close to the velocity involved in a particular stroke. Leg strength for jumping in basketball would probably best be developed by applying overload in the movement pattern of the actual jump.

Organizing a Strength Training Program

This section presents basic guidelines concerning strength training. People without previous experience in strength training should follow a program designed to produce all-around improvements in muscular strength. Appendix E illustrates basic "free-weight" exercises that can be done with minimal equipment. The exercises are designed to strengthen and tone the neck, arms, shoulders, chest, abdomen, back, buttocks, and legs.

THE WARM-UP

The value of warm-up or preliminary exercise in preventing muscle and joint injuries, as well as in improving performance, has been frequently and perhaps justifiably challenged over the years. Although the scientific basis for recommending a warm-up on these grounds is not conclusive, we feel it would be unwise to completely ignore warm-ups until there is more substantial evidence justifying their elimination. Furthermore, evidence is now available to indicate that moderate preliminary exercise improves the cardiovascular response to subsequent strenuous exercise. It appears that adjustments in blood flow within the heart muscle to a sudden and vigorous bout of exercise are not instantaneous and even healthy individuals may show poor oxygen supply to the heart under such conditions. However, with a prior warm-up of 2 minutes of easy jogging, the adjustments in blood flow and oxygen supply are much more favorable. Any sequence of calisthenic and flexibility exercises can be used as a warm-up, as well as running in place or other moderate and rhythmic exercises. The warm-up exercises illustrated in Figure 9-2 serve this purpose and can be completed in a few minutes. These exercises will gradually increase circulation and body flexibility, and may help deter muscle and joint injury.

The stretching or flexibility exercises should be done slowly and smoothly until you feel a mild tension on your muscles. The goal is not to complete many repetitions of the particular exercise, but rather to *hold* the stretching movement. A reasonable goal to achieve is to hold the stretch for about 10 seconds in the beginning; as flexibility improves, individuals should increase the duration of the static stretch to 30 seconds. Stretching that employs fast bouncing and jerky movement that use the body's momentum can strain or tear muscles and may actually set up a reflex action that will resist the muscle's stretching.

THE LOWER BACK

The lower back is one of the areas of the body most susceptible to injury. Many people lose considerable time at work, suffer chronic discomfort, and spend large amounts of money on orthopedists and chiropractors in an attempt to alleviate the pain caused by problems with the lower back. In fact, it has been estimated that one-half of the United States work force will suffer from back problems at some point during their career! In 1979, for example, accidents led to 245 milllion lost workdays, of which 200 million days were attributable to back injuries. The causes of this malady are not always apparent and the cure is elusive. However, many orthopedists feel the prime factors in "low back syndrome" are *muscular weakness*, especially in the abdominal region, and *poor joint flexibility* in the back and legs. Both strengthening and flexibility exercises are commonly prescribed for the prevention of and rehabilitation from chronic low back strain.

The use of strength training exercises poses a dilemma. If done properly, such training can provide an excellent means for strengthening the muscles of the abdomen and lower back. As is often the case, however, many people, attempting to lift too much weight, perform the exercises improperly. As a result additional muscle groups are recruited, the spinal column is placed in improper alignment, especially with the arching of the back, and lower back strain results. A seemingly simple exercise such as a sit-up, if done improperly with the legs stiff, the back arched and the head thrown back, can place tremendous strain on the lower spine (sit ups should always be done with the knees flexed). Pressing and curling exercises with weights, if performed with excessive hyperextension or arch to the back may cause a muscle strain or spinal pressure that can trigger lower back pain. For these reasons, those who begin a program of strengthening exercises are urged to do all exercises correctly in the manner described. One should never sacrifice proper execution to lift a heavier load or "squeeze out" an additional repetition. The extra weight lifted through improper technique will not facilitate strengthening the desired muscle groups, and may precipitate injury to the lower back.

SELECTING THE PROPER WEIGHT

In the beginning stages of a program, people should not attempt to see how much weight they can lift. This serves little purpose in improving strength and greatly increases the likelihood of muscle or joint injury. *It is unnecessary to exercise at maximum levels to develop muscular strength.* A resistance or load that represents between 60 and 80% of a muscle group's maximum strength or

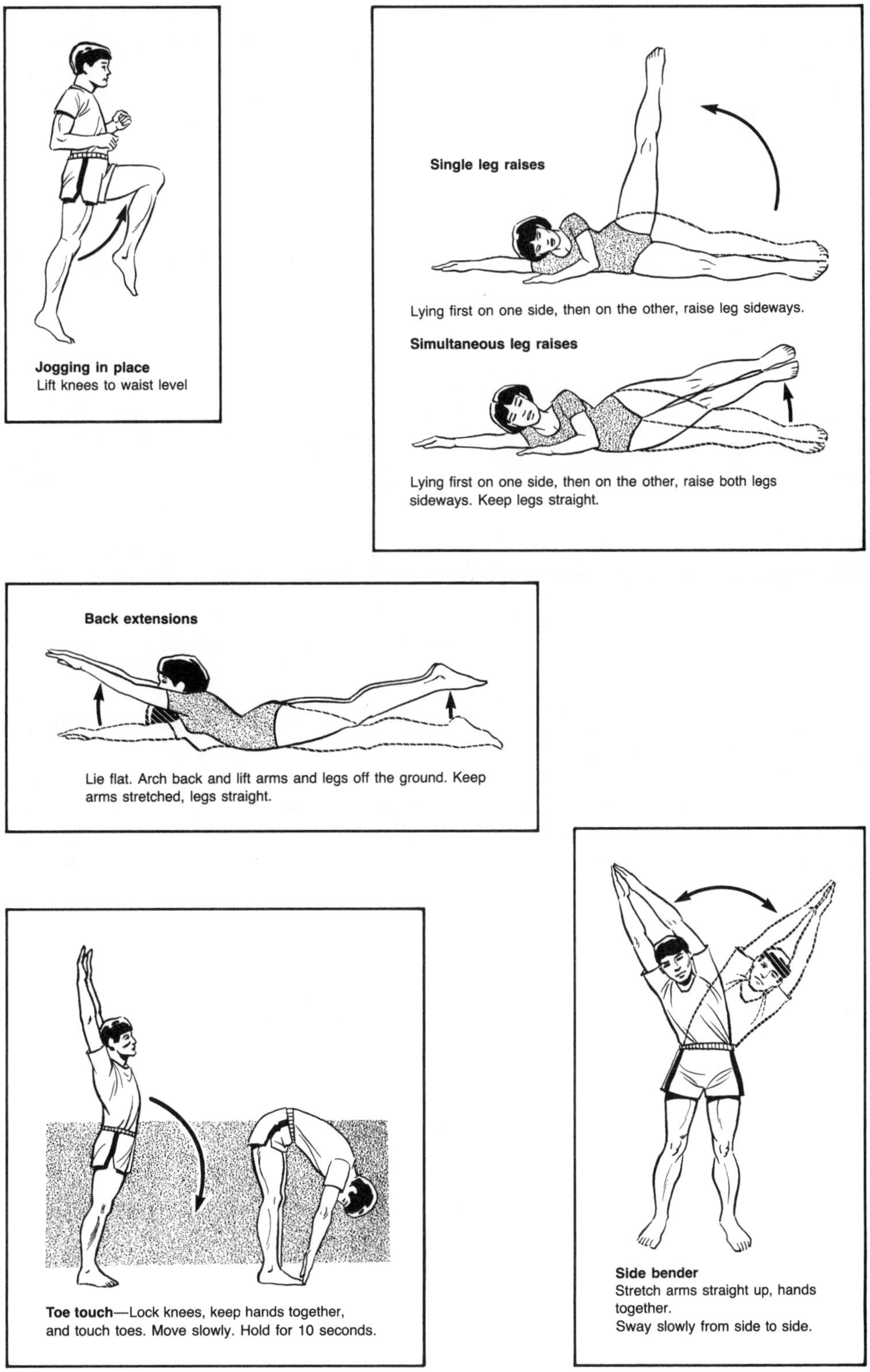
Jogging in place
Lift knees to waist level
Single leg raises
Lying first on one side, then on the other, raise leg sideways.
Simultaneous leg raises
Lying first on one side, then on the other, raise both legs sideways. Keep legs straight.
Back extensions
Lie flat. Arch back and lift arms and legs off the ground. Keep arms stretched, legs straight.
Toe touch—Lock knees, keep hands together, and touch toes. Move slowly. Hold for 10 seconds.
Side bender
Stretch arms straight up, hands together.
Sway slowly from side to side.

Figure 9-2. *Examples of calisthenic and flexibility exercises that can be performed as part of a "warm-up" prior to muscle training.*

force generating capacity is usually sufficient overload to produce gains in strength. When using barbells, weighted plates or pully and cam machines, such a resistance permits the completion of between 6 and 8 repetitions of a particular exercise. Our experience with barbells has shown that beginners should attempt to complete 12 repetitions of an exercise. The amount of weight lifted during 12 repetitions will not place an excessive strain on the muscles during the beginning phase of the muscular conditioning program. If the weight selected for the 12 repetitions feels "too easy," a heavier weight should be used. If the exerciser cannot do 12 repetitions, the weight is too heavy. This is a trial and error process and it may take several exercise sessions before a proper starting weight is selected.

After 5 or 6 exercise sessions the muscles will have adapted to the exercise, and the exerciser will have learned the correct movements involved in lifting. The number of repetitions should now be reduced to between 6 and 8 and the resistance increased accordingly. When the exerciser can complete 8 repetitions, add more weight. This additional weight will undoubtedly reduce the number of repetitions he or she can do. This is exactly the desired outcome. Eight repetitions should be achieved within several exercise sessions, and again, you will need to add more weight. This is one overload method that is generally used in weight training to increase the strength of a particular group of muscles. For a general strength conditioning program, select exercises that overload a variety of muscle groups. If strength training is geared to sports performance, specific exercises should be chosen that closely resemble the movements in the particular skill.

The exercises should be performed in the same order on each workout day. This is because many exercises involve more than one muscle group, and some fatigue may result from a previous exercise. By maintaining the same order of exercise, the cumulative fatigue effect should remain relatively constant. In scheduling workouts, consistency is the key to achieving a successful training effect. This does not mean that workouts should be scheduled every day. *From the relatively limited information available, at least 2 or 3 exercise sessions each week are necessary to continue strength improvements.* Some people exercise 5 or 6 days a week. However, with this protocol different muscle groups are usually exercised on alternate days, so in reality, a specific muscle group is still only trained 2 or 3 days a week.

SIX STEPS IN PLANNING THE WORKOUT

Step 1. Establish the primary aims and objectives of the strength training program. Strengthening exercises are performed for many different reasons: improved sports performance, development and maintenance of muscular tone or firmness, aesthetic enhancement, or fun and pleasure. Whatever the reason, include exercises that will help meet personal objectives. You should use a variety of exercises for an all-around strength conditioning program, with exercises for the neck, arms, forearms, shoulders, abdomen, back, chest, buttocks, and legs.

Step 2. Determine the length of time available for exercise. Work schedules and other restraints often pose limitations on the number of exercises that someone can complete during a workout. A minimum of about 15 minutes is usually required to complete a series of basic exercises. This includes the rest intervals as well as the time spent in actual exercise.

Step 3. Determine the available facilities and equipment. It is not necessary to purchase expensive equipment; many household items can be used to provide muscular overload, and often people can construct equipment with minimal expense. The exercises shown in Figure 9-3 rely on common household and store

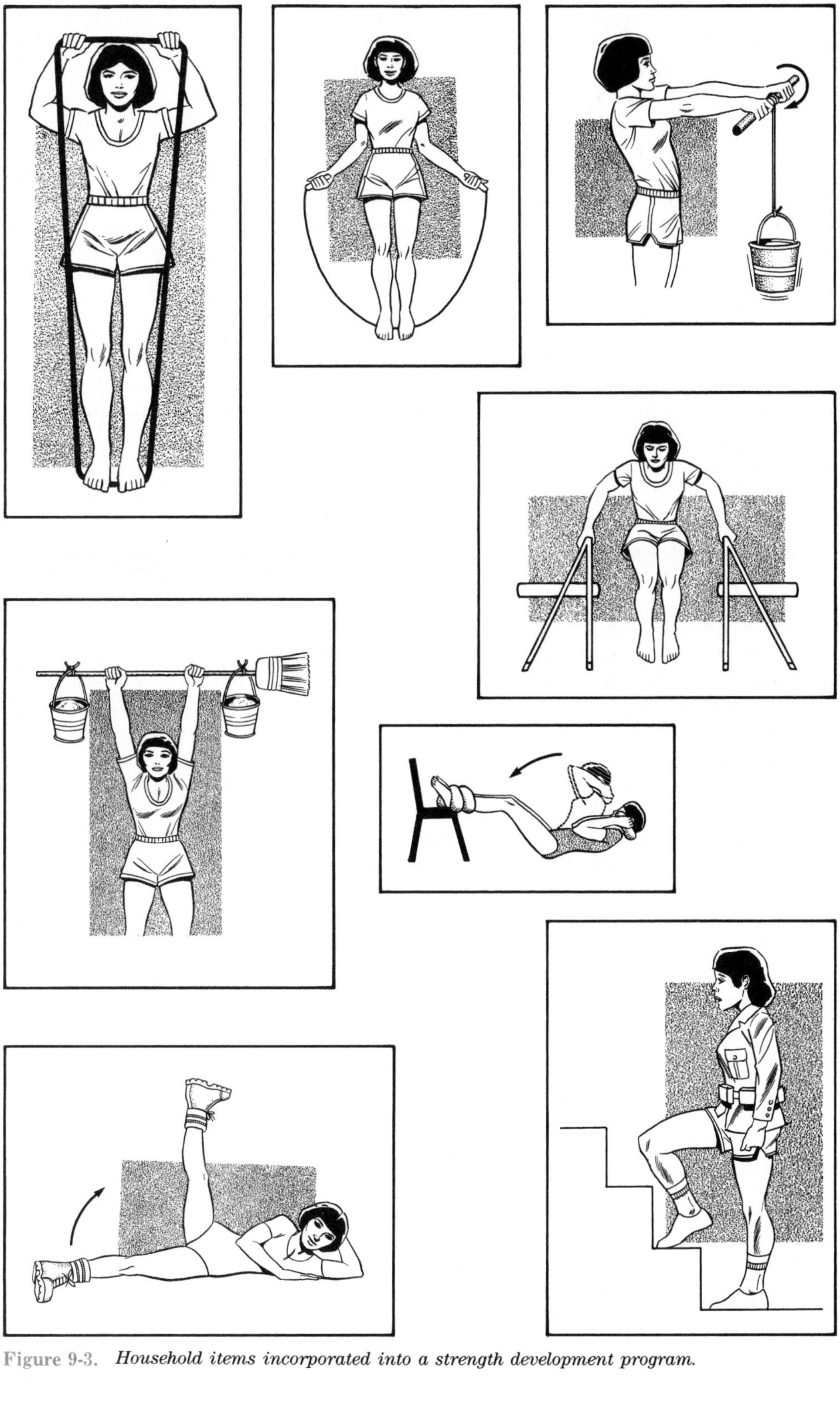

Figure 9-3. *Household items incorporated into a strength development program.*

items to construct strength training equipment. Weights can be made by filling plastic cleanser containers with water or filling socks and other clothes with sand. A broom or mop handle can serve as a bar to which these heavy objects can be attached. Ski boots, telephone books, bricks wrapped in a towel, and other objects can also provide the resistance to muscular contraction. Of course, barbells and dumbbells are the easiest to use and are relatively inexpensive. Chairs, table tops, and other household furniture items can take the place of standard gymnasium equipment. A piece of clothesline can be used as a jump rope.

Step 4. Selection of the exercises. A variety of exercises for strengthening the large muscle groups of the body are presented in Appendix E. These exercises represent basic "isotonic" exercises that should meet the needs of most people interested in toning the muscles and improving muscular strength. The exercises have been placed into one of three groups: (A) exercises for the neck, arms, and shoulders, (B) exercises for the chest, abdomen, and back, and (C) exercises for the buttocks and legs. In cases where exercises are illustrated without equipment, adaptations can be made by including weights. The shaded areas within each figure denote the muscle groups primarily affected by the exercise.

Step 5. Arrange an *exercise circuit,* similar to that described for circuit weight training. When arranging the exercises in a proper sequence, it is important not to perform consecutively two exercises that involve the same muscle groups. This way the possible transfer of fatigue effects will be minimized. For example, two exercises for the arms should be separated by other exercises that do not require the use of the arms in the same pattern of movement. Figure 9-4 illustrates the basic model of the circuit for hydraulic resistance exercise. In this example, there are 10 different exercise stations, with one exercise performed at each station. Because the principle of circuit exercise is universal in nature, the type of strengthening equipment used in the circuit is not the crucial element. Any type of equipment can be used from homemade cement "barbells" to the latest machines controlled by computers.

Each exercise may consist of any number of repetitions desired. Initially, when working with weights, 12 to 15 repetitions of each exercise are done until the proper load or resistance is established. After several weeks, add additional weights until a target number of 6 to 8 repetitions is achieved. The goal of this circuit could be simply to complete the desired exercises in the time available for the workout. When the target number of repetitions is achieved, add more weight. Another objective might be to perform the required number of repetitions of each exercise in the sequence within a *target time* previously established according to individual needs. For example, suppose the 10 exercise stations, each with one exercise to be performed 12 times, are to be completed twice. Initially, it may require 20 minutes to complete two circuits. This would then become the target time, and each exercise day the objective would be to complete two circuits within this time limit. As physiologic conditioning progresses, the target time will be achieved more easily. Once this occurs, several methods can be used to maintain a *progressive overload.* For example, a faster target time might be established. Other modifications could include the use of heavier weights while maintaining the 20-minute target time, or attempting to complete one additional circuit during the 20-minute exercise period. Thus circuits for the development of muscular strength can achieve overload by the manipulation of three variables: increase the load or resistance, increase the repetitions of exercise in the circuit, or decrease the target time. Each variable can be manipulated separately or in combination to ensure progressive overload.

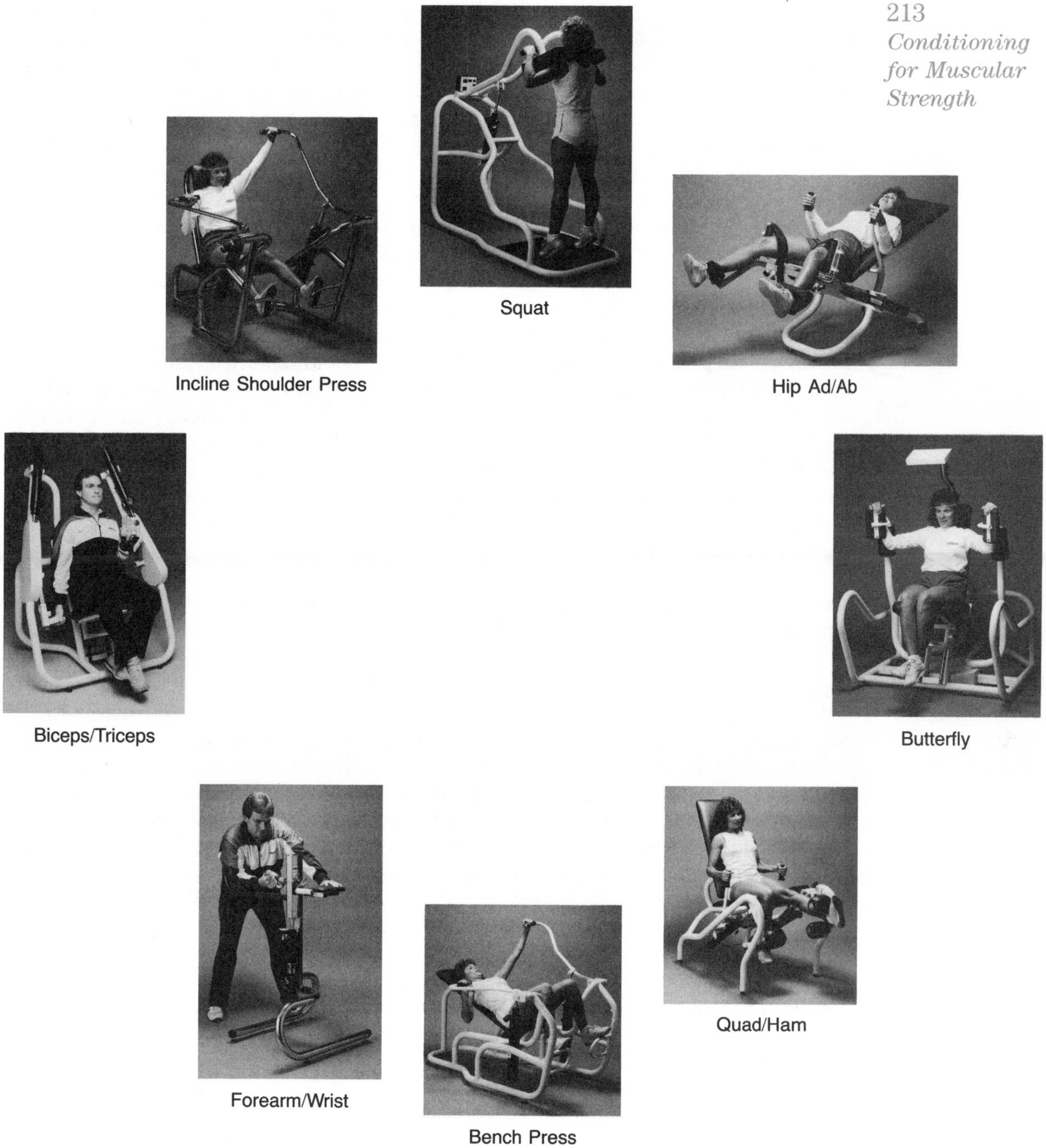
Squat
Incline Shoulder Press
Hip Ad/Ab
Biceps/Triceps
Butterfly
Quad/Ham
Forearm/Wrist
Bench Press

Figure 9-4. *Arrangement of an exercise circuit using hydraulic exercise devices. Each exercise should be designed for a different group of muscles. After completing an exercise at one station, the exerciser performs the next exercise in the circuit. To provide variety, music can be used to signal the start and end of each exercise and rest break. Louder volume can signal the start of exercise, and softer volume can signify the end of the rest period before proceeding to the next exercise. A reasonable exercise time is 20–30 seconds with a 20–40 second rest. At our own facilities, we use an exercise to rest ratio of 20:30 (20 seconds exercise, 30 seconds rest, 20 seconds exercise, and so on throughout the circuit). People usually complete 2 complete circuits, performing as many reps as they can during each exercise period. (Photos courtesy of Hydra-Fitness Industries, Belton, TX).*

It is also possible to apply the principle of overload to exercises that require little or no equipment. This is done by increasing the difficulty and thus the strenuousness of the exercise. For example, the conventional push-up can be made more difficult by changing the body position from horizontal (starting position on the level) to a slant by placing the feet on a 12- to 16-inch bench. The same can be done for sit-ups. Place the feet on the seat of a chair; hands are clasped behind the neck. Attempt to curl up until the elbows touch the knees, and then return to the starting position. This type of "incline" sit-up can be made even more strenuous if a weight is held across the chest or behind the head. A dumbbell, weight plate, or any other object that can be conveniently held will provide additional resistance to movement, and hence, will serve as an appropriate overload as fitness improves.

Step 6. The last step in planning the exercise workout involves the most efficient use of the available facilities. This is usually not a problem in gymnasiums or health clubs where specialized equipment and facilities are available. For those who exercise in their homes the situation is quite different and necessitates other solutions. In small or confined areas, progressing from one station to the next may not be possible. In this case, many exercises would have to be performed in one or two small areas. Sometimes, however, the constraints of exercising in a limited space makes a person more aware of the potential for using other available facilities, such as hallways, staircases, washrooms, dorm lounges, garages, or nearby parks and walk-ways.

We are aware of a muscular training and cardiovascular conditioning circuit arranged by a man who lived in a high rise apartment. He exercised 4 days a week, completing 3 circuits, each circuit consisting of 8 stations and 10 repetitions per station. Station 1 was sit-ups, done on the bedroom floor with knees bent and feet supported under the bed. He held a 10-pound weight behind his head. Station 2 consisted of pull-ups on a bar in the bathroom doorway. The exerciser wore a jacket filled with 20 pounds of sand. Station 3 was rope skipping in the hallway. To increase the intensity of this cardiovascular exercise, the exerciser wore ski boots while jumping at a rate of 100 skips a minute. Station 4 involved raising and lowering the body with the arms supported between two kitchen chairs, wearing the 20-pound jacket. Station 5 was performed on the living room floor. The exercise consisted of raising and lowering each leg while lying supported on the side, with a knee-high sock filled with 15 pounds of sand attached around the ankle. Station 6 was a chest press performed while lying supine on the floor, using a broom barbell with weights of plastic containers filled with 26 pounds of cement. Station 7 consisted of back extensions performed while lying face down over the edge of a coffee table with the feet secured under a rope tied around the table top, with a 10-pound weight held behind the head. Station 8 involved quickly descending and then ascending 5 flights of stairs. On the first and second circuit, stair climbing was done as fast as possible. Going up the stairs on the last circuit, the man hopped up each stair keeping his feet together, with only a minimal rest between floors!

Additional Reading

Caiozzo, V.J., et al.: Training-induced alterations of the in vivo force-velocity relationship of human muscle. *Journal of Applied Physiology: Respiration, Environmental, Exercise Physiology. 51:*750, 1981.

Costill, D.L., et al.: Adaptations in skeletal muscle following strength training. *Journal of Applied Physiology: Respiration, Environmental, Exercise Physiology. 46:*96, 1979.

Davies, K.J.A., et al.: Biochemical adaptation of mitochondria, muscle, and whole-animal respiration to endurance training. *Archives of Biochemistry and Biophysics. 209:*539, 1981.

Edstrom, L. and L. Grimby: Effect of exercise on the motor unit. *Muscle and Nerve. 9:*104, 1986.

Gettman, L.R. and M.L. Pollock: Circuit weight training: a critical review of its physiological benefits. *Physician and Sportsmedicine. 9:*44, 1980.

Gettman, L.R., et al.: A comparison of combined running and weight training with circuit weight training. *Medicine and Science in Sports and Exercise. 14:*229, 1982.

Goldberg, A.L., et al.: Mechanism of work induced hypertrophy. *Medicine and Science in Sports. 7:*185, 1975.

Gollnick, P.D. et al.: Fiber number and size in overloaded anterior latissimus dorsi muscle. *Journal of Applied Physiology. 54:*1292, 1983.

Gonyea, W.J. et al.: Exercise induced increases in muscle fiber number. *European Journal of Applied Physiology. 55:*137, 1986.

Gregor, R.J., et al.: Skeletal muscle properties and performance in elite female track athletes. *European Journal of Applied Physiology. 47:*355, 1981.

Hortobagyi, T. et al.: Effects of intense "stretching" flexibility training on the mechanical profile of the knee extensors and on the range of motion of the hip joint. *International Journal of Sports Medicine. 6:*317, 1985.

Hurley, B.F., et al.: Effects of high intensity strength training on cardiovascular function. *Medicine and Science in Sports and Exercise. 16:*483, 1984.

Ikai, M., and A.H. Steinhaus: Some factors modifying the expression of human strength. *Journal of Applied Physiology. 16:*157, 1961.

Katch, F.I., et al.: Relationship of maximal leg force and leg composition to treadmill and bicycle ergometer maximum oxygen uptake. *Medicine and Science in Sports. 6:*38, 1974.

Katch, F.I., and G. Danielson: Bicycle ergometer endurance in women related to maximal force, leg volume, and body composition. *Research Quarterly. 47:*366, 1976.

Katch, F.I., et al.: Evaluation of acute cardiorespiratory responses to hydraulic resistance exercise. *Medicine and Science in Sports and Exercise. 17:*168, 1985.

Katch, F.I. and S. Drumm: Effects of different modes of strength training on body composition and anthropometry. *Clinics in Sports Medicine. 5:*413, 1986.

Knuttgen, H.G.: Human performance in high intensity exercise with concentric and eccentric muscle contractions. *International Journal of Sports Medicine. 7:*6, 1986.

Larsson, L.: Physical training effects on muscle morphology in sedentary males at different ages. *Medicine and Science in Sports and Exercise. 14:*203, 1982.

Larsson, L. and P.A. Tesch: Motor unit fibre density in extremely hypertrophied skeletal muscles in man. Electrophysiological signs of muscle fibre hyperplasia. *European Journal of Applied Physiology. 55:*130, 1986.

Lortie, G. et al.: Relationships between skeletal muscle characteristics and aerobic performance in sedentary and active subjects. *European Journal of Applied Physiology. 54:*471, 1985.

Luthi, J.M. et al.: Structural changes in skeletal muscle tissue with heavy-resistance exercise. *International Journal of Sports Medicine. 7:*123, 1986.

MacDougall, J.D. et al.: Muscle ultrastructural characteristics of elite power lifters and bodybuilders. *European Journal of Applied Physiology. 48:*117, 1982.

MacDougall, J.D. et al.: Muscle fiber number in biceps brachii in body builders and control subjects. *Journal of Applied Physiology. 57:*1399, 1984.

McArdle, W.D., and G.F. Foglia: Energy cost and cardiorespiratory stress of isometric and weight training exercise. *Journal of Sports Medicine and Physical Fitness. 9:*23, 1969.

McCartney, N. et al.: Muscle power and metabolism in maximal intermittent exercise. *Journal of Applied Physiology. 60:*1164, 1986.

Nutter, J. and W.G. Thorland: Body composition and anthropometric correlates of isokinetic leg extension strength of young adult males. *Research Quarterly for Exercise and Sport. 58:*47, 1987.

O'Toole, M.L. et al.: The ultraendurance triathlete: a physiological profile. *Medicine and Science in Sports and Exercise. 19:*45, 1987.

Pels, A.E. et al.: Effects of leg press training on cycling, leg press, and running peak cardiorespiratory measures. *Medicine and Science in Sports and Exercise. 19:*66, 1987.

Saltin, B. et al.: Fiber types and metabolic potentials of skeletal muscles in sedentary man and endurance runners. *Annals of New York Academy of Sciences. 301:*3, 1977.

Simoneau, J.A. et al.: Skeletal muscle histochemical and biochemical characteristics in sedentary male and female subjects. *Canadian Journal of Physiology and Pharmacology. 63:*30, 1985.

Weltman, A.W. et al.: The effects of hydraulic resistance strength training in pre-pubertal males. *Medicine and Science in Sports and Exercise. 18:*629, 1986.

Wilmore, J.H.: Alterations in strength, body composition, and anthropometric measurements consequent to a 10-week weight training program. *Medicine and Science in Sports. 6:*133, 1974.

Winter, D.A. et al.: Errors in the use of isokinetic dynamometers. *European Journal of Applied Physiology. 46:*397, 1981.

10

Conditioning for Anaerobic and Aerobic Power

AN IMPORTANT ASPECT of many forms of physical activity is the necessity to generate energy rapidly. Because such energy release is almost instantaneous, sufficient oxygen cannot be delivered to the muscles quickly enough to match the energy requirements. Even if oxygen was available immediately, it could not be metabolized fast enough to be of much use. Thus, success in sprinting through the line in football, "spiking" in volleyball, or beating out an infield hit in softball depends in part on the capacity to generate energy anaerobically.

The importance of the capacity for rapid energy metabolism is clearly seen in a sport like football, where each play requires short periods of all-out, intense effort. Likewise, a maximum effort is required in sprint running and swimming, weightlifting, and during the "kick" phase of a middle distance run or swim. The apparent steady state sports such as basketball, tennis, field hockey, lacrosse, and soccer also involve sprinting, dashing, darting, and stop-and-go, in which the capacity to generate short bursts of anaerobic power plays an important role. Too often, coaches of sports such as basketball or soccer place considerable importance on the development of cardiovascular or aerobic capacity in their conditioning programs at the sacrifice of vigorous anaerobic conditioning. It is true that these sports require a relatively steady release of energy for a considerable period of time. However, in those crucial situations that demand an all-out effort, the relative capacity of the athlete's anaerobic energy system may be poor and the player or team will be unable to perform at full potential. On the other hand, training the anaerobic capacity of endurance athletes such as marathon runners or channel swimmers would be wasteful because the contribution of these energy systems to successful performance is minimal. Success in endurance activities necessitates a highly trained oxygen transport or aerobic energy system and a well-conditioned heart and vascular system capable of circulating large quantities of blood for long durations.

Figure 10-1 summarizes the predominant energy systems required in common physical activities. Keep in mind that the three energy systems, the ATP-CP system,

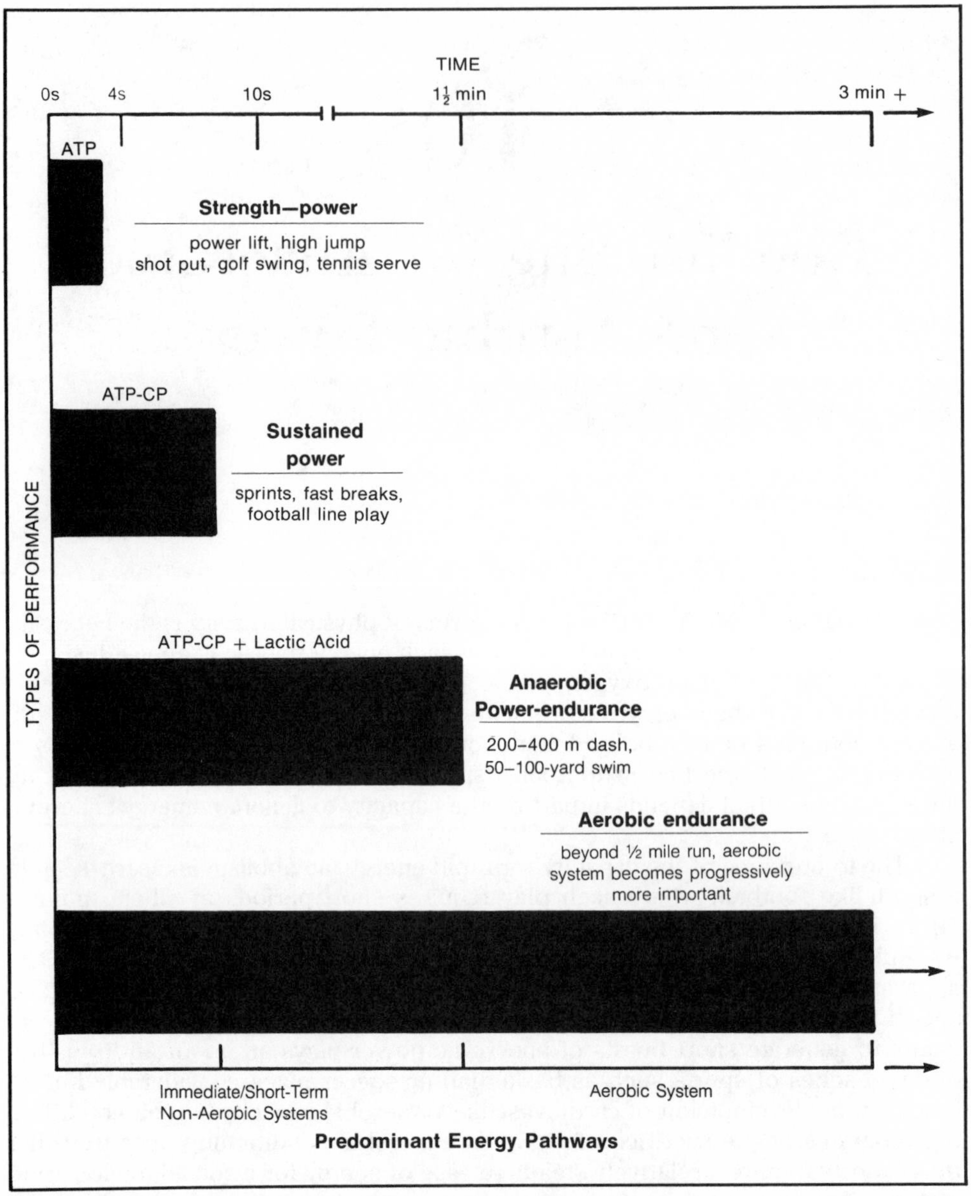
TIME
0s
4s
10s
1½ min
3 min +
ATP
Strength—power
power lift, high jump
shot put, golf swing, tennis serve
ATP-CP
Sustained power
sprints, fast breaks,
football line play
TYPES OF PERFORMANCE
ATP-CP + Lactic Acid
Anaerobic Power-endurance
200–400 m dash,
50–100-yard swim
Aerobic endurance
beyond ½ mile run, aerobic
system becomes progressively
more important
Immediate/Short-Term
Non-Aerobic Systems
Aerobic System
Predominant Energy Pathways

Figure 10-1. *Classification of activities based on duration of performance and the predominant energy pathways.*

the lactic acid system, and the oxygen or aerobic system are often operative simultaneously during physical activity. However, their relative contributions to the total energy requirement during an exercise may differ markedly. This contribution in the energy continuum is related directly to the length of *time* and *intensity* a specific activity is performed. With an intense, maximum burst of energy as in the tennis serve, golf swing, volleyball spike and even the 60- or 100-yard dash, the energy is provided anaerobically and supplied almost exclusively by the stored high energy phosphates, ATP and CP. In a performance that lasts between 10 and 90 seconds, as in a 100-yard swim or 220-yard run, the energy is still supplied predominantly by anaerobic reactions. In this case, however, the energy from lactic acid production plays a much more important role, and the training program for such activities must be of sufficient intensity and duration to stimulate lactic acid production as well as to overload the ATP-CP energy system. As the intensity of an activity diminishes somewhat and the duration extends to between 2 and 4 minutes, dependence upon energy from the phosphate stores decreases, while energy release from aerobic or oxygen-consuming reactions becomes more important. In wrestling, boxing, ice hockey, an 880-yard or 1-mile run, or a full-court press in basketball, the portion of energy required from anaerobic sources depends predominantly on a person's capacity and tolerance for lactic acid. In these activities aerobic energy metabolism occupies a role of equal importance. After 4 minutes of continuous exercise, an activity becomes more dependent on aerobic energy; in a marathon run or long-distance swim, the body is powered almost exclusively by the energy from aerobic reactions. It is clear, therefore, that in training for a particular sport or fitness goal, the activity must be evaluated in terms of its energy components. After this careful analysis, a proportionate allocation of time should be devoted to the overload or training of each of the particular energy systems.

Anaerobic Conditioning

The capacity to perform all-out exercise of up to 90-second duration depends mainly on anaerobic energy metabolism. As was the case with training to improve muscular strength, you must apply the overload principle in conditioning the anaerobic energy systems to improve this energy-generating capacity significantly.

THE ANAEROBIC ENERGY SYSTEMS

In Chapter 3 we presented the energy reactions at rest and during exercise in some detail. Recall that anaerobic energy is generated from the breakdown of the high-energy phosphates ATP and CP, as well as in the reactions of glycolysis, where glucose is ultimately transformed into lactic acid.

The Phosphate Pool

During the first 6 seconds of all-out exercise, energy is made available from the breakdown of the energy currency ATP and the energy reservoir CP. Energy is released almost immediately in these reactions and does not require oxygen. Sports such as football and weightlifting rely almost exclusively on energy derived from the phosphate pool. In these kinds of activities, developing the capacity of the ATP-CP energy system to the fullest should be of paramount importance.

Maximum overload of the phosphate pool can be achieved by engaging specific muscles in maximum bursts of effort for 5 or 10 seconds. A sprint swimmer might swim intervals of 20 to 25 yards, while the sprint runner could achieve a similar overload in the leg muscles by running sprints of 60 to 100 yards. A football lineman, on the other hand, might sprint for only 5 to 30 yards on any one play. To increase the intensity of the overload during this relatively short but intense exercise period, the player might run with a weighted belt or vest, or sprint up hills or stairs. Because the high energy phosphates supply the energy for such intense, intermittent exercise, only small amounts of lactic acid will be produced and recovery will be quite rapid. Thus, a subsequent exercise bout can begin after only a brief rest period. In training to enhance the ATP-CP energy capacity of specific muscles, the individual should undertake numerous bouts of intense, short-duration exercise. *The training activities selected must engage the muscles for which the person desires improved anaerobic power.*

Lactic Acid

As the duration of all-out effort extends beyond 10 seconds, dependence on anaerobic energy from the phosphates decreases, while the quantity of anaerobic energy generated increases in the reactions of glucose to lactic acid. To improve capability for more prolonged anaerobic energy release via the lactic acid energy system, the physiologic conditioning program must provide for increasing the degree of overload on this means of energy metabolism. This form of training is physiologically and psychologically taxing and requires considerable motivation. Repeat bouts of up to 1 minute of maximum running, swimming, or cycling, stopped 30 to 40 seconds before exhaustion, will cause lactic acid to increase to near maximum levels and overload this energy system. To assure that maximum levels of lactic acid are produced during each training session, the exercise bout should be repeated several times after 1 to 2 minutes of recovery. Each repeated work level will cause a "lactate stacking" that will result in higher levels of lactic acid than just one bout of all-out effort to the point of voluntary exhaustion. Of course, it is critical to use the specific muscle groups that need this enhanced anaerobic capacity. A backstroke swimmer should train by swimming backstroke, a cyclist must bicycle, and the basketball or football player must rapidly perform various movements and direction changes that are similar to those required by the demands of the sport.

When the body produces large amounts of lactic acid, recovery time from the exercise can be considerable. For this reason, this form of anaerobic power training should occur at the end of the conditioning session. Otherwise, fatigue from the high intensity, anaerobic training would carry over and perhaps hinder the efficiency of aerobic training. Remember, however, that if previous exercise is above the steady state aerobic level and lactic acid accumulates, its rate of removal will be facilitated if you maintain a moderate level of activity during recovery.

Aerobic Conditioning

The current interest in physiologic conditioning has resulted to a large degree from the desire of many people to improve their ability to sustain physical activity without fatigue. In most cases the desire is directed toward sports participation, although a variety of recreational, leisure, household, and occupational activities require a continuous and fairly high level of energy expenditure. Participation in swimming, jogging, tennis, hiking, bicycling, and many other forms of activity all require a cardiovascular system conditioned to supply adequate oxygen to the exercising muscles.

In the following discussion of aerobic conditioning we present a relatively simple method for evaluating a person's present physiologic status for aerobic exercise. Also, we present a program of activities that can be used to overload the aerobic energy system.

THE AEROBIC ENERGY SYSTEM

Continuous exercise performed for longer than 2 minutes requires energy from both anaerobic and aerobic metabolic reactions. The energy demands in the early stages of exercise are met by the anaerobic breakdown of the high energy phosphates, and by the initial phase of carbohydrate metabolism where glucose is transformed into pyruvic acid. However, the energy liberated from these anaerobic reactions is quite limited, supplying only enough energy to power an all-out run or swim for about 60 to 90 seconds. If exercise continues beyond this time, additional energy for the resynthesis of the phosphates must be supplied by reactions that require oxygen. Under aerobic conditions, pyruvic acid from carbohydrate metabolism, as well as the food fragments from fat and protein, are changed into various substances with the resulting formation of carbon dioxide, water, and large amounts of energy. The energy released from the complete breakdown of food is used to resynthesize the high energy phosphate ATP. If the supply of oxygen is adequate to meet the energy requirements, then exercise can be continued in a steady state and the feelings of discomfort from fatigue are minimal. On the other hand, if oxygen delivery or utilization is inadequate, anaerobic energy metabolism will exceed the energy generated from aerobic reactions, lactic acid will quickly accumulate, and fatigue will set in. Therefore, the intensity at which exercise can be sustained for relatively long periods of time depends on the body's capability for aerobic metabolism. This capacity depends in turn on the functional capacity of the support systems for oxygen transport—the heart, lungs, and vascular system. The terms "endurance fitness," "cardiovascular fitness," and "aerobic fitness" refer to the body's ability to generate ATP aerobically.

A USEFUL METHOD TO EVALUATE YOUR CARDIOVASCULAR CAPACITY

As we discussed in Chapter 3, a low heart rate during exercise and a small increment in heart rate with more vigorous exercise generally reflect a high level of cardiovascular fitness; this can be attributed to a large stroke volume of the heart. Because more blood can be pumped with each heart beat, a smaller increase in heart rate is required to deliver a specific quantity of blood with its complement of oxygen to the exercising muscles. The *step up test* provides a convenient means by which heart rate response can evaluate the efficiency of the cardiovascular response to aerobic exercise. Suppose, for example, three people perform 3 minutes of step up exercise on a bench to the cadence of a metronome. Figure 10-2 illustrates the heart rate response of each subject during the 3 minutes of stepping.

During the first minute of stepping the heart rate increases rapidly and then starts to level off. Subject A, a varsity basketball player, reaches a heart rate of 120 beats per minute at the end of 3 minutes, while the heart rate of subject B, a physical education major, is 142 beats per minute. For subject C, a sedentary college student, the heart rate response to this exercise is 170 beats per minute. It is clear that the cardiovascular stress of bench stepping for student C is considerably

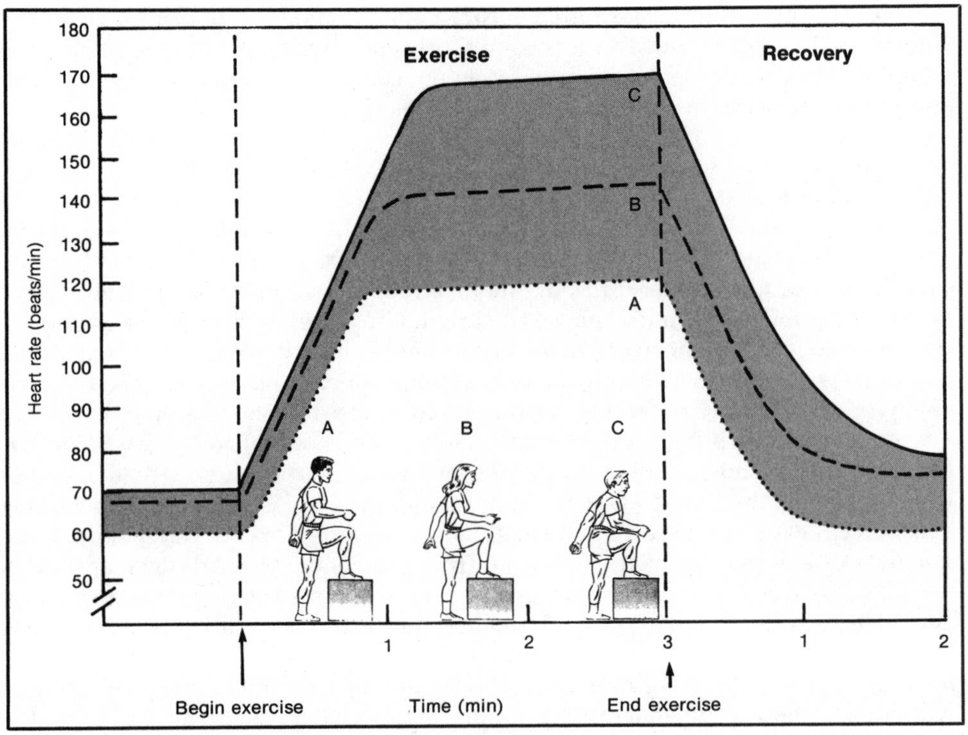
180
170
160
150
140
130
120
110
100
90
80
70
60
50
Heart rate (beats/min)
Exercise
Recovery
C
B
A
A
B
C
1
2
3
1
2
Begin exercise
Time (min)
End exercise

Figure 10-2. *Heart rate response of three people during a stepping exercise and in recovery.*

greater than for the other two students, especially student A, whose increase in heart rate is minimal. It is reasonable to conclude that cardiovascular capacity is greatest for the athlete, less for the physical education major, and relatively poor for the sedentary student.

One problem in applying the principles discussed above to a nonlaboratory situation is how to determine the exercise heart rate. The most accurate way to obtain heart rate during exercise is to monitor the electrical activity of the heart preceding each beat with an electrocardiographic monitor or ECG. An alternative is to record the heart rate during recovery, when the subject stops stepping. Figure 10-2 also shows the pattern of *heart rate recovery* of the three subjects for the 2 minutes immediately following the bench-stepping exercise. Notice that on completion of exercise, heart rate decreases rapidly during the first 30 seconds of recovery. Following this, the heart rate continues to decline but at a much slower rate. After 2 minutes heart rates have essentially returned to resting values. The most noticeable differences in heart rate between subjects A, B, and C are observed in the period immediately following exercise. Thus, if recovery heart rate is measured as soon as exercise stops, it is still fairly easy to discriminate between subjects in terms of their heart rate response during the stress of the exercise test.

THE QUEENS COLLEGE STEP TEST

Using a simple step up test, we have measured the "cardiovascular capacity" in thousands of male and female college students at Queens College in New York. To measure large numbers of students at the same time, stepping was done using the bottom step of the gymnasium bleachers that was 16¼ inches high. For women, the stepping cadence was set by a metronome at 88 beats per minute, or 22 complete step-ups; for men, it was set at 96 beats or 24 steps per minute. One complete stepping cycle on the bench represented 4 beats on the metronome, "up-up-down-down." Following a demonstration, students were given 15 seconds of practice stepping to adjust to the cadence of the metronome. The test was then begun and continued for 3 minutes. On completion of stepping the students remained standing while the pulse was counted at the carotid artery for a 15-second interval beginning 5 seconds after the end of stepping. This 15-second pulse rate value was then multiplied by 4 to express the heart rate score in beats per minute. Table 10-1 presents the percentile rankings for the various heart rate scores for men and women. Accompanying these scores are the corresponding values for maximal oxygen consumption that were *predicted* from the heart rate values. We will present the basis for this prediction of aerobic capacity shortly.

Please note that in comparing someone's heart rate response to the stepping exercise to that of the students measured at Queens College, you must follow the exact procedures for administering the test. The stepping cadence *must* be 22 steps per minute for women and 24 steps per minute for men. The bench height *must* be 16¼ inches and recovery heart rate *must* be measured during the 5- to 20-second interval at the end of exercise. If this isn't done, the resulting prediction may be inaccurate.

Table 10-1. *Percentile rankings for recovery heart rate and predicted maximal oxygen consumption for male and female college students.*

PERCENTILE RANKING	RECOVERY HR, FEMALE	PREDICTED MAX $\dot{V}O_2$ (ml/kg · min)	RECOVERY HR, MALE	PREDICTED MAX $\dot{V}O_2$ (ml/kg · min)
100	128	42.2	120	60.9
95	140	40.0	124	59.3
90	148	38.5	128	57.6
85	152	37.7	136	54.2
80	156	37.0	140	52.5
75	158	36.6	144	50.9
70	160	36.3	148	49.2
65	162	35.9	149	48.8
60	163	35.7	152	47.5
55	164	35.5	154	46.7
50	166	35.1	156	45.8
45	168	34.8	160	44.1
40	170	34.4	162	43.3
35	171	34.2	164	42.5
30	172	34.0	166	41.6
25	176	33.3	168	40.8
20	180	32.6	172	39.1
15	182	32.2	176	37.4
10	184	31.8	178	36.6
5	196	29.6	184	34.1

MEASUREMENT OF PULSE RATE

The accurate measurement of heart rate is essential in evaluating the response to the step test and comparing scores to established norms. Locating the pulse at rest requires some practice. The pulse can be easily located after exercise by pressing softly at the carotid artery along the trachea in the neck. Do not press too hard because this can slow your actual heart rate. Following exercise, the surge of blood from the heart distends this artery and the pulse is located easily. The recovery pulse rate can also be used to estimate the heart rate *during* exercise. In this case you should use the *immediate* 10-second recovery period. Then multiply the number of beats counted during the 10-second interval by 6 to express the heart rate per minute. The heart rate measured during the 10 seconds immediately after exercise only decreases by about 3%, or the equivalent of 4 to 6 beats per minute if the exercise heart rate is between 160 and 180 beats per minute.

PREDICTION OF MAXIMAL OXYGEN UPTAKE

It is reasonable to expect that a person with a low heart rate during the step test is in better "condition" than someone whose heart rate on the same test was relatively high. To evaluate the validity of this expectation, laboratory studies were conducted on a sample of men and women who were part of the larger norm study of the Queens College Step Test. Maximal oxygen consumption was measured for each subject using treadmill test procedures. Each subject's maximal oxygen consumption was then plotted in relation to the corresponding recovery heart rate score obtained on the step test. Figure 10-3 illustrates these results for the sample of women.

It was clear that a definite relationship existed. Subjects with higher maximal oxygen uptakes tended to have lower heart rate recovery scores on the step test. Although there was considerable variability about a line drawn through these points, a knowledge of maximal oxygen consumption could be obtained from recovery heart rate on the step test. We therefore derived the mathematical equation to describe the "best fit" line that passed through the scores for recovery heart rate and maximal oxygen consumption. The equations predicting maximal oxygen con-

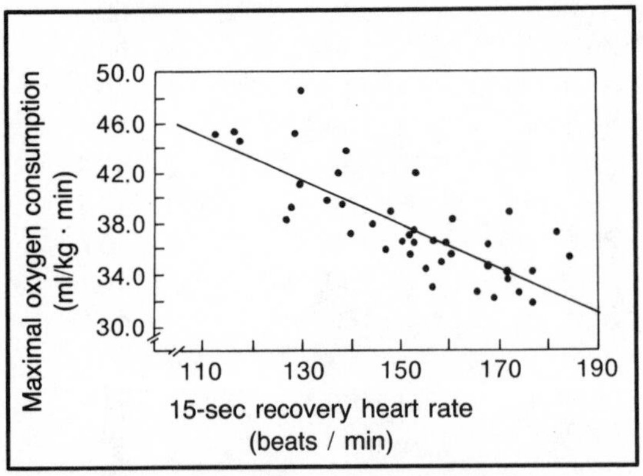
Maximal oxygen consumption (ml/kg · min)
50.0
46.0
42.0
38.0
34.0
30.0
110
130
150
170
190
15-sec recovery heart rate (beats / min)

Figure 10-3. *Scattergram and line of "best fit" relating step-test heart rate score and maximal oxygen consumption in college women.*

sumption from heart rate recovery for the men and women were as follows:

Men: max $\dot{V}O_2$ = 111.33 − (0.42 × step-test pulse rate, beats · min)
Women: max $\dot{V}O_2$ = 65.81 − (0.1847 × step-test pulse rate, beats · min)

The predicted maximal oxygen uptake value is expressed in relation to body weight as milliliters of oxygen consumed per kilogram of body weight per minute. This is written as ml/kg · min.

The above equations provide a reasonably accurate method for predicting maximal oxygen consumption from step test recovery heart rate for *college-aged* men and women. For example, suppose recovery heart rate following the Queens College Step Test for a woman was 156 beats per minute. Substituting this heart rate score in the equation would predict a maximal oxygen consumption of 37.0 ml/kg · min. A heart rate value of 172 beats per minute for a college-aged male results in a predicted maximal oxygen update of 39.1 ml/kg · min. To simplify these conversions, Table 10-1 presents the predicted maximal oxygen uptake values determined from recovery heart rate scores.

Ideally, the most accurate measurement of maximal oxygen uptake would take place in the laboratory, where fairly sophisticated equipment is used. This type of test would require near maximal physical effort from the subject. While the step test prediction method certainly does not possess the accuracy required for research purposes, it does provide a valid method for classification purposes. The step test method presented in this section gives as good an estimate of maximal oxygen consumption as that obtained with other submaximal tests that require the bicycle ergometer or treadmill, or performance in a running test on a track. You can evaluate the predicted maximal oxygen uptake score by comparing this value with the aerobic capacity classifications in Table 10-2. Although such classifica-

Table 10-2. *Aerobic capacity classification based on gender and age.*

	MAXIMAL OXYGEN CONSUMPTION (ml/kg · min)				
AGE	LOW	FAIR	AVERAGE	GOOD	HIGH
Women					
20–29	28	29–34	35–40	41–46	47
30–39	27	38–33	34–38	39–45	46
40–49	25	26–31	30–37	38–43	44
50–65	21	22–28	27–34	35–40	41
Men					
20–29	37	38–41	42–50	51–55	56
30–39	33	34–37	38–42	43–50	51
40–49	29	30–35	36–40	41–46	47
50–59	25	26–30	31–38	39–42	43
60–69	21	22–25	26–33	34–37	38

tions are subjective, they have been constructed from average values for aerobic capacity of hundreds of trained and sedentary men and women measured in this country and abroad.

THE TECHUMSEH STEP TEST: A VALID ALTERNATIVE

A step test has been developed for use with adult men and women of *all ages.* While a heart rate score on this test cannot be transposed into a value for maximal oxygen uptake, the recovery heart rates are valid for showing relative fitness for aerobic exercise. The fitness classifications have been constructed from average values based on a large sample from Techumseh, Michigan, a representative midwestern community. Because the norms are applicable to a broad range, the test is attractive from a practical standpoint because the work level is relatively moderate and the stepping surface is the approximate height of most stairs.

The test can be performed alone, but it is much easier with a partner. Find a stair or stool *8 inches high.* The correct stepping height is important and can easily be achieved by adjusting the stepping or floor surface with a board or similar hard, flat object. As with all standardized step tests, the correct stepping cadence is crucial, so practice briefly to make sure that you step up and down *twice* within a 5-second span, or *24 complete step-ups each minute for 3 minutes.* You can have your partner chant "Up, up; down, down; up, up; down, down" within a 5-second span to establish the proper cadence. Each new sequence starts at 5, 10, 15, 20, and so on. For more precision, set a metronome at *96 beats per minute* giving one footstep per beat.

Once you master the cadence, either time yourself or have someone else signal you when to begin and stop. At the completion of 3 minutes of stepping, remain standing and locate your pulse. Exactly 30 seconds after stopping, measure your pulse for 30 more seconds. The number of pulse beats, from 30 seconds after stepping to the 1-minute post-exercise period, is your heart rate score. Refer to Table 10-3 to obtain your cardiovascular fitness classification for your age and gender.

Although a bench of different height than that used in either the Queens College or Techumseh step tests will not permit the comparison of heart rate scores with the norms, you can still determine a person's heart rate response to a standard exercise stress. The heart rate response can then serve as the frame of reference for evaluating cardiovascular adaptation to a particular program of physiologic conditioning. As the circulatory system becomes more efficient in delivering blood and oxygen, the exercise heart rate as well as the heart rate in recovery will decrease. *The important consideration is that the procedures for administering a step test prior to the start and during the program must be identical each time the test is taken.*

FACTORS THAT AFFECT AEROBIC CONDITIONING

As shown in Figure 10-4, there are two major goals of aerobic conditioning: (1) to enhance the capacity of the central circulation for delivering blood, and (2) to develop the "metabolic machinery" to consume oxygen within the specific muscles.

Five factors should be considered to achieve success in aerobic conditioning: (1) the person's initial level of cardiovascular capacity, (2) the frequency of training, (3) duration of training, (4) intensity of training, and (5) the application of

Table 10-3. *Step test classifications based on 30-second recovery heart rate for men and women.*

	AGE			
CLASSIFICATION	20–29	30–39	40–49	50 & OLDER
Men		**Number of Beats**		
Outstanding	34–36*	35–38	37–39	37–40
Very good	37–40	39–41	40–42	41–43
Good	41–42	42–43	43–44	44–45
Fair	43–47	44–47	45–49	46–49
Low	48–51	48–51	50–53	50–53
Poor	52–59	52–59	54–60	54–62
Women				
Outstanding	39–42*	39–42	41–43	41–44
Very good	43–44	43–45	44–45	45–47
Good	45–46	46–47	46–47	48–49
Fair	47–52	48–53	48–54	50–55
Low	53–56	54–56	55–57	56–58
Poor	57–66	57–66	58–67	59–66

*Thirty-second heart rate is counted beginning 30 seconds after exercise stops.
Based on information in H.J. Montoye, *Physical Activity and Health: An Epidemiologic Study of an Entire Community* (Englewood Cliffs, N.J.: Prentice-Hall, 1975).

proper overload to the specific muscles to function under improved aerobic conditions.

1. Initial Level of Cardiovascular Capacity

As a general rule, the amount of improvement through physiologic conditioning depends largely on the person's initial state of cardiovascular capacity. Stated in simple terms, if you rate low at the start, there is room for significant improve-

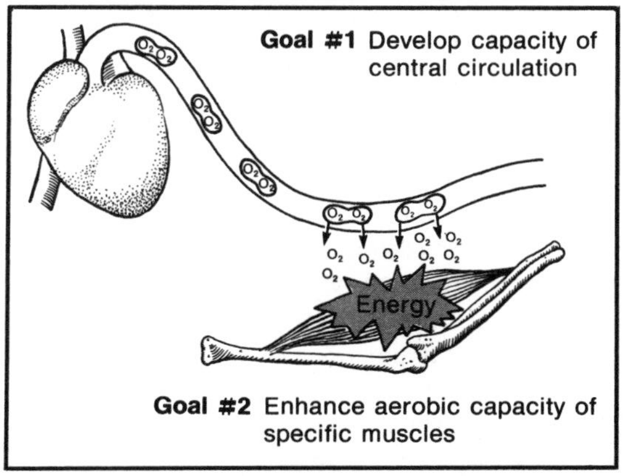
Goal #1 Develop capacity of central circulation
Energy
Goal #2 Enhance aerobic capacity of specific muscles

Figure 10-4. *Two major goals of aerobic conditioning.*

ment. On the other hand, if your aerobic capacity is already close to that of a world class endurance athlete, there is relatively little room to advance and the absolute amount of improvement may be small. However, a 5% improvement in physiologic function for an elite athlete is just as important as a 40% increase for a sedentary person. As a broad guideline, individuals classified as average in terms of maximal oxygen consumption generally show an improvement of about 10 to 15% from an aerobic conditioning program. Although fewer studies have been conducted with women, it appears that the amount of improvement in aerobic capacity that can be expected from training is similar to that of men.

The preceding discussion represents a generalization based on average values for cardiovascular improvement reported in the literature. Individual differences determined by genetic factors also play an important role in influencing the amount of improvement in aerobic capacity as a result of training. This makes it quite difficult to predict exactly how much improvement can be expected based on a subject's pretraining test results. Due to inherited traits, some people possess a relatively high aerobic capacity without having had any previous experience in physiologic training or conditioning programs. Some physiologists contend that a highly developed and efficient aerobic capacity is as much determined by the "choice" of parents as by participation in programs of vigorous aerobic conditioning.

2. Frequency of Training

In general, it is necessary to exercise at least 2 days a week to bring about adaptive changes in the aerobic systems. This was also true in training for muscular strength. Of course, it is possible to locate one or two research studies that report a significant improvement in cardiovascular capacity as a result of training only 1 day a week. The subjects in those studies, however, had been quite sedentary prior to training and for them any form of overload, even though infrequent, would stimulate cardiovascular improvement. In contrast, the majority of experiments dealing with the optimal frequency of training indicates that a training response occurs if exercise is performed 2 or preferably 3 times each week for at least 6 weeks. Interestingly several studies have shown that the improvements resulting from running or cycling 4 or 5 times a week were either no greater or only slightly greater than when the same exercise was performed only 3 times a week. It seems that an extra investment of time may not be that profitable in terms of producing changes in physiologic function, at least as measured by maximal oxygen uptake. *On the other hand, if exercise is used as a means for weight control, you should give strong consideration to exercising 5 or 6 days a week because this frequency of exercise can represent a considerable caloric expenditure when compared with training only 2 days a week.*

3. Duration of Training

One of the most common inquiries concerning exercise participation deals with the optimal duration of the daily workout. For example, are 10 minutes twice as beneficial as 5 minutes of jogging? Would a relatively fast run of 2 or 3 minutes that is repeated several times be recommended over a run performed at a slightly slower pace yet continued for 20 to 30 minutes? Precise answers to these questions are difficult because the mechanisms underlying the improvement in aerobic capacity are still not clearly understood. What is known, however, is that both *continuous* as well as *intermittent* overload are effective in improving aerobic capacity. Even a single 3- to 5-minute bout of vigorous exercise performed three times a week will improve aerobic capacity. Similarly, performing less exhausting but steady-state exercise for 20 minutes or longer will also increase the pumping ability of the heart as well as the metabolic capacity of the specific slow twitch muscle fibers. Most competitive endurance runners and swimmers spend from 2 to 3 hours or more per training session in activities geared to enhance the capacity of their physiologic systems.

4. Intensity of Training

Intensity of training is the most critical factor related to successful aerobic conditioning. The intensity of exercise reflects both the caloric requirements of the activity and the specific energy sources required. Intensity can be expressed in several ways: (1) as calories consumed, (2) as a percentage of maximal oxygen consumption, and (3) as a particular heart rate or some percentage of maximum heart rate, or (4) in terms of multiples of the resting metabolic rate required to perform the work. *By far, the most practical means of assessing and understanding the strenuousness of exercise is by means of the exercise heart rate.* Many researchers have used exercise heart rate to structure a training program and evaluate the effectiveness of various training intensities. In general, for college-age people the exercise must be of sufficient intensity to produce an increase in heart rate to at least 130 to 140 beats per minute. This is equivalent to about 50 to 55% of the maximum aerobic capacity, or about *70% of the maximum exercise heart rate.* This intensity of exercise appears to be the minimal stimulus required to provide cardiovascular improvement. Although this level of cardiovascular stress represents the *threshold* intensity for training improvement, more intense exercise is even more effective.

In one study, subjects who trained at a heart rate of 180 beats per minute made greater gains in endurance capacity than groups that trained at rates of 150 and 120 beats per minute. This does not mean that exercise must be strenuous in order to obtain positive results. On the contrary, an exercise heart rate of 140 beats per minute (70% of maximum heart rate for young adults) represents only moderately intense exercise that can safely be continued for a long period of time with little or no discomfort. This training level is frequently referred to as "conversational exercise"; it is sufficiently intense to stimulate a training effect yet not so strenuous that it limits a person from talking during the workout. *It is unnecessary to exercise above this heart rate in order to improve physiologic capacity.* Recall that as cardiovascular capacity improves heart rate gradually becomes reduced. Consequently the exercise level will have to increase periodically to achieve a threshold heart rate, or whatever target rate has been selected.

Within the framework of available research as well as the recommendations of the American College of Sports Medicine, an aerobic training program should be conducted 3 days a week utilizing 20 to 30 minutes of continuous exercise of sufficient intensity to expend about 300 kcal. This is usually assured by exercising at a pulse rate of about 70% of maximum pulse.

5. Specificity of Training

Another common inquiry concerning exercise participation deals with the question of whether swimming, cycling, or running is most effective in developing aerobic capacity. The usual answer is that each would probably be equally effective as a training stimulus, since all three provide an adequate overload to the central circulation. In fact, champion athletes in each of these activities are noted for their high maximal oxygen uptakes. Recall, however, that *two* physiologic capacities must be developed through an aerobic conditioning program. The first is the central circulation (heart and vascular system), that can be trained in a variety of "big muscle" activities such as running, swimming, rowing, and bicycling, *as long as a threshold heart rate is achieved during the training.* The second and equally important factor is the development of the aerobic metabolic capacity of the specific muscles. Activities like jogging, walking, and running broadly meet the two requirements of aerobic training for those activities that require a predominant use of the legs; that is, the central circulation can be overloaded and the lower leg musculature is used. One could raise the question, however, of whether training in running would improve one's aerobic capacity for swimming, or vice versa. Although the answers are far from definitive, the results from recent experiments have shown that improvement resulting from aerobic training is not as general as once thought.

In a study conducted in one of our laboratories, 20 men trained on a bicycle ergometer 20 minutes a day, 3 times a week, for 8 weeks. The training intensity was set at 85% of maximum heart rate. Each subject's maximal oxygen consumption was determined in the laboratory on both the treadmill and bicycle ergometer before and after the training program. Maximal oxygen uptake improved 7.8% as a result of the conditioning program of bicycle exercise when the subjects were measured on the bicycle test. However, when the subjects were measured during treadmill running, the improvement in aerobic capacity averaged only 2.6%. These results indicated that improvement in physiologic capacity was specific to the mode of exercise; there was little improvement in aerobic capacity with measured running, but a significant improvement when the test apparatus was the same as that used during training.

In another experiment of a similar nature, swimming was used as the means for aerobic conditioning. Fifteen men trained 1 hour a day, 3 days a week for 10 weeks. Training heart rates averaged between 85 and 95% of each subject's maximum heart rate. All subjects were measured during treadmill running, an exercise involving predominantly the leg muscles, and swimming, which uses the muscles of the arms and upper body. The results indicated complete specificity in the improvement in aerobic capacity with swim training. While improvements in maximal oxygen consumption averaged 11% when the subjects were measured while swimming, no improvement was demonstrated while running on the treadmill. This was surprising, since we had expected at least a minimal improvement on the running test due to the intense nature of the overload placed on the central circulation during the swim training. Apparently, there was no "transfer" in aerobic capacity from swim training to running.

At our present state of knowledge it is reasonable to advise that in training the aerobic systems for a specific activity such as rowing, swimming, or cycling, the method of training *must* overload the appropriate muscles required by the activity, as well as provide an exercise stress for the heart and vascular system. In each of the above examples, the appropriate overload would consist of training in the actual activity.

Developing an Aerobic Conditioning Program

In this section we present a method for gauging the intensity of training. We will also discuss the advantages and possible limitations of aerobic conditioning through intermittent and continuous training procedures.

Regardless of your present physical condition, there are some basic guidelines to follow as you begin your aerobic exercise program. These guidelines are based on both research and common sense, and are designed to help you achieve fitness effectively and enjoyably. The person who "pulls" a muscle or develops painful cramps early in an exercise program usually has violated one of the rules of intelligent conditioning.

1. *Start Slowly:* It is important to emphasize this point. Any sudden burst of vigorous activity following a few years of sedentary living could cause injury. While it is normal to experience minor muscle aches and twinges of joint pain with the initiation of an exercise program, it is not normal to experience severe muscular discomfort or excessive cardiovascular strain. Anyone who has experienced such discomfort knows that there is no greater discouragement to a program of regular exercise.
2. *Warm-Up:* Before you start any exercise program, it is important to stretch your muscles gently and limber up. There are numerous warm-up and calisthenic exercises you can do (your own favorites included), to limber up joints and stretch muscles. You should also run in place, jog on a treadmill, skip rope, or cycle on a stationary bicycle. The important point is to perform a variety of big muscle exercises in a rhythmic, moderate, and continuous manner so your pulse attains between 50 and 60% of its maximum.
3. *Dress Sensibly:* Wear loose-fitting, light cotton exercise attire (T-shirt, shorts, sweat socks and comfortable shoes). Above all, be comfortable and allow sweat to evaporate freely.
4. *Allow a Cool-Down Period:* After having exercised for 30 minutes or so, allow 5 to 10 minutes to gradually slow down before stopping. This allows metabolism to slowly progress back to normal levels. More importantly, however, a gradual cool down prevents blood from pooling in the large veins of the previously exercised muscles. Such *venous pooling* will bring about a drop in blood pressure to cause less blood to circulate to the brain and heart. Insufficient blood flow can cause dizziness, nausea, and even fainting, while a reduction in blood to the heart muscle may precipitate a series of irregular heart beats and trigger a dangerous cardiac episode.

DETERMINATION OF TRAINING INTENSITY

The intensity of training is probably the most important factor for increasing aerobic capacity. The term "intensity" is quite relative, however. What could pose a considerable exercise stress for one person might well be below the threshold intensity of 70% of maximum heart rate for the marathon runner. Thus it is necessary to evaluate a particular exercise task in terms of the stress it places on each person's aerobic systems. Several methods have been proposed for this purpose.

In one method the actual oxygen consumption during exercise is determined. For example, if jogging at 5.5 miles per hour requires an oxygen consumption of 33 ml/kg · min and the jogger's maximal oxygen consumption is 60 ml/kg · min, this particular exercise would represent an aerobic stress of 55% of the maximal aerobic capacity. For another person with a lower aerobic capacity of 40 ml/kg · min, the oxygen cost of jogging at 5.5 miles per hour would still be approximately 33 ml/kg · min, yet this person would be exercising at 83% of maximum. To provide a similar overload for the first jogger, the pace of jogging would have to be increased to about 8.6 miles per hour (48 ml O_2/kg · min). The strenuousness of any exercise is relative and depends on the present level of physiologic condition.

Although the assessment of exercise intensity by the direct measurement of oxygen consumption is quite accurate, it is impractical to measure oxygen consumption without a fairly extensive laboratory. An alternative is to use *exercise heart rate* to classify an exercise in terms of its relative intensity or strenuousness. This makes it possible to personalize an exercise program and regulate the intensity of exercise to keep pace with changes in physiologic capacity.

Train at a Percentage of Maximum Heart Rate

To train at a predetermined percentage of maximum heart rate requires a knowledge of what the heart rate would be during near-exhausting exercise. Someone's *actual* maximum heart rate can be determined immediately following 3 or 4 minutes of all-out running or swimming. This procedure is inadvisable, however, because such intense exercise is difficult and requires considerable motivation and could be dangerous for people predisposed to coronary heart disease. For this reason we recommend that people consider themselves "average," and use the age-predicted average maximum heart rates shown in Table 10-4. As a general rule, maximum heart rate is approximately 220 beats per minute minus the person's age. In addition to the average age-adjusted maximum heart rates, Figure 10-5 illustrates the "training sensitive zone" that represents the threshold level of 70% and the upper level of 90% of maximum heart rate for each age group. *Conditioning of the aerobic systems will occur as long as the exercise heart rate is within this zone.*

Suppose a 30-year-old man wishes to train at moderate intensity, yet still be at or above the threshold level. A training heart rate would be selected that is equal to

Table 10-4. *Age-predicted maximum heart rate and "training sensitive zone" for submaximal exercise.*

AGE, YEARS	AGE-PREDICTED MAXIMUM HEART RATE	TRAINING SENSITIVE ZONE: LOWER LIMIT 70% HEART RATE	TRAINING SENSITIVE ZONE: UPPER LIMIT 90% HEART RATE
15	210	147	189
20	200	140	180
25	195	136	175
30	190	133	171
35	185	129	166
40	180	126	162
45	173	121	156
50	166	116	149
55	160	112	144
60	155	108	139
65	150	105	135

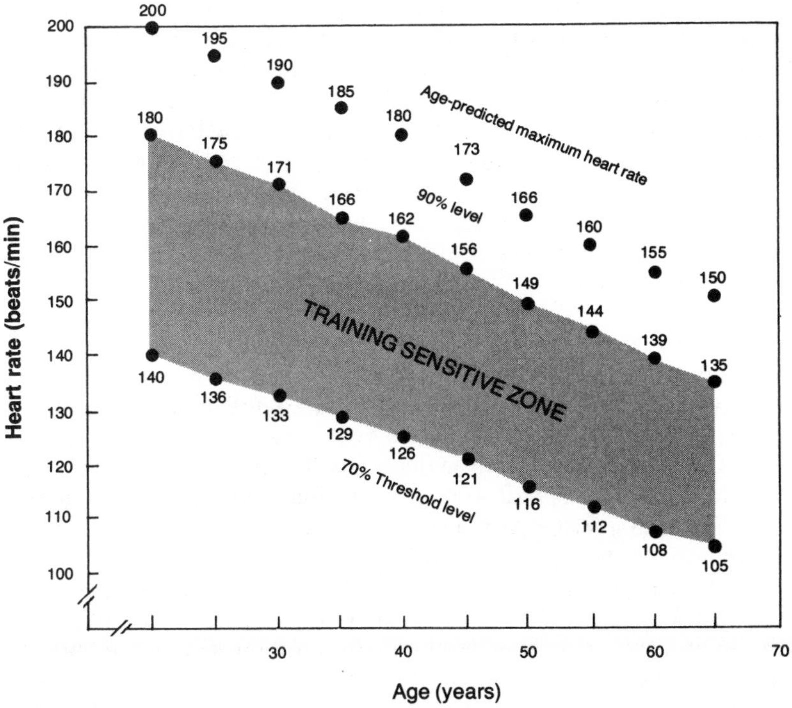
Heart rate (beats/min)
Age (years)
Age-predicted maximum heart rate
90% level
TRAINING SENSITIVE ZONE
70% Threshold level
200
195
190
185
180
173
166
160
155
150
180
175
171
166
162
156
149
144
139
135
140
136
133
129
126
121
116
112
108
105
100
110
120
130
140
150
160
170
180
190
200
30
40
50
60
70

Figure 10-5. *Maximal heart rate and target zone for use in aerobic exercise training programs.*

70% of the age-predicted maximum heart rate, or a target exercise heart rate of 133 beats per minute (0.70 × 190). For a 54-year-old woman, on the other hand, the target heart rate would be 116 beats per minute (0.70 × 166). By trial and error each person can arrive at a walking, jogging, or cycling speed that would produce the desired target heart rate.

In carrying out this trial-and-error procedure, the person should exercise moderately for 3 to 5 minutes, counting pulse rate for 10 seconds immediately afterwards. If the exercise is not intense enough to produce the target heart rate, he repeats the same exercise but at a faster pace: jogging instead of walking, pedaling faster or switching to a lower gear while cycling, or swimming faster, covering a greater distance within a specified time. If the 30-year-old man wants to increase his training intensity to 85% of maximum, his exercise heart rate would have to be increased to 161 beats per minute to work at the same relative training intensity of 85% of maximum (0.85 × 190) as the "typical" 30-year-old man.

Adjust for Swimming and Other Upper Body Exercise

In one of our laboratories, we compared the cardiovascular response to running and swimming in trained and untrained subjects. In both activities the cardiovascular and metabolic adjustments to exercise were quite similar. The maximum heart rate of swimming, however, averaged about 13 beats per minute lower than that of running. This occurred in both trained and untrained subjects, and could probably be attributed to the utilization of the arms primarily during exercise as well as the influence of the horizontal body position during swimming and the cooler temperature of the water. Therefore, if you select swimming or other forms of upper body exercise such as arm cranking as the training exercise, consider the decrease in maximum heart rate that occurs in this form of work in establishing the appropriate exercise intensity. We recommend that an average of 13 beats per minute be subtracted from the age-predicted maximum heart rate values in Figure 10-5. Consequently, a 25-year-old person wishing to swim at 80% of maximum heart rate would select a swimming speed that produced a heart rate of about 146 beats per minute $(0.80) \times (195-13)$. This represents more accurately the appropriate training heart rate for swimming.

Is Less Intense Exercise Effective?

The recommendation for training at 70% of maximum heart rate as the threshold for aerobic improvements is a *general guideline* for establishing effective yet comfortable exercise levels. It is now clear that even less intense exercise will produce meaningful fitness gains for many individuals. While 20 to 30 minutes of continuous exercise at the 70% level will stimulate a training effect, exercise at the lower intensity of 60% for 45 minutes will also prove beneficial. A lower exercise intensity is offset by a longer exercise duration. The important point is that regardless of the exercise level you select, more is not necessarily better, and excessive amounts of exercise increase your chance for bone, joint, and muscle injury. As is pointed out in the next chapter, achievement of the cardiovascular benefits of exercise do not require heroic levels of weekly physical activity. Far too many people unfortunately push themselves adhering to the slogan, "no pain, no gain." For most purposes, 30 minutes of regular exercise performed within the training sensitive zone, 3 to 4 times a week, is probably all that's required.

CONTINUOUS EXERCISE TRAINING

Continuous training involves steady state exercise performed at either moderate or high intensity for a sustained period. With this form of training, it is only necessary to exercise at least 20 minutes at or above the threshold heart rate. This can be done with activities such as swimming, cycling, stationary and forward running, rope skipping or stepping up and down on a bench. By its very nature, continuous exercise training is submaximum and can be engaged in for considerable time in relative comfort. This form of training is therefore suitable for people just beginning an exercise program. It is certainly a more pleasant method of training the oxygen transport system than the more intense interval training discussed in the next section. Continuous exercise training can be maintained at the threshold intensity of 70% maximum heart rate or increased to 85 or even 90% of maximum heart rate.

Continuous exercise training is desirable for endurance athletes because it allows them to train at nearly the same intensity as in actual competition. A champion middle-distance runner may run 5 miles continuously in 26 minutes during workouts at a heart rate of 180 beats per minute; this pace would not be exhausting but would still nearly duplicate race conditions. By finishing each exercise session with several all-out sprints stopped 30 to 40 seconds before exhaustion, the athlete can also train the anaerobic system that does play a small role in such middle-distance events, especially at the race's finish. The marathon runner will train at a slightly slower pace than the middle-distance champion because much longer distance must be run in practice as well as in competition. To provide some relief from this relatively high-intensity, continuous running, exercise can also be performed continuously at a lesser intensity but for longer durations. In this way distance runners can run between 100 to 200 miles during a week of training.

INTERVAL EXERCISE TRAINING

Many activities carried out in daily life in general, and in sports in particular, are intermittent and characterized by periods of intense activity interspersed with periods requiring only a moderate to low level of energy expenditure. Interval training is based on the concept that the correct spacing of work and rest periods enables someone to accomplish a tremendous amount of exercise over a considerable period of time with minimal fatigue. The rest-to-work intervals can vary from a few seconds to several minutes or more. The training prescription can vary in terms of the intensity and duration of the exercise interval, the length of the recovery period, and the number of repetitions. The apparent value of interval training is that intermittent exercise permits high intensity training for long periods of actual exercise at a given intensity. For example, running continuously at a "4-minute mile" pace would exhaust most people within 1 or 2 minutes. However, running at this speed for only 15 seconds followed by a 30-second rest period would enable many people to run 4 minutes at this near record pace. Of course this is not equivalent to a 4-minute mile; but during 4 minutes of running, 1 mile would have been run even though the combined work and rest intervals would have taken 11 minutes and 30 seconds.

The rationale for interval training also has a sound basis in physiologic fact. In the above example of the continuous run at a 4-minute mile pace a major portion of energy would be supplied through the anaerobic production of lactic acid. Within a minute or two the lactic acid levels would rise precipitously and cause exhaustion. On the other hand, intermittent exercise performed for 20 seconds or less would allow a severe load to be imposed on the muscles and oxygen transport systems before lactic acid accumulates appreciably. In this way the oxygen debt incurred during the work interval would be predominantly "alactic" in nature and recovery would take place quickly. The work interval could then begin again after only a brief rest period.

In interval training as in other forms of physiologic conditioning, *the intensity of exercise should be geared to the particular energy systems the person desires to train.* Sprint runners and swimmers should train by running or swimming for short distances at maximum intensity and near race pace. In training for longer distances the exercise interval should be at least 1 minute. A longer work interval will engage the aerobic systems, while shorter exercise intervals place a greater overload on the anaerobic energy systems. Generally you can use pulse rate to gauge the intensity of exercise as well as the length of the recovery period. Fast running for about 1 minute will elevate heart rate close to maximum levels. When heart rate decreases to 120 beats per minute after exercise, physiologic recovery is sufficient to begin another exercise. Only a short rest period should be used when the exercise intervals are less than 90 seconds because during this brief exercise period, oxygen consumption does not have enough time to adjust to the demands of the exercise. For this reason the succeeding exercise interval should begin before recovery is completed. This will ensure that the circulatory and metabolic stress will reach maximum levels even though the exercise intervals are short. With longer periods of intermittent exercise there is sufficient time for metabolic and circulatory adjustments; for this reason, the duration of the rest interval is not as crucial.

At present, there is insufficient evidence for a claim as to the superiority of either continuous or interval exercise training for enhancing aerobic capacity. Either training procedure will succeed; they can probably be used interchangeably.

Maintaining Aerobic Fitness

An interesting question concerns the optimal frequency, duration, and intensity of exercise required to *maintain* the improved aerobic fitness attained through training. Recent studies reveal that if the exercise intensity is maintained, the frequency and duration of training can be reduced considerably without any decrements in aerobic performance (6 day a week training reduced to 2 days; 40 minutes a day training reduced to 13 minutes). However, a small reduction in exercise intensity, keeping training frequency and duration constant, would cause a corresponding decline in aerobic fitness.

Exercising During Pregnancy

With a considerable number of women involved in physically demanding occupations and active lifestyles, there is growing interest as to: (a) the degree that pregnancy affects the metabolic cost and physiologic strain by exercise, (b) the effects of exercise on the fetus, and (c) the course of pregnancy including final outcome and ease of delivery.

It is generally observed that the cardiovascular responses during exercise follow normal response patterns and that pregnancy offers no greater physiologic strain to the mother during moderate exercise other than that provided by the additional weight gain and possible encumbrance of fetal tissue. In fact, if body weight is supported during exercise, as in stationary bicycling, the exercise response for heart rate and oxygen consumption during pregnancy is essentially identical to that observed prior to and following birth.

Studies of uterine blood flow during exercise in various species of mammals indicate that in healthy animals, oxygen supply to the developing fetus is maintained during moderate to heavy levels of maternal exercise. However, in animals with one umbilical artery tied off to restrict placental circulation, there is a significant *reduction* in fetal oxygen supply. The researchers concluded that vigorous maternal exercise was well tolerated by the fetus, but could be potentially harmful to a fetus with some limitation of the umbilical circulation.

It appears that for a previously active, healthy woman during an uncomplicated pregnancy, moderate aerobic exercise does not produce circulatory alterations that compromise fetal oxygen supply. Because vigorous exercise probably diverts some blood from the uterus, that could pose some hazard for a fetus with restricted placental blood flow, it would be prudent for a pregnant woman to exercise in moderation, especially if the pregnancy is comprised to any degree. Because an elevation in maternal core temperature could comprise the dissipation of heat from the fetus through the placenta, it is recommended that during warm weather, pregnant women should exercise in the cool part of the day, for shorter intervals, while maintaining regular fluid intake.

Although regular aerobic exercise can serve an important role in maintaining the functional capacity, optimal body weight, and general well being of a pregnant woman, it remains unclear whether extremes of maternal exercise are beneficial to the developing fetus, or if exercise enhances the course of pregnancy including labor, delivery, and outcome.

Additional Reading

American College of Sports Medicine: The recommended quantity and quality of exercise for developing and maintaining fitness in healthy adults. *Medicine and Science in Sports. 10:*7, 1978.

Clapp, J.F., III and S. Dickstein: Endurance exercise and pregnancy outcome. *Medicine and Science in Sports and Exercise. 16:*556, 1984.

Clausen, J.P.: Effect of physical training on cardiovascular adjustments to exercise in man. *Physiological Reviews. 57:*779, 1977.

Costill, D.L.: *Inside Running: Basics of Sports Physiology.* Indianapolis, Benchmark Press, 1986.

Coyle, E.F. et al.: Time course of loss of adaptations after stopping prolonged intense endurance training. *Journal of Applied Physiology. 57:*1857, 1984.

Dudley, G.A. and R. Djamil: Incompatibility of endurance- and strength-training modes of exercise. *Journal of Applied Physiology. 59:*1446, 1985.

Gergley, T. et al.: Specificity of arm training on aerobic power during swimming and running. *Medicine and Science in Sports and Exercise. 16:*349, 1984.

Greer, N.L. and F.I. Katch: Validity of palpation recovery pulse rate following four intensities of bench step exercise. *Research Quarterly for Exercise and Sport. 53:*340, 1982.

Hickson, R.C., et al.: Reduced training intensities and loss of aerobic power, endurance, and cardiac growth. *Journal of Applied Physiology. 58:*492, 1985.

Hoppeler, H. et al.: Endurance training in humans: aerobic capacity and structure of skeletal muscle. *Journal of Applied Physiology. 59:*320, 1985.

Jarrett, J.C. and W.N. Spellacy: Jogging during pregnancy: an improved outcome? *Obstetrics and Gynecology. 61:*705, 1983.

Katch, V.L. et al.: Biological variability in maximum aerobic power. *Medicine and Science in Sports and Exercise. 14:*21, 1982.

Knuttgen, H.G. and K. Emerson, Jr.: Physiological response to pregnancy at rest and during exercise. *Journal of Applied Physiology. 36:*549, 1974.

Legge, B.J., and E.W. Banister: The Astrand-Rhyming nomogram revisited. *Journal of Applied Physiology. 61:*1203, 1986.

Magel, J.R. et al.: Specificity of swim training on maximum oxygen uptake. *Journal of Applied Physiology. 38:*151, 1975.

McArdle, W.D. et al.: Specificity of run training on $\dot{V}O_2$ max and heart rate changes during running and swimming. *Medicine and Science in Sports. 10:*16, 1978.

Ready, A.E. and H.A. Quinney: Alterations in anaerobic threshold as the result of endurance training and detraining. *Medicine and Science in Sports and Exercise. 14:*292, 1982.

Ruten Franz, J.: Longitudinal approach to assessing maximal aerobic power during growth: the European experience. *Medicine and Science in Sports and Exercise. 18:*270, 1986.

Sawka, M.N. et al.: Alactic capacity and power. *European Journal of Applied Physiology. 45:*109, 1980.

Scheuer, J. and C.M. Tipton: Cardiovascular adaptations to training. *Annual Review of Physiology. 39:*221, 1977.

Stamford, B.A. et al.: Exercise recovery above and below anaerobic threshold following maximal work. *Journal of Applied Physiology. 51:*840, 1981.

Thorland, W.G. et al.: Strength and anaerobic responses of elite female sprint and distance runners. *Medicine and Science in Sports and Exercise. 19:*56, 1987.

Withers, R.T. et al.: Specificity of the anaerobic threshold in endurance trained cyclists and runners. *European Journal of Applied Physiology. 47:*93, 1981.

11

Aging, Exercise, and Cardiovascular Health

THERE IS NO QUESTION that the physiologic and exercise performance capabilities of older people are generally below those of younger counterparts. What is uncertain is the degree that these differences are attributable to true biologic aging or simply the result of environmental factors and disuse brought on by social constraints that alter the lifestyles and activity opportunities for people as they grow older. No longer can older men and women be stereotyped as sedentary with little or no initiative to pursue active lifestyles. The past decade has seen a tremendous upswing in participation by so-called "senior citizens" in a broad range of physical activity experiences and exercise programs. *Research clearly demonstrates that if an active lifestyle is continued into later years, a relatively high level of function is retained and vigorous activities can be engaged in safely and successfully.*

Aside from the positive effects of exercise in maintaining physiologic function, it now appears that physical activity is protective against the ravages of this nation's greatest killer, *coronary heart disease.* Individuals in physically active occupations have a 2- to 3-fold *lower* risk of heart attack than those in sedentary jobs. Furthermore, the chances of surviving a heart attack are much greater for those with a physically demanding job or life-style that includes frequent, vigorous physical activity.

Despite the inherent problems in heart disease research, there is considerable evidence to support the contention that evolution is not keeping pace with automation. Regular physical activity can favorably modify some of the important risk factors related to heart disease. Elevated blood pressure can be lowered by participation in a regular program of aerobic conditioning; body weight, body fat, and elevated blood lipids can be favorably modified with prudent exercise and diet; the blood clotting mechanism can become normalized with exercise training, which might reduce the changes of a blood clot forming on the roughened surface of the coronary arteries. Research with animals has demonstrated an improved blood supply to the heart muscle as a result of regular exercise. If such an adaptation in the heart's circulation actually takes place in humans, then regular exercise may retard the heart disease process or maintain an adequate supply of blood to the heart muscle to compensate for those channels already narrowed by fatty deposits on the vascular walls. More than likely, these vascular adaptations would reduce the chance of heart attack and decrease the severity of damage to the heart muscle should a vessel become clogged.

From a practical standpoint, a lifestyle that includes vigorous physical exercise may be effective in preventing or at least slowing down the cumulative effects of the highly atherogenic American diet and a sedentary and stressful environment. Regardless of genetics, age, and life circumstances, individuals can significantly enhance their chances for a healthy life by adapting sound health habits that include regular exercise. In the sections that follow, we explore several aspects of the aging process with special emphasis on exercise and its relation to cardiovascular disease.

Aging and Bodily Function

Figure 11-1 shows that the various measures of bodily function generally improve rapidly during childhood to reach a maximum between age 20 and 30 years; thereafter, there is a gradual decline in functional capacity with advancing years. While the trend with age is generally similar for the physically active person, physiologic function is attained at about 25% higher levels for each age category, so that a 50-year-old active man or woman may attain the functional capabilities of a 20-year-old counterpart. Although all measures eventually decline with age, not all decline at the same rate and there is considerable variation from person to person

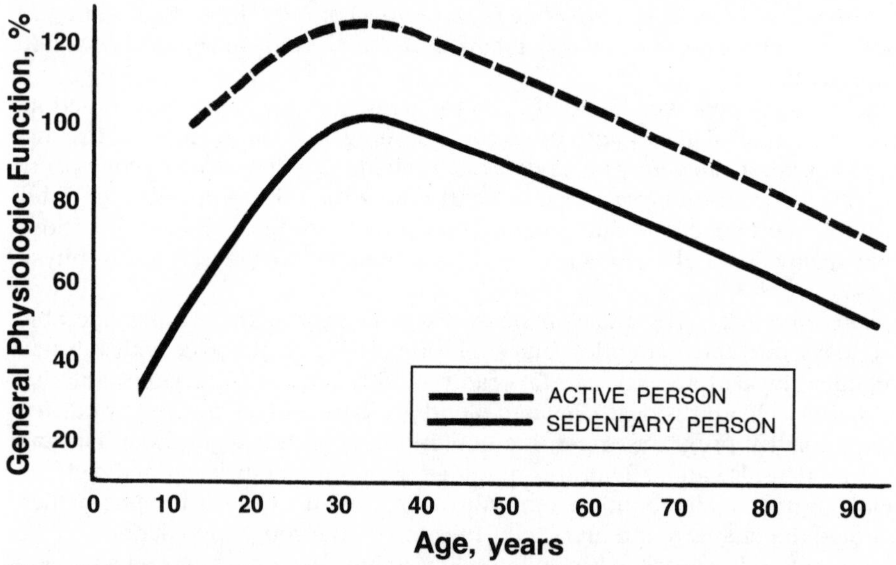
General Physiologic Function, %
120
100
80
60
40
20
ACTIVE PERSON
SEDENTARY PERSON
0
10
20
30
40
50
60
70
80
90
Age, years

Figure 11-1. *Generalized curve to illustrate changes in physiologic function with age. All comparisons are made against the 100% value achieved by the 20- to 30-year-old sedentary person.*

and from system to system within the same person. Nerve conduction velocity, for example, declines only 10 to 15% from 30 to 80 years of age, whereas resting cardiac index (ratio of cardiac output to surface area) and joint flexibility decline 20 to 30%; maximum breathing capacity at age 80 is about 40% that of a 30-year-old. Brain cells die at a constant rate until age 60, while the liver and kidneys lose about 40 to 50% of their function between ages 30 and 70. By age 70, the average female has lost about 30% of her bone mass, while men at this age have lost only about 15%.

Because longitudinal exercise studies on the same subjects are lacking, it is not known whether long-term exercise participation can change the actual rate of decline in physiologic function or "override" deterioration in function that normally occurs with increasing age.

MUSCULAR STRENGTH

Maximum strength of men and women is generally achieved between the ages of 20 and 30 years when muscular cross-sectional area is usually the largest. Thereafter, there is a progressive decline in strength for most muscle groups so that between age 20 to 70 years there is a 30% reduction in overall strength. This is due primarily to a 3 to 5% reduction in muscle mass (actual loss of muscle fibers) each decade due to a loss of total muscle protein brought about by inactivity, aging, or both. Indirect evidence indicates that habitual physical training facilitates protein retention and strength maintenance. Research *shows clearly* that older adults can increase muscular strength and endurance with regular overload, strength-type training.

FLEXIBILITY

With advancing age, connective tissue (cartilage, ligaments, and tendons) becomes stiffer and more rigid which reduces joint flexibility. What is not certain, however, is the degree that biologic aging per se causes these changes or the impact with which sedentary living or degenerative disease affects the tissues that comprise a specific joint. What is clearly known is that appropriate exercises that move joints through their full range of motion can increase flexibility by as much as 20 to 50% in men and women at all ages.

NERVOUS SYSTEM

The cumulative effects of aging on central nervous system function are exhibited by a 37% decline in the number of spinal cord axons, a 10% decline in nerve conduction velocity, and a significant loss in the elastic properties of connective tissue. Such changes partially explain the age-related decrements in neuromuscular performance. When reaction time is partitioned into a central processing time and muscle contraction time, it is the central processing time that is affected most by the aging process. Thus, aging largely affects the ability to detect a stimulus and process the information to produce a response. Since reflexes such as the knee jerk reflex do not involve processing in the brain, they are less affected by the aging process than voluntary responses. While there is an aging effect on the nervous system in terms of reaction time, *physically active groups (be they young or old) move significantly faster than a corresponding age group that is less physi-*

cally active. These observations suggest that an active life-style may *significantly* and *positively* affect movement function at any age. It is tempting to speculate that the biologic aging of certain neuromuscular functions can be somewhat retarded by regular participation in physical activity.

CARDIOVASCULAR FUNCTION

Maximal oxygen consumption and endurance performance show a steady decline in men and women after age 20 and by age 65, aerobic endurance has decreased by about 35%. The heart's ability to pump blood decreases about 8% per decade during adulthood. This is due to various age-related decrements in physiologic functions related to oxygen transport. A clear change is a progressive decline in the maximal heart rate. A rough approximation of the change in maximal heart rate with age is expressed by the following relationship:

$$\text{max HR (beats / min)} = 220 - \text{age (years)}$$

Regular exercise, however, appears to retard this age-related decline in maximal heart rate. Also contributing to a reduced blood flow capacity with age is a reduction in the heart's stroke volume that may reflect changes in myocardial contractility. Other age-related changes in the cardiovascular system include a reduction of blood flow capacity to peripheral tissues, a narrowing of the arteries that supply blood to the heart (by middle-age arterial blood vessels are about 30% narrower), and a decrease in the elasticity of major blood vessels.

BODY WEIGHT AND BODY FAT

The accumulation of excess fat usually begins early in childhood or develops slowly in adulthood. Middle-aged men and women invariably weigh more than college-aged counterparts of the same height—and this weight difference is due to differences in *body fat.* In the Western world, the average 20-year-old male will gain between one-half to one pound of fat each year until the sixth decade of life. In one study, the fat content of 27 adult men increased an average of 14 pounds over a 12-year period, from age 32 to 44. This was equal to the group's total gain in body weight over the duration of the study. The extent to which such gains in body fat during adulthood represent a normal biologic pattern is unknown. However, observations of older individuals who maintain physically active lifestyles suggests that this pattern can be reduced significantly.

After age 60, there is a reduction in total body weight even though there is an increase in body fat. This occurs because in the upper age group, many of the grossly overweight people have died so there are just not many heavy subjects to be measured. Also, lean body weight does tend to decrease with age. This is largely due to the aging skeleton becoming demineralized and porous; concurrently, the quantity of muscle mass is reduced. The degree to which regular physical activity can retard these changes in body density with age is also unknown.

A major limitation of age-trend studies is that the same subjects are not followed over time, but rather different subjects in different age categories are evaluated at the same time. From such cross-sectional data, one attempts to generalize as to expected age-related changes for an individual. Sometimes these generalizations are misleading. For example, today's 70- and 80-year-olds are generally shorter than 20-year-old college students. This does not necessarily mean that we get shorter as we grow older (although this does happen to some extent). Rather, the young adults of this generation are better nourished than their 80-year-old counterparts were at the age of 20 and thus achieve optimal growth. In terms of body fat changes, the limited longitudinal data from the same subjects tend to support the trends noted in cross-sectional studies.

Regular Exercise: A Fountain of Youth?

It is unclear whether changes in physiologic function are a direct result of the aging process per se or of a lack of habitual physical activity. *In fact, sedentary living may bring about losses in functional capacity that are as great as the effects of aging itself!* Results from training studies show no loss in aerobic capacity over a 10-year period for middle-aged men who were regular participants in running and swimming programs. In fact, at age 55, these active men had maintained the same values for blood pressure, body weight, and maximal oxygen consumption they had when measured at age 45.

While exercise may not necessarily be a "fountain of youth," researchers are finding that regular, moderate physical activity not only retards the loss in functional capacity associated with aging and disuse, but often reverses the loss regardless of when in life a person becomes active. Some researchers maintain that a 30-minute program of rapid walking performed by an older person 3 or 4 times a week can turn back the biologic clock some 10 years. Research with the elderly shows that exercise among 60 and 70 year old individuals improves fitness to levels associated with men and women 20 to 30 years younger! Improvements have been noted in muscular strength, body composition, joint flexibility (stiff joints are often the result of disuse, not arthritis), aerobic capacity, pulmonary and neural function, heart disease risk profile, and resistance to depression. Evidence is also accumulating that regular exercise can conserve and actually retard the loss of bone mass in the elderly, thus staving off the ravages of osteoporosis that afflicts both women and men.

Does Exercise Improve Health and Extend Life?

Over the years, medical experts have debated whether a lifetime that incorporates regular exercise contributes to good health and perhaps longevity compared to the sedentary "good life". Because older fit individuals have many of the functional characteristics of younger people, one could argue that improved physical fitness and a vigorous lifestyle may retard the aging process and confer some protection to health in later life. In an early study of exercise and longevity, former Harvard oarsmen exceeded their predicted longevity by 5.1 years per man. While other research supported these findings, these studies were plagued with methodologic problems, including inadequate record keeping, small sample size, improper statistical procedures for estimating expected longevity, and an inability to account for other important factors such as socioeconomic background, body type, cigarette smoking, and family background.

One group of researchers attempted to overcome many of the limitations of earlier research in their study of the diseases and longevity of former college athletes. Because collegiate athletes usually have a longer involvement in habitual physical activity prior to entering college than non-athletes, and since they *may* remain more physically active after college, this seemed to be an excellent group to study to provide insight concerning exercise and longevity.

Figure 11-2 shows there was essentially no difference in the longevity of the ex-athletes compared to non-athletes. Some degree of equality in genetic background existed between the groups because there was similarity in the average age at death of grandparents, parents, and siblings of ex-athletes and non-athletes. Such findings suggest that participation in athletics as a young adult does not necessarily ensure increased longevity in later years. It is still possible, however, that regular physical activity practiced *throughout life* offers protection in terms of health and longevity. Certainly, if aerobic type-endurance exercise can reduce the risk of early heart disease, then regular physical activity at a sufficient level of intensity should have a positive effect on longevity.

Recent research concerning the lifestyles and exercise habits of 17,000 Harvard alumni who entered college between 1916–1950 gives strong evidence that only *moderate* aerobic exercise, equivalent to jogging about 3 miles a day, promotes good health and may actually add years to life. Men who expended about 2000 kcal of exercise on a weekly basis had one-quarter to one-third lower death rates than classmates who did little or no exercise. To achieve 2000 kcal in weekly exercise would require moderate activity such as a daily 30-minute walk, run, cycle, swim, cross-country ski, or aerobic dance. The results of these long term studies can be summarized as follows:

> Regular exercise counters the life-shortening effects of cigarette smoking and excess body weight. Even for people with high blood pressure (a primary heart disease risk), those who exercised regularly reduced their death rate by one-half.

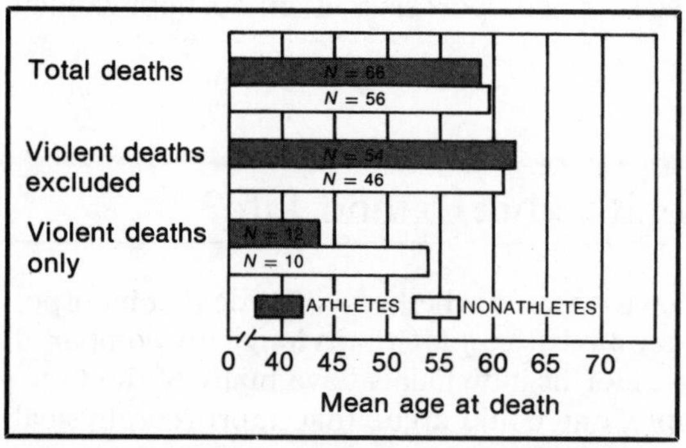
Total deaths
N = 68
N = 56
Violent deaths excluded
N = 54
N = 46
Violent deaths only
N = 12
N = 10
ATHLETES
NONATHLETES
0 40 45 50 55 60 65 70
Mean age at death

Figure 11-2. *Age at death of athletes and nonathletes. None of the differences between the groups are statistically significant. (From Montoye, H.J. et al.: The Longevity and Morbidity of College Athletes. Indianapolis, Indiana, Phi Epsilon Kappa, 1957.)*

People who exercised regularly had a reduced risk of dying from any of the major diseases. This is illustrated clearly in Figure 11-3.

Genetic tendencies toward an early death were countered by regular exercise. For individuals who had one or both parents die before age 65 (another significant health risk), a lifestyle that included regular exercise reduced the risk of death by 25%. A 50% reduction in mortality rate was observed for those whose parents lived beyond 65 years.

Within limits, the person who exercised more had an improved health profile. For example, the mortality rates were 21% lower for men who walked 9 or more miles a week than men who walked 3 miles or less. Exercising in light sport activities increased life expectancy 24% over men who remained sedentary. For the perspective of energy expenditure, the life expectancy of Harvard alumni increased steadily from an exercise energy expenditure of 500 kcal per week to 3500 kcal; this was equivalent of 6 to 8 hours of strenuous exercise. In addition, active men lived an average of 1 to 2 years longer than sedentary classmates. Beyond weekly exercise of 3500 kcal, there were *no additional* health or longevity benefits. In fact, when exercise was carried to extremes, the men had higher death rates than their more moderately active colleagues.

It should be kept in mind that Harvard alumni are a special group (mainly white, male, affluent) who may not represent the general population. The authors conclude, "There is a widespread and long-standing popular belief that adequate

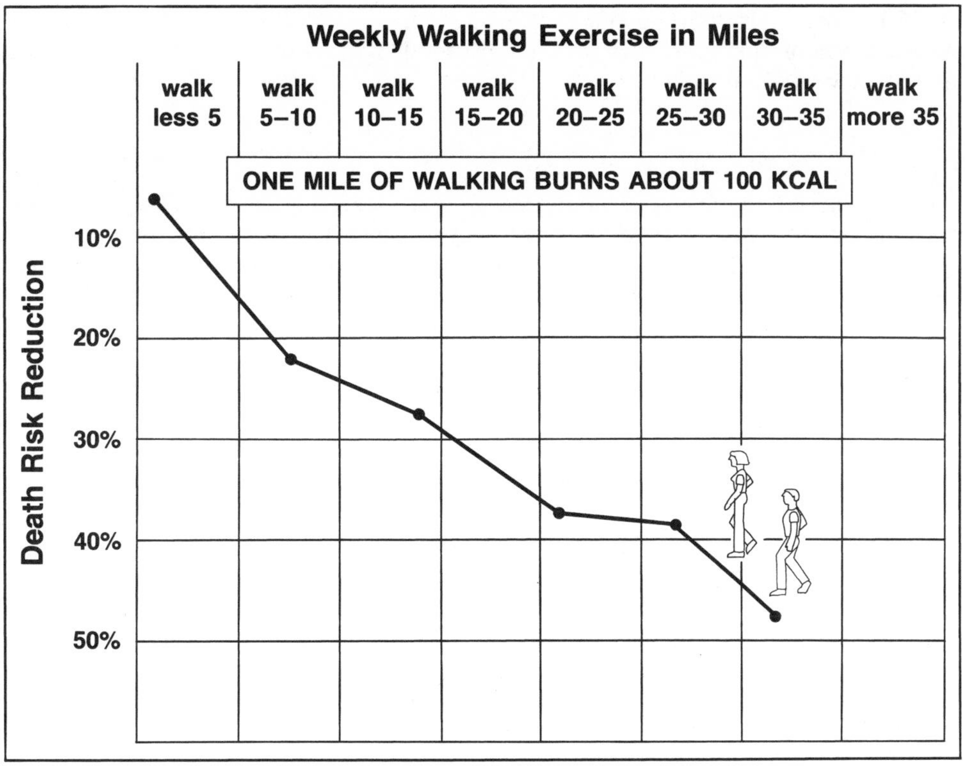
Weekly Walking Exercise in Miles
walk less 5
walk 5–10
walk 10–15
walk 15–20
walk 20–25
walk 25–30
walk 30–35
walk more 35
ONE MILE OF WALKING BURNS ABOUT 100 KCAL
Death Risk Reduction
10%
20%
30%
40%
50%

Figure 11-3. *Reduced risk of death with regular exercise.*

physical exercise is necessary to preserve life and its desirable qualities into old age. Discussions of this thesis date back to antiquity and have intensified in recent times. The present study adds new evidence to support this view."

Coronary Heart Disease

Diseases of the cardiovascular system have reached epidemic proportions in the United States and other affluent, high-technology industrialized nations. Figure 11-4 illustrates that 50% of the total deaths in the United States are caused by diseases of the heart and blood vessels. Stated in a somewhat more graphic fashion, as many as 1,500,000 Americans may have a heart attack this year and about one-third of them will die. Between ages 55 and 65, about 13 of every 100 men and 6 of every 100 women die from CHD. While the death rates for women lag about 10 years behind those of men, the gap is closing fast, especially with the upswing in cigarette smoking by women. Although recent years have shown a slight decline in mortality from CHD, it is still the greatest single killer and the most common cause of premature death. It is estimated that 63.4 million Americans have cardiovascular disease. For every American who dies of cancer, nearly 3 die of heart-related disease. The economic cost attributable to such health disasters—medical costs, loss of earnings and productivity—is staggering—85 billion dollars a year in 1987—not to mention the emotional impact of a loss of a loved one in the prime of life! For 1987, the total cost worked out to $361 for each adult and child in the United States. The economic costs are on the rise. In 1985, the total was $72.1 billion, and in 1986, it was $78.6 billion!

THE HEART'S BLOOD SUPPLY

Although literally tons of blood may flow through the heart each day, none of its nourishment passes directly into the heart muscle. This is because there are no direct circulatory channels to the cardiac muscle within the heart's chambers. Instead the heart muscle has an elaborate circulatory network of its own. As shown in Figure 11-5, these vessels form visible, crownlike arterial network, called the *coronary circulation,* on top of the heart. Openings for the two coronary arteries are situated in the aorta at a point where the freshly oxygenated blood leaves the left ventricle to be distributed through the body. These arteries then curl around the heart's surface; the *right coronary artery* supplies predominantly the right atrium and ventricle, whereas the greatest volume of blood flows in the *left coronary artery* to supply the tissue of the left atrium and ventricle and a small part of the right ventricle. These vessels divide and eventually form a dense capillary network within the heart muscle.

The driving force of the heart pushes a portion of blood into the coronary arteries with each heartbeat. This blood is distributed throughout the heart's vascular network to the individual muscle fibers. The blood supply to the heart is so profuse that at least one capillary supplies each of the heart's muscle fibers. After the blood passes through the capillaries, it empties into the right atrium via the coronary veins. Exercise produces increased pressure in the aorta that causes a proportionately greater flow of oxygenated blood to be forced into the coronary circulation.

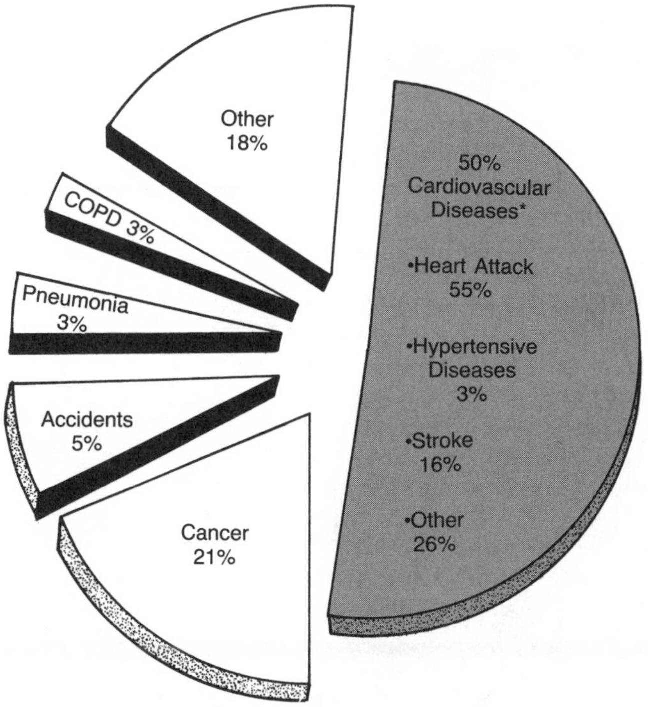
Other
18%
COPD 3%
Pneumonia
3%
Accidents
5%
Cancer
21%
50%
Cardiovascular
Diseases*
•Heart Attack
55%
•Hypertensive
Diseases
3%
•Stroke
16%
•Other
26%

*Based on data from the American Heart Association, "1987 Heart Facts". The total cost of cardiovascular disease in 1987 is estimated at $85.2 billion dollars!

Leading Causes of Death
United States: 1981 Estimate

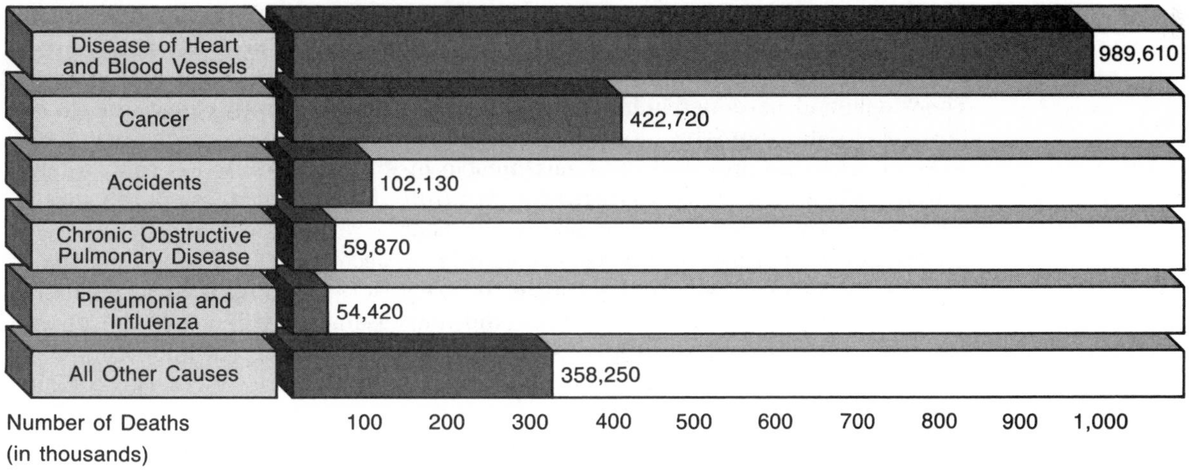
Disease of Heart and Blood Vessels
989,610
Cancer
422,720
Accidents
102,130
Chronic Obstructive Pulmonary Disease
59,870
Pneumonia and Influenza
54,420
All Other Causes
358,250
Number of Deaths
(in thousands)
100 200 300 400 500 600 700 800 900 1,000

Source: Modified from the National Center for Health Statistics, U.S. Public Health Service, DHHS

Figure 11-4. *Leading causes of death in the United States: 1981 Estimates. COPD is chronic obstructive lung disease.*

A LIFE-LONG PROCESS

As shown in Figure 11-6, CHD involves long-term degenerative changes in the inner lining of the arteries that supply the heart muscle. These vessels become congested with either lipid-filled plaques or fibrous scar tissue or both. Almost all

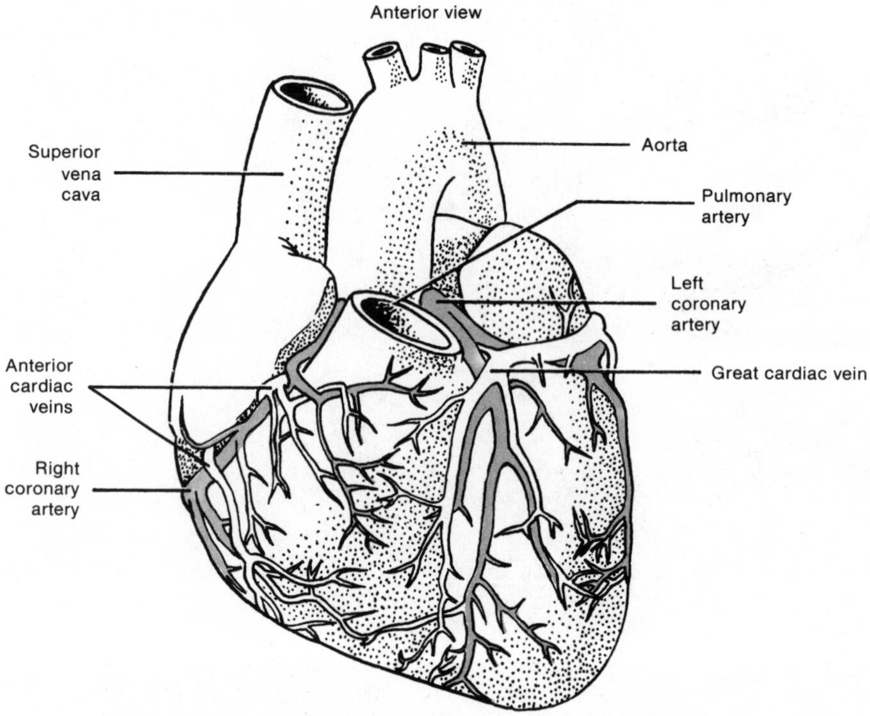
Anterior view
Superior
vena
cava
Aorta
Pulmonary
artery
Left
coronary
artery
Great cardiac vein
Anterior
cardiac
veins
Right
coronary
artery

Figure 11-5. *The coronary circulation. Arteries are shaded dark and veins are unshaded.*

people show some evidence of CHD, and it can be quite severe in seemingly healthy young adults.

The degenerative process of *atherosclerosis* begins in childhood and progresses silently for decades. There seems to be little harm, however, until there is marked arterial narrowing and the heart becomes poorly supplied with oxygen. The roughened, hardened lining of the coronary artery frequently causes the slowly flowing blood to clot. This blood clot may plug one of the smaller coronary vessels. In such cases, a portion of the heart muscle dies and the person is said to have suffered a heart attack or *myocardial infarction.* If the blockage is not too severe, but blood flow is still reduced below the heart's requirement, the person may experience temporary chest pains termed *angina pectoris.* These pains are usually felt during exertion because this causes the greatest demand for myocardial blood flow. Such anginal attacks provide painful and dramatic evidence of the importance of adequate oxygen supply to this vital organ. Generally, death occurs from CHD when there is advanced obstruction in several major blood vessels that supply the heart muscle.

Scientists are not sure exactly how fatty-type deposits or plaques develop. Many feel this lumpy thickening of the arterial wall begins as a fatty streak on the vessel's inner lining. It is often argued that this process is in some way facilitated by consuming a diet high in cholesterol and saturated fat. The deposition of fatty material eventually leads to calcification and fibrotic changes so that the arterial walls become narrower, rigid and hard, making blood flow more difficult. It has also been suggested that changes in cellular characteristics of the vessel's smooth muscle wall initiate the atherosclerotic process. These changes cause cellular mu-

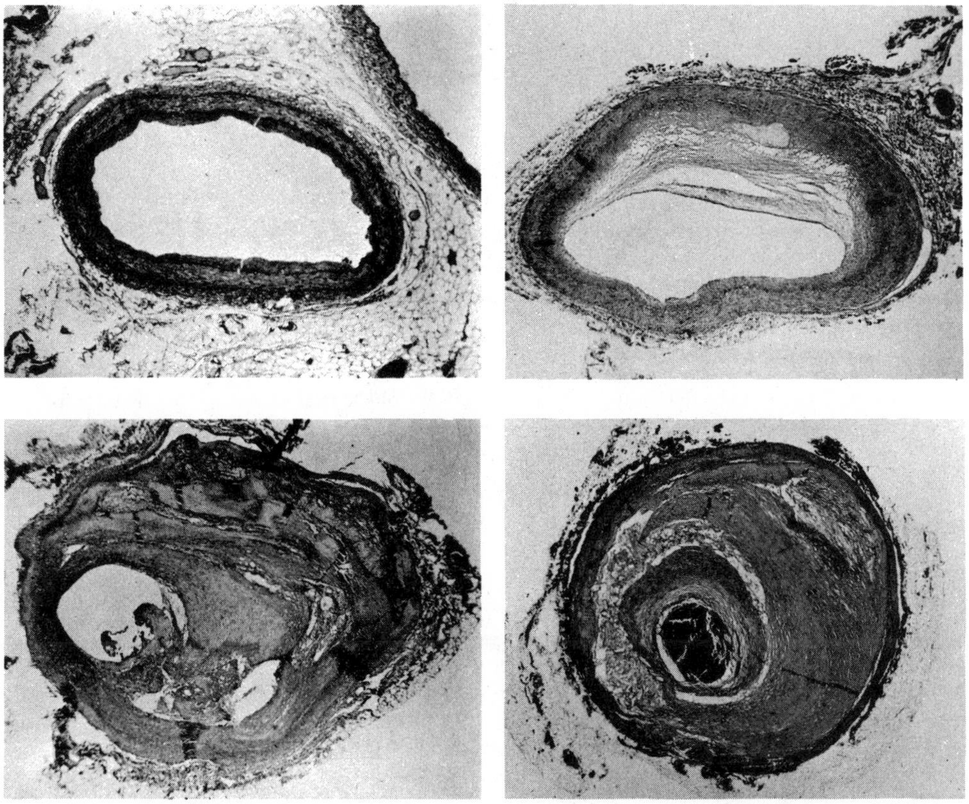

Figure 11-6. *Progressive narrowing of a normal coronary artery. During this degeneration process fatty deposits accumulate on the arterial wall. The wall becomes roughened and loses its elasticity, and the size of the opening becomes smaller. If the opening becomes too narrow, blood flows so slowly that it coagulates forming a clot. This plugs the artery depriving the heart muscle of vital blood to cause a heart attack.*

tation of smooth muscle cells and proceed in a manner similar to the development of a benign tumor. Abnormal cell division may be triggered by a sequence of repetitive injury to the arterial wall brought on by environmental factors such as diet, cigarette smoking, and high blood pressure.

RISK FACTORS FOR HEART DISEASE

Significant information has been gathered over the past 35 years on the natural history and dynamics of heart disease. By studying the incidence of heart attacks, chest pain, and sudden death in previously healthy people in large representative communities such as Framingham, Massachusetts, scientists have uncovered specific factors that contribute either directly or indirectly to the probability of getting this disease. From this, the relative importance of each factor has been established. *In general, the greater the risk factor the more likely it is that the coronary arteries are diseased or will become diseased in the near future.* This is not to say that a specific risk factor is the cause of the disease, as numerous factors may be acting and interacting in a cause and effect manner. However, based on the total evidence presently available it is prudent to assess these factors on a personal basis and make efforts to modify each within reasonable limits. In fact, part of the reason for the decline in CHD since the mid 1960s may be that people are taking charge of their lifestyles and altering modifiable risk factors in favorable directions. The following is a list of the more frequently implicated CHD risk factors: (1) age and gender; (2) elevated blood lipids; (3) hypertension; (4) cigarette smoking; (5) physical inactivity; (6) obesity; (7) diabetes mellitus; (8) diet; (9) heredity; (10) personality and behavior patterns; (11) high uric acid levels; (12) pulmonary function abnormalities; (13) race; (14) electrocardiographic abnormalities during rest and exercise; and (15) tension and stress. The significant heart disease risk factors including those that can and cannot be modified as well as important contributing factors are:

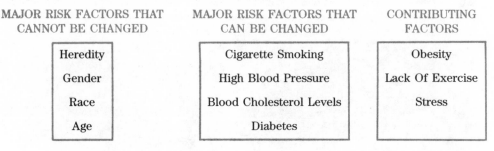

MAJOR RISK FACTORS THAT CANNOT BE CHANGED	MAJOR RISK FACTORS THAT CAN BE CHANGED	CONTRIBUTING FACTORS
Heredity	Cigarette Smoking	Obesity
Gender	High Blood Pressure	Lack Of Exercise
Race	Blood Cholesterol Levels	Stress
Age	Diabetes	

It is difficult to determine quantitatively the importance of a single CHD risk factor in comparison to any other because many of the factors are interrelated. For example, blood lipid abnormalities, diabetes, heredity, and obesity often go hand-in-hand. Compounding such observations is the often observed finding that physical training generally lowers body weight, body fat, and blood lipids. Also, certain groups are generally exposed to less psychologic stress because of the nature of their occupation or cultural setting.

The factors of age, gender, and heredity are predetermined and cannot be controlled or remedied. Based on careful risk factor evaluation, however, three "treatable" factors—serum lipids, blood pressure, and cigarette smoking—stand out as potent, consistent CHD risk factors. Of somewhat less predictive value than these three *primary risk factors* are the risk factors of obesity, personality type, and physical inactivity. It must be noted that although these factors are closely associated with CHD, the associations do not necessarily infer causality. It still remains to be shown that modification of each of the risk factors offers effective protection from the disease. Until definite proof is demonstrated, however, logic causes us to assume that elimination or reduction of one or more risk factors will cause a corresponding decrease in the probability of contracting CHD.

AGE, GENDER, AND HEREDITY

The likelihood of developing CHD generally increases rapidly with age. For a white American male between the ages of 25 and 35 the chances of dying from heart disease is 10 in 100,000; this increases to 1000 in 100,000 between the ages of 55 and 64. At most ages women fare much better than men. For example, a middle-aged man stands about 6 times the chances of dying from a heart attack as a woman of similar age. However, American women still lead all other countries in heart disease rates and the specific "sex advantage" is reduced greatly in older age. This has led some to speculate that some of this CHD protection for women may be provided by hormonal differences between the genders. The age risk factor is due in large part to the fact that other associated risk factors such as hypertension, elevated blood lipids, and glucose intolerance become more prevalent in older years. Although the cause is not known, heart attacks that strike at an early age appear to run in families.

BLOOD LIPIDS

The precise mechanism by which elevated blood fats (lipids) affect the development of CHD is not fully understood. Nevertheless, the overwhelming evidence links high levels of blood lipids with increased incidence of CHD. For example, the American Heart Association estimates that a man with a blood cholesterol level above 250 mg/dl of blood has about 3 times the risk of heart attack as a man with cholesterol below 200 mg/dl. In many cases, these elevated lipids are related to consuming diets high in saturated fats and cholesterol, as well as to excess body fat and lifestyles that are too stressful and physically inactive.

Cholesterol and triglycerides are the two most common lipids associated with CHD risk. These fats are not soluble in water so they do not circulate freely in the blood plasma. Rather, they are transported in combination with a carrier protein to form a *lipoprotein.* This lipoprotein can vary in size depending on how much protein and fat it contains. Serum cholesterol represents the total cholesterol contained in the different lipoproteins. Although it is proper to refer to an elevation in blood lipids as *hyperlipidemia,* it is more meaningful to evaluate and discuss the different types of *hyperlipoproteinemia.*

The distribution of cholesterol among the various types of lipoproteins is a more powerful predictor of heart disease than simply the total quantity of plasma lipids. This partially explains how one person with a high total serum cholesterol may not develop CHD, while another with a lower cholesterol level develops the disease. As shown in Figure 11-7, a high level of *high-density lipoproteins* (HDL, that comprise the smallest portion of lipoproteins but contain the largest quantity of protein and least amount of cholesterol) is associated with a lower heart disease risk. In contrast, elevated levels of the cholesterol-rich, *low-density lipoproteins* (LDL) represent an increased risk. In fact, data from the Framingham study suggest that very high levels of HDL may actually confer longevity.

Although much controversy exists as to the precise role of lipoproteins in heart disease, it is generally believed that the LDL are the means for transporting fat throughout the body for delivery to the cells, including those of the smooth muscle walls of the arteries. Here it ultimately becomes involved in the artery-narrowing process of atherosclerosis. Whereas LDL carries cholesterol to the tissues, HDL may act as a scavenger gathering cholesterol from cells (including arterial walls) and returning it to the liver where it is metabolized and excreted in the bile. It is also possible that HDL may retard cholesterol buildup in the cells by interfering with the binding and subsequent uptake of LDL at the cell membrane of the peripheral tissue.

Research is currently progressing to clarify whether HDL is truly protective and what factors can raise them. For one thing, cigarette smoking has adverse effects of the HDL patterns, while moderate alcohol consumption may improve the lipoprotein profile. *It is encouraging from an exercise perspective that HDL levels are elevated in endurance athletes and may be favorably altered in sedentary people who engage in aerobic training.* Concurrently, the LDL are lowered so the net result is a considerably improved ratio of HDL to LDL or HDL to total cholesterol. This exercise effect appears to be independent of whether or not the diet is

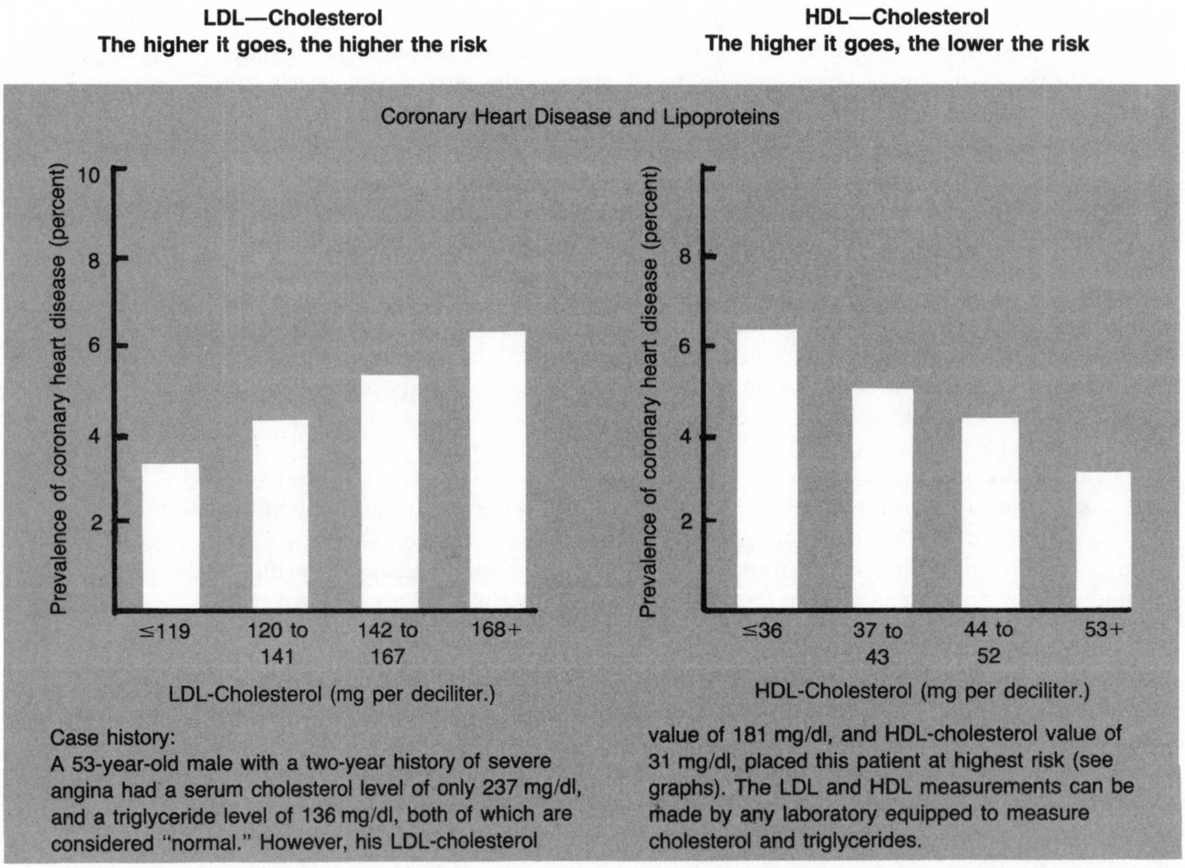
LDL—Cholesterol
The higher it goes, the higher the risk
HDL—Cholesterol
The higher it goes, the lower the risk
Coronary Heart Disease and Lipoproteins
Prevalence of coronary heart disease (percent)
10
8
6
4
2
≤119
120 to 141
142 to 167
168+
LDL-Cholesterol (mg per deciliter.)
Prevalence of coronary heart disease (percent)
8
6
4
2
≤36
37 to 43
44 to 52
53+
HDL-Cholesterol (mg per deciliter.)
Case history:
A 53-year-old male with a two-year history of severe angina had a serum cholesterol level of only 237 mg/dl, and a triglyceride level of 136 mg/dl, both of which are considered "normal." However, his LDL-cholesterol value of 181 mg/dl, and HDL-cholesterol value of 31 mg/dl, placed this patient at highest risk (see graphs). The LDL and HDL measurements can be made by any laboratory equipped to measure cholesterol and triglycerides.

Figure 11-7. *Coronary heart disease and lipoproteins. (Courtesy CPC International, Best Foods Division.)*

low in fat or whether or not the exerciser is overweight. The effect of regular endurance-type exercise on the blood lipid profile is certainly a strong argument for incorporating vigorous physical activity into a total program of health maintenance and preventive medicine.

The important factors that may affect the level of blood cholesterol as well as the lipoprotein fractions are:

Favorable Effects

- Weight loss through food restriction
- Regular aerobic exercise
- Intake of high fiber foods, particularly water soluble fibers such as in beans, legumes, and oat bran
- Increased polyunsaturated to saturated fatty acid ratio in diet as well as monounsaturated fat
- Increased intake of unique polyunsaturated fats in fish oils
- Moderate alcohol consumption

Unfavorable Effects

- Cigarette smoking
- Diet high in saturated fat and preformed cholesterol
- Emotionally stressful situations
- Certain oral contraceptives

HYPERTENSION

For individuals whose arteries have become "hardened" because fatty materials have deposited within their walls (or because the vessel's connective tissue layer has thickened), or whose arterial system offers excessive resistance to blood flow in the periphery due to nervous strain or kidney malfunction, systolic pressure at rest may be as high as 250 or even 300 mm Hg. The diastolic or run-off pressure may also be elevated above 90 mm Hg. Such high blood pressure, called *hypertension,* imposes a chronic, excessive strain on the normal functioning of the cardiovascular system. It has been estimated that 1 out of every 5 persons will have abnormally high blood pressure sometime during their lives. Presently, more than 37 million Americans have systolic pressures over 140 mm Hg or diastolic pressures over 90 mm Hg. These values form the *borderline* limits for the classification of high blood pressure. Uncorrected chronic hypertension can lead to heart failure, heart attack, stroke, or kidney failure.

Hypertension is often called the silent killer because it generally progresses unnoticed for decades before it deals its deadly blow. It is also a mysterious killer because the cause is unknown in more than 90 percent of the cases. Statistics indicate that the optimal blood pressure for longevity is about 110 mm Hg systolic and 70 mm Hg diastolic. Anything higher results in an increased risk for disease. For example, a man with a systolic blood pressure above 150 mm Hg has more than 2 times the risk of heart disease as a man with 120 mm Hg.

Hypertension can often be reduced by altering factors over which we have direct control. If you are overweight, reduce; if you smoke, stop, because the nicotine may constrict peripheral blood vessels and elevate blood pressure. Reduce salt intake as sodium can cause the body to retain fluid that boosts blood pressure. High blood pressure can also be effectively treated by relatively safe drugs (called diuretics) that reduce fluid volume.

Further encouraging news is that *both systolic and diastolic blood pressure can be significantly lowered with a regular program of exercise.* In patients with documented coronary artery disease and in "borderline" hypertensive patients, the effects of exercise training on blood pressure were impressive. For middle-aged male patients resting systolic pressure decreased from 139 to 133 mm Hg following 4 to 6 weeks of training. In addition, during submaximal exercise, systolic pressure decreased from 173 to 155 mm Hg, whereas diastolic pressure was also reduced from 92 to 79 mm Hg. Consequently, mean arterial blood pressure during exercise was reduced by approximately 14% following training. Based on available evidence, a prudent recommendation is to have your blood pressure checked periodically and include exercise in most therapeutic programs to manage hypertension.

CIGARETTE SMOKING

In terms of health status, the more a person smokes, the less healthy he or she is likely to be in the future. Cigarette smoking may be one of the best predictors of CHD. In fact, the probability of death from heart disease for smokers is almost twice as great as for non-smokers. Essentially, the more you smoke, the deeper you inhale, the stronger the cigarette in terms of tars and noxious byproducts, the greater your risk. In addition, smokers are nearly 5 times as likely to have a stroke as non-smokers. The increase in death rate from heart disease among women in this country almost parallels their increased consumption of cigarettes. Surprisingly, this CHD risk for men and women is associated with 2 to 3 times more deaths than the excess mortality of cigarette smokers due to lung cancer!

It is generally observed that the smoking risk acts independently of other risk factors. At the same time, however, if other risk factors are present, the multiple risks interact in an *additive* way and cigarette smoking may even accentuate the influence of other risks. The interaction of the three primary CHD risk factors when elevated in the same person is shown in Figure 11-8. With one risk factor, a 45-year-old man's chances of CHD during the year is about 2 times that of a man with no risks. With three risk factors present, the man's chance of chest pain, heart attack, or sudden death is 5 times higher than if there were no risk factors present.

OBESITY

Approximately 40% of all Americans are considered too heavy because their body weight is at least 10% above their ideal weight. This is not necessarily an adult problem as, for many, the onset of obesity begins in the first and second decades of life. The average male and female in the United States is about 9 pounds heavier than their 1960 counterparts, even though the nation's per capita caloric intake has steadily *decreased* over this 30-year period. Such facts further support the position that the "creeping obesity" in our society may be more due to physical *inactivity* than overeating.

It is difficult to determine quantitatively the importance of excess body fat per se as a risk to good health. However, the death rate for men who weigh 30% more than they should is nearly 70% higher than those of normal weight. The overfat condition is often associated with multiple risk factors such as hypertension and elevated serum lipids. In addition, an obese person usually consumes a highly atherogenic diet, that is, one that is high in saturated fats and cholesterol. It certainly appears that extra pounds can mean a greater chance of developing high

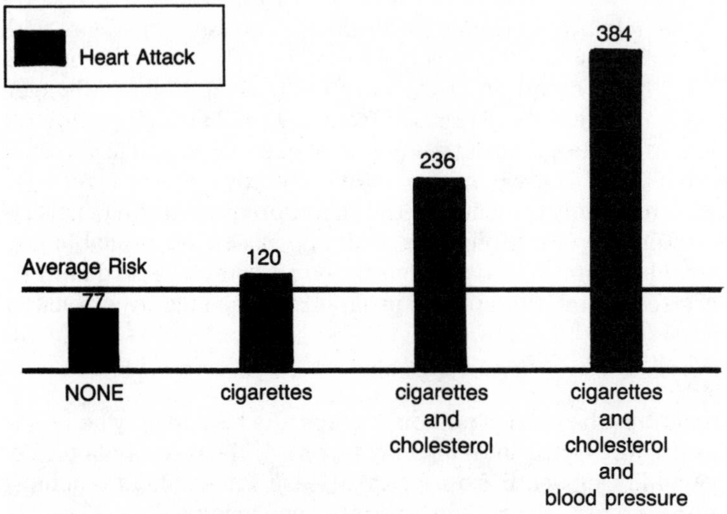
Heart Attack
384
236
Average Risk
120
77
NONE
cigarettes
cigarettes and cholesterol
cigarettes and cholesterol and blood pressure

Figure 11-8. ***Combining the risk factors. Persons with combinations of risk factors have experienced even more problems with coronary artery disease than those with fewer numbers. How risk factors are combined is an important consideration. Example is for a 45-year-old male. Modified from Heart Facts 1987, Dallas, TX, by permission of American Heart Association, Inc. #55-005-K, 1978.***

blood pressure as well as hyperlipidema, impaired glucose tolerance, and abnormal uric acid values. In the presence of these factors, obesity assumes a much stronger role as a health risk.

Weight loss and accompanying fat reduction generally contribute to normalizing cholesterol and triglyceride levels and have a beneficial effect on blood pressure. In fact, the normally observed relationship between age and blood pressure is partially explained because as we grow older, we have a tendency to put on weight. Although being too fat may not be a primary CHD risk factor, its role as a secondary and contributing factor in heart disease cannot be denied.

PERSONALITY AND BEHAVIOR PATTERNS

There appears to be a distinct type of personality that is susceptible to heart disease. The *coronary-prone* behaviors that typify what psychologists call the Type A personality reflect a lifestyle characterized as hard-driving, ambitious, impatient, short-tempered, hostile, and restless. Unrelenting pressures, drives, deadlines, anxieties, depression, and a constant struggle against the limitations of time are all part of this *stress syndrome*—with its accompanying recurrent and excessive stimulation of the body's "fight or flight" hormonal response that may be detrimental to the health of the heart. The opposite style of behavior, exemplified by the equally-capable, easy going, coronary-resistant Type B personality, is under no time pressure. This personality type is essentially categorized by the absence of Type A behaviors. Generally, one is neither all Type A nor all Type B, but rather a blend of both types of behavior patterns.

The precise manner of how personality traits and behaviors influence the development of CHD is unknown, let alone whether one's basic personality "type" can be significantly altered to influence a disease process. However, it does seem desirable to recognize, manage, and effectively channel excess stress in one's daily life. To this end, exercise blended with the techniques of behavior modification is a positive step in channeling potentially harmful behaviors into ones that will have positive "spin off." Regular exercise is an excellent way to vent tension and reduce external and internal stressors.

PHYSICAL INACTIVITY

Information on the role of physical activity in protecting one from CHD is sometimes contradictory but generally encouraging. Physically active people generally have fewer clinical symptoms of heart disease. When a heart attack does strike, their chances for survival are much greater than those of their inactive counterparts. In a 9-year study of Californians, sedentary men and women were more than twice as likely to die prematurely compared to those who exercised frequently. In terms of health status, those who reported even mild exercise were better off than completely sedentary people.

Such findings are circumstantial and must be viewed with caution for several reasons. For one thing, comparisons are often made between active and sedentary people with the assumption that other factors (blood lipids, hypertension, cigarette smoking, occupational status, body fatness) are essentially equal. This assumption is frequently not met. It is also possible that people with strong constitutions who are "destined" to live longer select active occupations or leisure-time pursuits. Likewise, as people detect certain symptoms of CHD, they move into a sedentary job or life-style. Thus at the time of death, they are rated as being inactive.

While the results from the latest studies argue strongly for regular physical activity, "critical or absolute proof" of the protective role of exercise against premature cardiovascular disease in humans is still lacking. Experiments with nonhuman primates, however, provide some direct evidence for the benefits of exercise. In one such study, monkeys were randomly assigned to a moderate, treadmill exercise program of running, 1 hour 3 times a week, or no exercise. Both groups were fed a relatively high fat diet. The exercised animals had significantly higher levels of HDL and lower LDL levels than their sedentary counterparts. Most importantly, they showed *no signs* of the coronary artery narrowing observed in the non-exercised group, and sudden death was observed *only* in the sedentary animals. Upon autopsy of all animals, the researchers noted that exercise was associated with substantially reduced overall atherosclerotic involvement. Exercise produced much larger and heavier hearts that were supplied with larger, healthy-appearing coronary arteries with less atherosclerosis. The conclusion was that moderate exercise may prevent or retard heart disease in primates.

While sufficient direct proof is lacking, the major weight of research on animals and humans indicates that regular exercise may operate against CHD in a variety of beneficial ways. These include:

1. Improved myocardial circulation and metabolism that protects the heart from hypoxic stress; this includes possible enhanced vascularization, as well as modest increases in cardiac glycogen stores and glycolytic capacity that could be beneficial when the heart's oxygen supply is compromised.
2. Enhanced mechanical or contractile properties of the myocardium; this may enable the conditioned heart to maintain or increase contractility during a specific challenge.
3. A more favorable blood clotting characteristic and other hemostatic mechanisms.
4. Normalized blood lipid profile, especially via an increase in HDL and lowering of LDL.
5. Favorably altered heart rate and blood pressure so the work of the myocardium is significantly reduced at rest and during exercise.
6. A more desirable body composition (higher lean to fat ratio).
7. A more favorable neural-hormonal balance that may conserve oxygen for the myocardium.
8. A favorable outlet for psychologic stress and tensions.
9. Increased ability to dissolve blood clots that could block a blood vessel to cause a stroke (brain) or myocardial infarction (heart).

In view of these findings, we wholeheartedly endorse vigorous exercise as a preventive and rehabilitative health measure.

ASSESS YOUR HEART DISEASE RISK—"RISKO"

Table 11-1 is a chart of risk factors that gives some idea of a person's chances for developing heart disease. This chart is a modified form of a more elaborate version generated from the more than 35 years of research on the natural history of

Relative Risk Category

SCORE	RELATIVE RISK CATEGORY
6–11	Risk well below average
12–17	Risk below average, OK
18–24	Average risk
25–31	Moderate risk
32–40	High risk
41–62	Very high risk, see your physician

Table 11-1. *CHD risk appraisal, RISKO*

AGE	10 to 20 1	21 to 30 2	31 to 40 3	41 to 50 4	51 to 60 6	61 to 70 and over 8
HEREDITY	No known history of heart disease 1	1 relative with cardiovascular disease Over 60 2	2 relatives with cardiovascular disease Over 60 3	1 relative with cardiovascular disease Under 60 4	2 relatives with cardiovascular disease Under 60 6	3 relatives with cardiovascular disease Under 60 7
WEIGHT	More than 5 lbs. below standard weight 0	−5 to +5 lbs. standard weight 1	6–20 lbs. over weight 2	21–35 lbs. over weight 3	36–50 lbs. over weight 5	51–65 lbs. over weight 7
TOBACCO SMOKING	Non-user 0	Cigar and/or pipe 1	10 cigarettes or less a day 2	20 cigarettes a day 4	30 cigarettes a day 6	40 cigarettes a day or more 10
EXERCISE	Intensive occupational and recreational exertion 1	Moderate occupational and recreational exertion 2	Sedentary work and intense recreational exertion 3	Sedentary occupational and moderate recreational exertion 5	Sedentary work and light recreational exertion 6	Complete lack of all exercise 8
CHOLES-TEROL OR FAT % IN DIET	Cholesterol below 180 mg/dl Diet contains no animal or solid fats 1	Cholesterol 181–205 mg/dl Diet contains 10% animal or solid fats 2	Cholesterol 206–230 mg/dl Diet contains 20% animal or solid fats 3	Cholesterol 231–255 mg/dl Diet contains 30% animal or solid fats 4	Cholesterol 256–280 mg/dl Diet contains 40% animal or solid fats 5	Cholesterol 281–300 mg/dl Diet contains 50% animal or solid fats 7
BLOOD PRESSURE	100 upper reading 1	120 upper reading 2	140 upper reading 3	160 upper reading 4	180 upper reading 6	200 or over upper reading 8
GENDER	Female under 40 1	Female 40–50 2	Female over 50 3	Male 4	Stocky male 6	Bald stocky male 7

Explanation of variables: *Heredity*—count parents, brothers, and sisters who have had a heart attack or stroke; *Smoking*—if you inhale deeply and smoke a cigarette way down, add one point to your score. Do not subtract because you think you do not inhale or smoke only a half inch on a cigarette; *Exercise*—lower your score one point if you exercise regularly and frequently; *Cholesterol/Saturated Fat Intake*—a cholesterol blood level is best. If you have not had a blood test recently, then estimate honestly the percentage of solid fats you eat. These are usually of animal origin—lard, cream, butter, and beef and lamb fat. If you eat much saturated fat, your cholesterol level will probably be high; *Blood Pressure*—if you have no recent reading but have passed an insurance or general medical examination, chances are you have a blood pressure level of 140 or less; *Gender*—this takes into account the fact that men have from 6 to 10 times more heart attacks than women of child-bearing age. (Adapted from the Michigan Heart Association.)

heart disease in the community of Framingham, Massachusetts. The assessment is for adult men and women of all ages. While this is certainly not a substitute for regular medical checkups, the information will be helpful in providing insight as to potential areas for concern. Many of these telltale characteristics are habits or the result of habits that can be controlled. *It certainly would be beneficial to help identify risk factors at an early age (perhaps at age 2 or 3!) to thwart the escalation of "silent" heart disease that is so prevalent in our highly mechanized, Western Society.*

To play RISKO, assign the appropriate numerical value that represents your present status for each category. Add up the scores in each category to determine your relative risk. Keep in mind that while there is nothing you can do as to your age, gender, and heredity risks, other factors such as blood pressure, tension, cigarette smoking, serum cholesterol, diet, exercise, and obesity can be modified.

Additional Reading

Amsterdam, E.A., et al.: (Eds): Exercise in Cardiovascular Health and Disease. New York, Yorke Medical Books, 1977.

Badenhop, D.T., et al.: Physiological adjustments to higher- or lower-intensity exercise in elders. *Medicine and Science in Sports and Exercise. 15:*496, 1983.

Blair, S.N. et al.: Changes in coronary heart disease risk factors associated with increased treadmill time. *American Journal of Epidemiology. 118:*352, 1983.

Bruce, R.A.: Exercise, functional aerobic capacity and aging—another viewpoint. *Medicine and Science in Sports and Exercise. 16:*8, 1984.

Crow, R.S. et al.: Risk factors, exercise fitness and electrocardiographic response to exercise in 12,866 men at high risk of symptomatic coronary heart disease. *American Journal of Cardiology. 57:*1075, 1986.

Ehsani, A.A. et al.: Effects of 12 months of intense exercise training on ischemic ST-segment depression in patients with coronary artery disease. *Circulation. 64:*1116, 1981.

Fisher, A.: The Healthy Heart. Virginia, Time-Life Books, 1981.

Friedman, M. and R. Rosenman: Type A Behavior and Your Heart. New York, Alfred A. Knopf, 1974.

Froelicher, V.: Exercise and health. *The American Journal of Medicine. 70:*987, 1981.

Hartung, G.H.: Jogging—The potential for prevention of heart disease. *Comprehensive Therapy. 6:*28, 1980.

Hartung, G.H. et al.: Effects of marathon running, jogging and diet on coronary risk factors in middle-aged men. *Preventive Medicine. 10:*316, 1981.

Hoeg, J.M., et al.: An approach to the management of hyperlipoproteinemia. *Journal of the American Medical Association. 255:*512, 1986.

Holloszy, J.O.: Exercise, health and aging: A need for more information. *Medicine and Science in Sports and Exercise. 15:*1, 1983.

Hurley, B.F. et al.: High density-lipoprotein cholesterol in body builders vs powerlifters. Negative effects of androgen use. *Journal of the American Medical Association. 252:*507, 1984.

Kramsch, D.M. et al.: Reduction of coronary atherosclerosis by moderate conditioning exercise in monkeys on an atherogenic diet. *New England Journal of Medicine. 305:*1483, 1981.

Leon, A.S. et al.: Effects of a vigorous walking program on body composition, and carbohydrate and lipid metabolism of obese young men. *American Journal of Clinical Nutrition. 32:*1776, 1979.

Montoye, H.J.: Physical Activity and Health: An Epidemiologic Study of an Entire Community. Englewood Cliffs, N.J., Prentice-Hall, 1975.

Morris, J.N. et al.: Vigorous exercise in leisure time: protection against coronary heart disease. *Lancet. 2:*1207, 1980.

NIH Consensus Development Conference: Lowering blood cholesterol to prevent heart disease. *Journal of the American Medical Association. 253:*2080, 1985.

Oster, G. and A.M. Epstein: Primary prevention and coronary heart disease: the economic benefits of lowering serum cholesterol. *American Journal of Public Health. 76:*647, 1986.

Paffenbarger, R.S., Jr., et al.: Energy expenditure, cigarette smoking, and blood pressure level as related to death from specific diseases. *American Journal of Epidemiology. 108:*12, 1978.

Paffenbarger, R.S., Jr., et al.: Physical activity, all-cause mortality, and longevity of college alumni. *New England Journal of Medicine. 314:*605, 1986.

Pollock, M.L. and D.H. Schmidt, (Eds.): Heart Disease and Rehabilitation. Boston, Houghton-Mifflin, 1979.

Posner, J.D.: Exercise capacity in the elderly. *American Journal of Cardiology. 57:*52C, 1986.

Puska, P.: Possibilities of a preventive approach to coronary heart disease starting in childhood. Acta Paediatrica Scandinavica Supplement. *318:*229, 1985.

Pyörälä, K.: Dietary cholesterol in relation to plasma cholesterol and coronary heart disease. *American Journal of Clinical Nutrition. 45:*1176, 1987.

Ransford, C.P.: A role for amines in the antidepressant effects of exercise: a review. *Medicine and Science in Sports and Exercise. 14:*1, 1982.

Rayssiguier, Y. and E. Gueux.: Magnesium and lipids in cardiovascular disease. *Journal of the American College of Nutrition. 5:*507, 1986.

Ross, R.: The pathogenesis of atherosclerosis—an update. *New England Journal of Medicine. 314:*488, 1986.

Seals, D.R., et al.: Endurance training in older men and women. I. Cardiovascular response to exercise. *Journal of Applied Physiology. 57:*1024, 1984.

Shephard, R.J.: Ischaemic Heart Disease and Exercise. Chicago, Year Book Medical Publishers Inc., 1981.

Shephard, R.J.: *Physical Activity and Aging.* Chicago, Year Book Medical Publishers, Inc., 1978.

Smith, E.L.: Exercise for prevention of osteoporosis: A review. *The Physician and Sportsmedicine. 3:*72, 1982.

Smith, E.L., and R.C. Serfass: *Exercise and Aging.* Hillside, N.J., Enslow Publishers, 1981.

Spirduso, W.W.: Physical fitness, aging, and psychomotor speed: A review. *Journal of Gerontology. 35:*850, 1980.

Stamler, J.: Diet and coronary heart disease. *Biometrics. 38:*95, 1982.

Toll, A. and Small, D.M.: Current concepts: Plasma high density lipoproteins. *New England Journal of Medicine. 229:*1232, 1978.

Vandervoort, A.A., et al.: Strength and endurance of skeletal muscle in the elderly. *Physiotherapy.* Canada. *38:*167, 1986.

General Readings (All Chapters)

American College of Sports Medicine: *Exercise and Sport Sciences Reviews.* Edited by K. Pandolf. Vol. 14. New York, Macmillan, 1986.

Astrand, P.O., and K. Rodahl: *Textbook of Work Physiology.* 2nd ed. New York, McGraw-Hill Book Co., 1977.

Brownell, K.D. and J.P. Foreyt (eds.). Handbook of Eating Disorders. Physiology, Psychology, and Treatment of Obesity, Anorexia, and Bulimia. Basic Books, Inc., New York, 1986.

Cioffi, L.A., W.P.T. Jones, and T.B. Van Itallie: *The Body Weight Regulatory System: Normal and Disturbed Mechanisms.* New York, Raven Press, 1981.

Costill, D.L.: *Inside Running: Basics of Sports Physiology.* Indianapolis, Benchmark Press, 1986.

Durnin, J.V.G.A., and R. Passmore: *Energy, Work and Leisure.* London, Hueneman Educational Books, 1967.

Food and Nutrition Board: *Recommended Dietary Allowances.* Washington, D.C., National Academy of Sciences, revised, 1980.

Galbo, H.: *Hormonal and Metabolic Adaptation to Exercise.* New York, G.T. Verlag, Inc., 1983.

Hamilton, E.M. and E. Whitney: *Nutrition. Concepts and Controversies.* St. Paul, West Publishing Company, 1985.

Haskell, W., J. Scala, and J. Whittam (Eds.): *Nutrition and Athletic Performance.* Palo Alto, Bull Publishing Co., 1982.

Jones, N.L., N. McCartney, and A.J. McComas, Eds.: *Human Muscle Power.* Champaign Human Kinetics Publishers Inc., 1986.

Katch, F.I., (Ed.): *Sport, Health, and Nutrition.* The 1984 Olympic Scientific Congress Proceedings, Vol. 2, Champaign, IL, Champaign Human Kinetics Publishers Inc., 1986.

Katch, F.I. and V.L. Katch: Optimal Health and Body Composition. In Shangold, M. and G. Mitkin (eds.). *Women, Exercise, and Sports Medicine.* Philadelphia, F.A. Davis, 1987.)

Komi, P.V.: *Exercise and Sport Biology.* Champaign, IL, Human Kinetics Publishers, 1982.

Krause, M.V., and M.A. Hunscher: *Food, Nutrition and Diet Therapy.* Philadelphia, W.B. Saunders Co., 1979.

Lehninger, A.L.: *Bioenergetics*, 2nd ed. Menlo Park, CA, W.A. Benjamin, 1971.

McArdle, W.D., F.I. Katch, and V.L. Katch: *Exercise Physiology. Energy, Nutrition, and Human Performance*, 2nd edition, Philadelphia, Lea & Febiger, 1986.

Pollock, M.D., et al.: *Health and Fitness Through Physical Activity.* New York, John Wiley & Sons, 1978.

Shephard, R.J.: *Physical Activity and Aging.* Chicago, Year Book Medical Publishers, Inc., 1978.

Skinner, J.: *Exercise Testing and Exercise Prescription for Special Cases. Theoretical Basis and Clinical Application.* Philadelphia, Lea & Febiger, 1987.

Smith, E. and R.C. Serfass: *Exercise and Aging.* Hillside, NJ, Enslow Publishers, 1981.

Vander, A.J. et al.: *Human Physiology: The Mechanisms of Body Function.* New York, McGraw-Hill Book Co., 1980.

Wasserman, K. et al.: *Principles of Exercise Testing and Interpretation.* Philadelphia, Lea & Febiger, 1987.

Watt, B.K., and A.L. Merrill: *Composition of Foods—Raw, Processed and Prepared.* Handbook no. 8, Washington, D.C., U.S. Department of Agriculture, 1963.

Williams, M.H.: *Nutritional Aspects of Human Physical and Athletic Performance.* Springfield, Charles C Thomas, 1976.

Williams, M.H.: *Lifetime Physical Fitness: A Personal Choice.* Dubuque, IA, Wm. C. Brown, 1985.

Worthington-Roberts, B.S.: *Contemporary Developments in Nutrition.* St. Louis, C.V. Mosby Co., 1981.

APPENDIX A

COMPUTERIZED MEAL AND EXERCISE PLAN

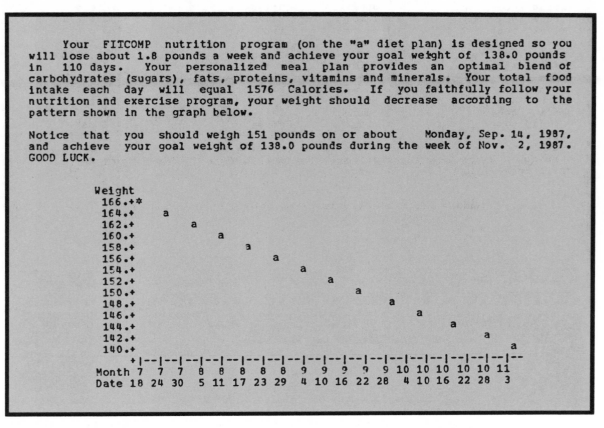

```
     Your  FITCOMP  nutrition  program (on the "a" diet plan) is designed so you
will lose about 1.8 pounds a week and achieve your goal weight of  138.0 pounds
in   110 days.   Your  personalized  meal  plan  provides  an  optimal  blend of
carbohydrates (sugars), fats, proteins, vitamins and minerals.  Your total  food
intake  each  day  will  equal  1576  Calories.   If  you faithfully follow your
nutrition and exercise program, your weight should  decrease  according  to  the
pattern shown in the graph below.

Notice  that  you  should weigh 151 pounds on or about    Monday, Sep. 14, 1987,
and  achieve  your goal weight of 138.0 pounds during the week of Nov.  2, 1987.
GOOD LUCK.

       Weight
        166.+*
        164.+   a
        162.+      a
        160.+         a
        158.+            a
        156.+               a
        154.+                  a
        152.+                     a
        150.+                        a
        148.+                           a
        146.+                              a
        144.+                                 a
        142.+                                    a
        140.+                                       a
            +|--|--|--|--|--|--|--|--|--|--|--|--|--|--|--|--|--|--|--
       Month 7  7  7  8  8  8  8  8  9  9  9  9  9 10 10 10 10 10 11
       Date 18 24 30  5 11 17 23 29  4 10 16 22 28  4 10 16 22 28  3
```

Example of weight loss curve. For this individual who initially weighed 165 lb, the desired weight loss was 27 lb.

Meat (amount for 70 calories)	
Canadian Bacon	1 ounce
Farmers cheese	1 ounce
Ricotta cheese	1 ounce
Mozzarella	1 ounce
Egg	1
Peanut butter	2 tbsp
Cottage cheese	1/4 cup
Tuna	1/4 cup
Salmon - canned	1/4 cup
Turkey	1 ounce
Chicken	1 ounce
Lamb shoulder	1 ounce
Lamb roast	1 ounce
Lamb chops	1 ounce
Lamb leg	1 ounce
Sirloin	1 ounce
Rump steak	1 ounce
Round steak	1 ounce
Tenderloin	1 ounce
Flank steak	1 ounce
Chuck steak	1 ounce
Veal - chops	1 ounce
Veal - cutlets	1 ounce
Pork Roast	1 ounce
Pork Chops	1 ounce
Pork - ham	1 ounce
Pork - leg	1 ounce
Ground round	1 ounce
Ground beef	1 ounce
Scallops	1 ounce
Shrimp	1 ounce
Fish-fresh/frzn	1 ounce
Cornish hen	1 ounce

Treats (amount for 80 calories)	
Popcorn (popped)	3 cup
Oatmeal cookies	1 1/2 2" dia
Choc chip cookie	1 1/2 2" dia
Chocolate fudge	1 sml pc
Candy bar, choc	1 small
Cupcake-icing	1 small

Alcohol (amount for 80 calories)	
Cognac	1 1/2 ounce
Wine red/white	3 1/2 ounce
Sherry	1 1/2 ounce
Port	1 1/2 ounce
Liquor	1 1/2 ounce
Beer	6 ounce
Ale	6 ounce

Fruit (amount for 40 calories)	
Papaya	3/4 cup
Apricot juice	1/2 cup
Prune juice	1/4 cup
Prunes	2
Pineapple juice	1/3 cup
Orange juice	1/2 cup
Banana	1/2 small
Apple juice	1/3 cup
Raisins	2 tbsp
Oranges	1 small
Dates	2
Cider - any kind	1/3 cup
Raspberries	1/2 cup
Apple	1 small
Tangarines	1 medium
Pineapple	1/2 cup
Nectarines	1 small
Watermelon	1 cup
Honeydew	1/6 small
Cantaloupe	1/4 small
Apple sauce	1/2 cup

Examples of food items selected from the questionnaire. The vegetable, bread and fat selections are not shown. The caloric values are a close approximation to actual values.

****

1576 Calorie Food Plan

Nutrient Composition

Carbohydrate...	261 grams or	64.% of your total calories
Protein........	71 grams or	17.% of your total calories
Fat............	35 grams or	19.% of your total calories

	Breakfast	Lunch	Dinner
Day 1	Cooked grits 1 1/2 cup Milk, skim 1 cup Cream - light 4 tbsp Apricot juice 1 cup	Bread-any kind 3 slice Milk, skim 1 cup Pork - ham 1 ounce Cauliflower 1/2 cup Raisins 6 tbsp	Candy bar, choc 1 small Mashed potato 1 cup Milk, skim 1 cup Veal - cutlets 2 ounce Rhubarb 1 1/2 cup Radishes no limit Diet Margarine 4 tsp Tangarines 2 medium

	Breakfast	Lunch	Dinner
Day 2	Toast 3 slice Milk, skim 1 cup Bacon - crisp 2 strip Prune juice 1/2 cup	Bread-any kind 3 slice Milk, skim 1 cup Peanut butter 2 tbsp Celery 1/2 cup Oranges 3 small	Beer 6 ounce Baked potato 1 small Milk, skim 1 cup Pork Roast 2 ounce Artichokes 1 1/2 cup Lettuce no limit Diet Margarine 4 tsp Pineapple 1 cup

This is an example of the first two days of a 1,576 calorie food plan. The usual procedure is to generate a 14-day plan; because foods are arranged as exchanges within a given food category, each exchange is assigned a specific calorie value. Therefore, one can exchange any one food within a food category with any other food in that category. In addition, any one complete breakfast, lunch, or dinner can be interchanged for any other breakfast, lunch, or dinner. This makes the number of food combinations for a given day equal to 14 factorial.

```
--------------------------------------------------------------------------
STEP Walk for 2 1/2 miles in 47 minutes 24 seconds(18 min 58 sec/mile)
  9  This exercise burns 280 calories.

     Cycle 3 1/2 miles in 19 minutes 26 seconds(10.80 miles/hour)
     Repeat this 2 times. This exercise burns 229 calories.

     Swim 275 yards in 9 minutes 50 seconds(27.96 yards/min)
     Repeat this 5 times. This exercise burns 290 calories.

     The following alternate activites will expend approximately the
     same number of calories as the aerobic activities above expend.
               Racquetball       for      51. minutes
               Circuit Training  for      22. minutes
               Squash            for      38. minutes
               Badminton         for      92. minutes
               Basketball        for      34. minutes
               Downhill Skiing   for      40. minutes
               Tennis            for      82. minutes
               Golf              for      47. minutes
               Aerobic Dancing   for      28. minutes
--------------------------------------------------------------------------
```

Example for Step 9 of the complementary beginner aerobic exercise plan to accompany the daily meal plans. With this program, individuals proceed to the next week's exercise after they complete their choice of exercise at least 3 times in the same week. Caloric expenditure represents average values for a particular body weight.

This kind of computer-generated output gives the person freedom to exchange activities for any given workout; it offers flexibility and variety in planning workouts to meet individual preferences. The major advantage, however, is the maintenance of caloric equivalency between the different activities that is linked with caloric input from the menus. If inclement weather prohibits jogging or cycling, then swimming or racquetball, for example, can be substituted without altering either the required calorie output (activity) or the required calorie input (food) side of the energy balance equation. In this way, the individual stays in phase with his or her tailor made weight loss curve. The exercise prescription is sensitive to individual differences because it considers age, gender, and current level of physical activity (relative fitness status).

HOW TO ORDER THE COMPUTERIZED MEAL AND EXERCISE PLAN

1. Send $16 (check, money order, or business, school or university purchase order only) to the following address:

   Computer Meal and Exercise Plan
   P.O. Box 431
   Amherst, Ma 01004

2. Make payable to: FITCOMP
3. Outside continental USA add $2 for postage and bank handling (total $18).

Please Note: Questionnaires are processed within 48 hours of receipt; you should receive the printout, under normal mail conditions, within 10 days. The $16 cost for the program applies until Dec. 31, 1991. Thereafter, price subject to change and availability. For updated information after this date, write to Computer Plan/Katch, McArdle, Lea & Febiger, 600 Washington Square, Philadelphia, Pa. 19106. The computer meal and exercise plan is an exclusive product of Fitcomp®, Fitness Technologies, Inc., P.O. Box 431, Amherst, MA 01004

More detailed information about the FITCOMP computerized meal and exercise plan can be found in the following article: Katch F.I. and V.L. Katch. Computer technology to evaluate body composition, nutrition, and exercise. *Preventive Medicine. 12:*619, 1983. See also Katch, F.I., Nutrition for the athlete. *In:* Welsh, R.P. and Shephard, R.J. (eds.). *Current Therapy in Sports Medicine.* B.C. Decker, Toronto, 1985.

COMPUTERIZED MEAL PLAN AND EXERCISE QUESTIONNAIRE

Please print with a ballpoint pen.

1. Name ______________________ (First) (Last)

2. Address ______________________ (Street Number and Name) (Apt. #)
______ ______ ______ City State Zip

3. Age ______ (years)

4. a. ______ Female b. ______ Male

5. Current body weight ______ (nearest pound)

6. Height (nearest $\frac{1}{4}$ in.) ___ feet ___ inches ___ fraction

7. How much you would like to weigh ______ (nearest pound)

8. Place an **X** next to the exercises you would like for your program. Select at least one from Group 1. Group 2 are optional.

9. Place an **X** next to the *one* section which best describes your current level of daily physical activity:
   a. ____ **Inactive:** You have a sit-down job and no regular physical activity.
   b. ____ **Relatively Inactive:** Three to four hours of walking or standing per day are usual. You have *no* regular organized physical activity during leisure time.
   c. ____ **Light Physical Activity:** You are sporadically involved in recreational activities such as weekend golf or tennis, occasional jogging, swimming or cycling.
   d. ____ **Moderate Physical Activity:** Usual job activities might include lifting or stair climbing, or you participate regularly in recreational/fitness activities such as jogging, swimming or cycling at least three times per week for 30 to 60 minutes each time.
   e. ____ **Very Vigorous Physical Activity:** You participate in *extensive* physical activity for 60 minutes or more at least four days per week.

Group 1. a. ____ Walking, Jogging, Running; b. ____ Swimming; c. ____ Cycling.

Group 2. d. ____ Racquetball; e. ____ Circuit Weight Training; f. ____ Squash; g. ____ Badminton; h. ____ Basketball;

i. ____ Downhill Skiing; j. ____ Tennis; k. ____ Golf; l. ____ Aerobic dancing.

FOOD PREFERENCE LIST

Select the foods you want as part of your daily diet from the Food Groups below. Mark an **X** in the box next to the food items you wish within each Group. You *must* select at least *one* item from Groups 1 through 18. To ensure menu variety, be sure to select all the foods you would like to eat. If you omit a choice from one of the required groups, the computer will make a selection for you. *Please Note:* The computer *cannot* make vegetarian menus. You may select none, or as many choices as you wish from Groups 19, 20 and 21—these are optional.

Group 1	A ☐ milk, skim	B ☐ milk, non-fat	C ☐ milk, 2%	
Group 2	A ☐ yogurt, skim milk B ☐ yogurt, 2% milk	C ☐ yogurt, regular milk D ☐ yogurt, fruit	E ☐ whole milk F ☐ choc. milk, non-fat	G ☐ buttermilk H ☐ ice milk
Group 3	A ☐ egg B ☐ mozzarella	C ☐ ricotta cheese D ☐ farmers cheese	E ☐ cheddar cheese F ☐ american cheese	G ☐ swiss cheese H ☐ canadian bacon
Group 4	A ☐ chicken B ☐ turkey C ☐ hot dog	D ☐ corned beef E ☐ salmon, canned F ☐ tuna	G ☐ crab, canned H ☐ oysters	I ☐ cottage cheese J ☐ peanut butter
Group 5	A ☐ chuck steak B ☐ flank steak C ☐ tenderloin	D ☐ round steak E ☐ rump steak F ☐ sirloin	G ☐ lamb leg H ☐ lamb chops	I ☐ lamb roast J ☐ lamb shoulder
Group 6	A ☐ cornish hen B ☐ fish, fresh and frzn. C ☐ shrimp D ☐ scallops	E ☐ ground beef F ☐ ground round G ☐ pork leg H ☐ pork/ham	I ☐ pork chops J ☐ pork roast K ☐ pork shoulder L ☐ veal shoulder	M ☐ veal cutlets N ☐ veal chops O ☐ veal roast
Group 7	A ☐ avocado B ☐ olives	C ☐ almonds D ☐ pecans	E ☐ peanuts, dry roast F ☐ walnuts	G ☐ cream cheese H ☐ bacon, crisp
Group 8	A ☐ diet margarine			
Group 9	A ☐ cream, light B ☐ french dressing	C ☐ 1000 island dressing D ☐ italian dressing	E ☐ mayonnaise F ☐ sour cream	G ☐ blue cheese dressing H ☐ tartar sauce
Group 10	A ☐ raisin bread B ☐ bagel C ☐ english muffin	D ☐ toast E ☐ bran flakes F ☐ cereal, dry	G ☐ puffed cereal H ☐ cooked cereal	I ☐ cooked grits J ☐ donut, plain
Group 11	A ☐ bread, any kind B ☐ cooked barley	C ☐ arrowroot crackers D ☐ graham crackers	E ☐ matzo F ☐ soda crackers	G ☐ plain muffin H ☐ cooked rice
Group 12	A ☐ cooked spaghetti B ☐ cooked noodles C ☐ cooked macaroni D ☐ beans, cooked E ☐ lentils, cooked	F ☐ corn, off cob G ☐ corn, on cob H ☐ lima beans I ☐ parsnips	J ☐ peas K ☐ baked potato L ☐ mashed potato M ☐ squash	N ☐ biscuit O ☐ corn bread P ☐ corn muffins Q ☐ yam
Group 13	A ☐ apple juice B ☐ banana C ☐ grapefruit juice	D ☐ grapefruit E ☐ grape juice F ☐ orange juice	G ☐ pineapple juice H ☐ prunes I ☐ prune juice	J ☐ apricot juice K ☐ papaya
Group 14	A ☐ apple B ☐ apricot C ☐ apricot, dried D ☐ blackberries	E ☐ blueberries F ☐ raspberries G ☐ strawberries H ☐ cider, any kind	I ☐ dates J ☐ mango K ☐ orange L ☐ peach	M ☐ pear N ☐ plum O ☐ raisins
Group 15	A ☐ apple sauce B ☐ cherries C ☐ grapes	D ☐ cantaloupe E ☐ honeydew	F ☐ watermelon G ☐ nectarine	H ☐ pineapple I ☐ tangerine
Group 16	A ☐ cucumber B ☐ vegetable juice	C ☐ tomato D ☐ tomato juice	E ☐ carrots F ☐ green pepper	G ☐ celery H ☐ cauliflower
Group 17	A ☐ asparagus B ☐ bean sprouts	C ☐ beets D ☐ broccoli	E ☐ brussel sprouts F ☐ cabbage	G ☐ eggplant
Group 18	A ☐ collards B ☐ kale C ☐ mustard greens D ☐ spinach	E ☐ turnip greens F ☐ mushrooms G ☐ okra	H ☐ string beans I ☐ artichokes J ☐ rutabaga	K ☐ sauerkraut L ☐ turnips M ☐ zucchini

Optional Choices

Group 19	A ☐ lettuce B ☐ radishes	C ☐ chicory D ☐ endive	E ☐ escarole F ☐ parsley	G ☐ watercress
Group 20	A ☐ ale B ☐ beer	C ☐ liquor D ☐ port	E ☐ sherry F ☐ wine, red/white	G ☐ cognac
Group 21	A ☐ cake, angel food B ☐ cake, fruit C ☐ cake, pound	D ☐ cupcake, with icing E ☐ candy bar, choc. F ☐ chocolate fudge	G ☐ marshmallows, reg. H ☐ choc. chip cookies I ☐ oatmeal cookies	J ☐ sugar cookies K ☐ pudding L ☐ popcorn, popped

APPENDIX **B**

Energy Expenditure in Household, Recreational, and Sport Activities (in kcal per min)

ACTIVITY	KG / LB	50 / 110	53 / 117	56 / 123	59 / 130	62 / 137	65 / 143	68 / 150
Archery		3.3	3.4	3.6	3.8	4.0	4.2	4.4
Badminton		4.9	5.1	5.4	5.7	6.0	6.3	6.6
Bakery, general (F)		1.8	1.9	2.0	2.1	2.2	2.3	2.4
Basketball		6.9	7.3	7.7	8.1	8.6	9.0	9.4
Billiards		2.1	2.2	2.4	2.5	2.6	2.7	2.9
Bookbinding		1.9	2.0	2.1	2.2	2.4	2.5	2.6
Boxing								
in ring		6.9	7.3	7.7	8.1	8.6	9.0	9.4
sparring		11.1	11.8	12.4	13.1	13.8	14.4	15.1
Canoeing								
leisure		2.2	2.3	2.5	2.6	2.7	2.9	3.0
racing		5.2	5.5	5.8	6.1	6.4	6.7	7.0
Card playing		1.3	1.3	1.4	1.5	1.6	1.6	1.7
Carpentry, general		2.6	2.8	2.9	3.1	3.2	3.4	3.5
Carpet sweeping (F)		2.3	2.4	2.5	2.7	2.8	2.9	3.1
Carpet sweeping (M)		2.4	2.5	2.7	2.8	3.0	3.1	3.3
Circuit training								
Hydra-Fitness		6.6	7.0	7.4	7.8	8.2	8.6	9.0
Universal		5.8	6.2	6.5	6.9	7.2	7.5	7.9
Nautilus		4.6	4.9	5.2	5.5	5.8	6.0	6.3
Free Weights		4.3	4.5	4.8	5.0	5.3	5.5	5.8
Cleaning (F)		3.1	3.3	3.5	3.7	3.8	4.0	4.2
Cleaning (M)		2.9	3.1	3.2	3.4	3.6	3.8	3.9
Climbing hills								
with no load		6.1	6.4	6.8	7.1	7.5	7.9	8.2
with 5-kg load		6.5	6.8	7.2	7.6	8.0	8.4	8.8
with 10-kg load		7.0	7.4	7.8	8.3	8.7	9.1	9.5
with 20-kg load		7.4	7.8	8.2	8.7	9.1	9.6	10.0

* Data from Bannister, E.W. and Brown, S.R.: The relative energy requirements of physical activity, IN H.B. Falls (ed.): Exercise Physiology. New York, Academic Press, 1968; Howley, E.T. and Glover, M.E.: The caloric costs of running and walking one mile for men and women. Medicine and Science in Sports 6:235, 1974; Passmore, R. and Durnin, J.V.G.A.: Human energy expenditure. Physiological Reviews 35:801, 1955. *Note:* Symbols (M) and (F) denote experiments for males and females, respectively. See p. 108 for instructions on how to use this appendix.

71 157	74 163	77 170	80 176	83 183	86 190	89 196	92 203	95 209	98 216
4.6	4.8	5.0	5.2	5.4	5.6	5.8	6.0	6.2	6.4
6.9	7.2	7.5	7.8	8.1	8.3	8.6	8.9	9.2	9.5
2.5	2.6	2.7	2.8	2.9	3.0	3.1	3.2	3.3	3.4
9.8	10.2	10.6	11.0	11.5	11.9	12.3	12.7	13.1	13.5
3.0	3.1	3.2	3.4	3.5	3.6	3.7	3.9	4.0	4.1
2.7	2.8	2.9	3.0	3.2	3.3	3.4	3.5	3.6	3.7
9.8	10.2	10.6	11.0	11.5	11.9	12.3	12.7	13.1	13.5
15.8	16.4	17.1	17.8	18.4	19.1	19.8	20.4	21.1	21.8
3.1	3.3	3.4	3.5	3.7	3.8	3.9	4.0	4.2	4.3
7.3	7.6	7.9	8.2	8.5	8.9	9.2	9.5	9.8	10.1
1.8	1.9	1.9	2.0	2.1	2.2	2.2	2.3	2.4	2.5
3.7	3.8	4.0	4.2	4.3	4.5	4.6	4.8	4.9	5.1
3.2	3.3	3.5	3.6	3.7	3.9	4.0	4.1	4.3	4.4
3.4	3.6	3.7	3.8	4.0	4.1	4.3	4.4	4.6	4.7
9.4	9.7	10.2	10.5	10.9	11.4	11.7	12.1	12.5	12.9
8.3	8.6	8.9	9.3	9.6	10.0	10.3	10.7	11.0	11.4
6.6	6.8	7.1	7.4	7.7	8.0	8.2	8.5	8.8	9.1
6.1	6.3	6.6	6.8	7.1	7.4	7.6	7.9	8.1	8.4
4.4	4.6	4.8	5.0	5.1	5.3	5.5	5.7	5.9	6.1
4.1	4.3	4.5	4.6	4.8	5.0	5.2	5.3	5.5	5.7
8.6	9.0	9.3	9.7	10.0	10.4	10.8	11.1	11.5	11.9
9.2	9.5	9.9	10.3	10.7	11.1	11.5	11.9	12.3	12.6
9.9	10.4	10.8	11.2	11.6	12.0	12.5	12.9	13.3	13.7
10.4	10.9	11.3	11.8	12.2	12.6	13.1	13.5	14.0	14.4

ACTIVITY	KG LB	50 110	53 117	56 123	59 130	62 137	65 143	68 150
Coal mining								
drilling coal, rock		4.7	5.0	5.3	5.5	5.8	6.1	6.4
erecting supports		4.4	4.7	4.9	5.2	5.5	5.7	6.0
shoveling coal		5.4	5.7	6.0	6.4	6.7	7.0	7.3
Cooking (F)		2.3	2.4	2.5	2.7	2.8	2.9	3.1
Cooking (M)		2.4	2.5	2.7	2.8	3.0	3.1	3.3
Cricket								
batting		4.2	4.4	4.6	4.9	5.1	5.4	5.6
bowling		4.5	4.8	5.0	5.3	5.6	5.9	6.1
Croquet		3.0	3.1	3.3	3.5	3.7	3.8	4.0
Cycling								
leisure, 5.5 mph		3.2	3.4	3.6	3.8	4.0	4.2	4.4
leisure, 9.4 mph		5.0	5.3	5.6	5.9	6.2	6.5	6.8
racing		8.5	9.0	9.5	10.0	10.5	11.0	11.5
Dancing								
Dancing (F)								
aerobic, medium		5.2	5.5	5.8	6.1	6.4	6.7	7.0
aerobic, intense		6.7	7.1	7.5	7.9	8.3	8.7	9.2
ballroom		2.6	2.7	2.9	3.0	3.2	3.3	3.5
choreographed		8.4	8.9	9.4	9.9	10.4	10.9	11.4
"twist," "wiggle"		5.2	5.5	5.8	6.1	6.4	6.7	7.0
Digging trenches		7.3	7.7	8.1	8.6	9.0	9.4	9.9
Drawing (standing)		1.8	1.9	2.0	2.1	2.2	2.3	2.4
Eating (sitting)		1.2	1.2	1.3	1.4	1.4	1.5	1.6
Electrical work		2.9	3.1	3.2	3.4	3.6	3.8	3.9
Farming								
barn cleaning		6.8	7.2	7.6	8.0	8.4	8.8	9.2
driving harvester		2.0	2.1	2.2	2.4	2.5	2.6	2.7
driving tractor		1.9	2.0	2.1	2.2	2.3	2.4	2.5
feeding cattle		4.3	4.5	4.8	5.0	5.3	5.5	5.8
feeding animals		3.3	3.4	3.6	3.8	4.0	4.2	4.4
forking straw bales		6.9	7.3	7.7	8.1	8.6	9.0	9.4
milking by hand		2.7	2.9	3.0	3.2	3.3	3.5	3.7
milking by machine		1.2	1.2	1.3	1.4	1.4	1.5	1.6
shoveling grain		4.3	4.5	4.8	5.0	5.3	5.5	5.8
Field hockey		6.7	7.1	7.5	7.9	8.3	8.7	9.1
Fishing		3.1	3.3	3.5	3.7	3.8	4.0	4.2
Food shopping (F)		3.1	3.3	3.5	3.7	3.8	4.0	4.2
Food shopping (M)		2.9	3.1	3.2	3.4	3.6	3.8	3.9
Football		6.6	7.0	7.4	7.8	8.2	8.6	9.0
Forestry								
ax chopping, fast		14.9	15.7	16.6	17.5	18.4	19.3	20.2
ax chopping, slow		4.3	4.5	4.8	5.0	5.3	5.5	5.8
barking trees		6.2	6.5	6.9	7.3	7.6	8.0	8.4
carrying logs		9.3	9.9	10.4	11.0	11.5	12.1	12.6
felling trees		6.6	7.0	7.4	7.8	8.2	8.6	9.0
hoeing		4.6	4.8	5.1	5.4	5.6	5.9	6.2
planting by hand		5.5	5.8	6.1	6.4	6.8	7.1	7.4
sawing by hand		6.1	6.5	6.8	7.2	7.6	7.9	8.3
sawing, power		3.8	4.0	4.2	4.4	4.7	4.9	5.1

71	74	77	80	83	86	89	92	95	98
157	163	170	176	183	190	196	203	209	216
6.7	7.0	7.2	7.5	7.8	8.1	8.4	8.6	8.9	9.2
6.2	6.5	6.8	7.0	7.3	7.6	7.8	8.1	8.4	8.6
7.7	8.0	8.3	8.6	9.0	9.3	9.6	9.9	10.3	10.6
3.2	3.3	3.5	3.6	3.7	3.9	4.0	4.1	4.3	4.4
3.4	3.6	3.7	3.8	4.0	4.1	4.3	4.4	4.6	4.7
5.9	6.1	6.4	6.6	6.9	7.1	7.4	7.6	7.9	8.1
6.4	6.7	6.9	7.2	7.5	7.7	8.0	8.3	8.6	8.8
4.2	4.4	4.5	4.7	4.9	5.1	5.3	5.4	5.6	5.8
4.5	4.7	4.9	5.1	5.3	5.5	5.7	5.9	6.1	6.3
7.1	7.4	7.7	8.0	8.3	8.6	8.9	9.2	9.5	9.8
12.0	12.5	13.0	13.5	14.0	14.5	15.0	15.5	16.1	16.6
7.3	7.6	7.9	8.2	8.5	8.9	9.2	9.5	9.8	10.1
9.6	10.0	10.4	10.8	11.2	11.6	12.0	12.4	12.8	13.2
3.6	3.8	3.9	4.1	4.2	4.4	4.5	4.7	4.8	5.0
11.9	12.4	12.9	13.4	13.9	14.4	15.0	15.5	16.0	16.5
7.3	7.6	7.9	8.2	8.5	8.9	9.2	9.5	9.8	10.1
10.3	10.7	11.2	11.6	12.0	12.5	12.9	13.3	13.8	14.2
2.6	2.7	2.8	2.9	3.0	3.1	3.2	3.3	3.4	3.5
1.6	1.7	1.8	1.8	1.9	2.0	2.0	2.1	2.2	2.3
4.1	4.3	4.5	4.6	4.8	5.0	5.2	5.3	5.5	5.7
9.6	10.0	10.4	10.8	11.2	11.6	12.0	12.4	12.8	13.2
2.8	3.0	3.1	3.2	3.3	3.4	3.6	3.7	3.8	3.9
2.6	2.7	2.8	3.0	3.1	3.2	3.3	3.4	3.5	3.6
6.0	6.3	6.5	6.8	7.1	7.3	7.6	7.8	8.1	8.3
4.6	4.8	5.0	5.2	5.4	5.6	5.8	6.0	6.2	6.4
9.8	10.2	10.6	11.0	11.5	11.9	12.3	12.7	13.1	13.5
3.8	4.0	4.2	4.3	4.5	4.6	4.8	5.0	5.1	5.3
1.6	1.7	1.8	1.8	1.9	2.0	2.0	2.1	2.2	2.3
6.0	6.3	6.5	6.8	7.1	7.3	7.6	7.8	8.1	8.3
9.5	9.9	10.3	10.7	11.1	11.5	11.9	12.3	12.7	13.1
4.4	4.6	4.8	5.0	5.1	5.3	5.5	5.7	5.9	6.1
4.4	4.6	4.8	5.0	5.1	5.3	5.5	5.7	5.9	6.1
4.1	4.3	4.5	4.6	4.8	5.0	5.2	5.3	5.5	5.7
9.4	9.8	10.2	10.6	11.0	11.4	11.7	12.1	12.5	12.9
21.1	22.0	22.9	23.8	24.7	25.5	26.4	27.3	28.2	29.1
6.0	6.3	6.5	6.8	7.1	7.3	7.6	7.8	8.1	8.3
8.7	9.1	9.5	9.8	10.2	10.6	10.9	11.3	11.7	12.1
13.2	13.8	14.3	14.9	15.4	16.0	16.6	17.1	17.7	18.2
9.4	9.8	10.2	10.6	11.0	11.4	11.7	12.1	12.5	12.9
6.5	6.7	7.0	7.3	7.6	7.8	8.1	8.4	8.6	8.9
7.7	8.1	8.4	8.7	9.0	9.4	9.7	10.0	10.4	10.7
8.7	9.0	9.4	9.8	10.1	10.5	10.9	11.2	11.6	12.0
5.3	5.6	5.8	6.0	6.2	6.5	6.7	6.9	7.1	7.4

ACTIVITY	KG LB	50 110	53 117	56 123	59 130	62 137	65 143	68 150
Forestry *(continued)*								
stacking firewood		4.4	4.7	4.9	5.2	5.5	5.7	6.0
trimming trees		6.5	6.8	7.2	7.6	8.0	8.4	8.8
weeding		3.6	3.8	4.0	4.2	4.5	4.7	4.9
Furriery		4.2	4.4	4.6	4.9	5.1	5.4	5.6
Gardening								
digging		6.3	6.7	7.1	7.4	7.8	8.2	8.6
hedging		3.9	4.1	4.3	4.5	4.8	5.0	5.2
mowing		5.6	5.9	6.3	6.6	6.9	7.3	7.6
raking		2.7	2.9	3.0	3.2	3.3	3.5	3.7
Golf		4.3	4.5	4.8	5.0	5.3	5.5	5.8
Gymnastics		3.3	3.5	3.7	3.9	4.1	4.3	4.5
Horse-grooming		6.4	6.8	7.2	7.6	7.9	8.3	8.7
Horse-racing								
galloping		6.9	7.3	7.7	8.1	8.5	8.9	9.3
trotting		5.5	5.8	6.2	6.5	6.8	7.2	7.5
walking		2.1	2.2	2.3	2.4	2.5	2.7	2.8
Ironing (F)		1.7	1.7	1.8	1.9	2.0	2.1	2.2
Ironing (M)		3.2	3.4	3.6	3.8	4.0	4.2	4.4
Judo		9.8	10.3	10.9	11.5	12.1	12.7	13.3
Jumping Rope								
70 per min		8.1	8.6	9.1	9.6	10.0	10.5	11.0
80 per min		8.2	8.7	9.2	9.7	10.2	10.7	11.2
125 per min		8.9	9.4	9.9	10.4	11.0	11.5	12.0
145 per min		9.9	10.4	11.0	11.6	12.2	12.8	13.4
Knitting, sewing (F)		1.1	1.2	1.2	1.3	1.4	1.4	1.5
Knitting, sewing (M)		1.2	1.2	1.3	1.4	1.4	1.5	1.6
Locksmith		2.9	3.0	3.2	3.4	3.5	3.7	3.9
Lying at ease		1.1	1.2	1.2	1.3	1.4	1.4	1.5
Machine-tooling								
machining		2.4	2.5	2.7	2.8	3.0	3.1	3.3
operating lathe		2.6	2.8	2.9	3.1	3.2	3.4	3.5
operating punch press		4.4	4.7	4.9	5.2	5.5	5.7	6.0
tapping and drilling		3.3	3.4	3.6	3.8	4.0	4.2	4.4
welding		2.6	2.8	2.9	3.1	3.2	3.4	3.5
working sheet metal		2.4	2.5	2.7	2.8	3.0	3.1	3.3
Marching, rapid		7.1	7.5	8.0	8.4	8.8	9.2	9.7
Mopping floor (F)		3.1	3.3	3.5	3.7	3.8	4.0	4.2
Mopping floor (M)		2.9	3.1	3.2	3.4	3.6	3.8	3.9
Music playing								
accordion (sitting)		1.6	1.7	1.8	1.9	2.0	2.1	2.2
cello (sitting)		2.1	2.2	2.3	2.4	2.5	2.7	2.8
conducting		2.0	2.1	2.2	2.3	2.4	2.5	2.7
drums (sitting)		3.3	3.5	3.7	3.9	4.1	4.3	4.5
flute (sitting)		1.8	1.9	2.0	2.1	2.2	2.3	2.4
horn (sitting)		1.5	1.5	1.6	1.7	1.8	1.9	2.0
organ (sitting)		2.7	2.8	3.0	3.1	3.3	3.4	3.6

71 157	74 163	77 170	80 176	83 183	86 190	89 196	92 203	95 209	98 216
6.2	6.5	6.8	7.0	7.3	7.6	7.8	8.1	8.4	8.6
9.2	9.5	9.9	10.3	10.7	11.1	11.5	11.9	12.3	12.6
5.1	5.3	5.5	5.8	6.0	6.2	6.4	6.6	6.8	7.1
5.9	6.1	6.4	6.6	6.9	7.1	7.4	7.6	7.9	8.1
8.9	9.3	9.7	10.1	10.5	10.8	11.2	11.6	12.0	12.3
5.5	5.7	5.9	6.2	6.4	6.6	6.9	7.1	7.3	7.5
8.0	8.3	8.6	9.0	9.3	9.6	10.0	10.3	10.6	11.0
3.8	4.0	4.2	4.3	4.5	4.6	4.8	5.0	5.1	5.3
6.0	6.3	6.5	6.8	7.1	7.3	7.6	7.8	8.1	8.3
4.7	4.9	5.1	5.3	5.5	5.7	5.9	6.1	6.3	6.5
9.1	9.5	9.9	10.2	10.6	11.0	11.4	11.8	12.2	12.5
9.7	10.1	10.6	11.0	11.4	11.8	12.2	12.6	13.0	13.4
7.8	8.1	8.5	8.8	9.1	9.5	9.8	10.1	10.5	10.8
2.9	3.0	3.2	3.3	3.4	3.5	3.6	3.8	3.9	4.0
2.3	2.4	2.5	2.6	2.7	2.8	2.9	3.0	3.1	3.2
4.5	4.7	4.9	5.1	5.3	5.5	5.7	5.9	6.1	6.3
13.8	14.4	15.0	15.6	16.2	16.8	17.4	17.9	18.5	19.1
11.5	12.0	12.5	13.0	13.4	13.9	14.4	14.9	15.4	15.9
11.6	12.1	12.6	13.1	13.6	14.1	14.6	14.6	15.6	16.1
12.6	13.1	13.6	14.2	14.7	15.2	15.8	16.3	16.8	17.3
14.0	14.6	15.2	15.8	16.4	16.9	17.5	18.1	18.7	19.3
1.6	1.6	1.7	1.8	1.8	1.9	2.0	2.0	2.1	2.2
1.6	1.7	1.8	1.8	1.9	2.0	2.0	2.1	2.2	2.3
4.0	4.2	4.4	4.6	4.7	4.9	5.1	5.2	5.4	5.6
1.6	1.6	1.7	1.8	1.8	1.9	2.0	2.0	2.1	2.2
3.4	3.6	3.7	3.8	4.0	4.1	4.3	4.4	4.6	4.7
3.7	3.8	4.0	4.2	4.3	4.5	4.6	4.8	4.9	5.1
6.2	6.5	6.8	7.0	7.3	7.6	7.8	8.1	8.4	8.6
4.6	4.8	5.0	5.2	5.4	5.6	5.8	6.0	6.2	6.4
3.7	3.8	4.0	4.2	4.3	4.5	4.6	4.8	4.9	5.1
3.4	3.6	3.7	3.8	4.0	4.1	4.3	4.4	4.6	4.7
10.1	10.5	10.9	11.4	11.8	12.2	12.6	13.1	13.5	13.9
4.4	4.6	4.8	5.0	5.1	5.3	5.5	5.7	5.9	6.1
4.1	4.3	4.5	4.6	4.8	5.0	5.2	5.0	5.5	5.7
2.3	2.4	2.5	2.6	2.7	2.8	2.8	2.9	3.0	3.1
2.9	3.0	3.2	3.3	3.4	3.5	3.6	3.8	3.9	4.0
2.8	2.9	3.0	3.1	3.2	3.4	3.5	3.6	3.7	3.8
4.7	4.9	5.1	5.3	5.5	5.7	5.9	6.1	6.3	6.6
2.5	2.6	2.7	2.8	2.9	3.0	3.1	3.2	3.3	3.4
2.1	2.1	2.2	2.3	2.4	2.5	2.6	2.7	2.8	2.8
3.8	3.9	4.1	4.2	4.4	4.6	4.7	4.9	5.0	5.2

ACTIVITY	KG LB	50 110	53 117	56 123	59 130	62 137	65 143	68 150
Music playing *(continued)*								
piano (sitting)		2.0	2.1	2.2	2.4	2.5	2.6	2.7
trumpet (standing)		1.6	1.6	1.7	1.8	1.9	2.0	2.1
violin (sitting)		2.3	2.4	2.5	2.7	2.8	2.9	3.1
woodwind (sitting)		1.6	1.7	1.8	1.9	2.0	2.1	2.2
Painting, inside		1.7	1.8	1.9	2.0	2.1	2.2	2.3
Painting, outside		3.9	4.1	4.3	4.5	4.8	5.0	5.2
Planting seedlings		3.5	3.7	3.9	4.1	4.3	4.6	4.8
Plastering		3.9	4.1	4.4	4.6	4.8	5.1	5.3
Printing		1.8	1.9	2.0	2.1	2.2	2.3	2.4
Racquetball		8.9	9.4	10.0	10.5	11.0	11.6	12.1
Running, cross-country		8.2	8.6	9.1	9.6	10.1	10.6	11.1
Running, horizontal								
11 min, 30 s per mile		6.8	7.2	7.6	8.0	8.4	8.8	9.2
9 min per mile		9.7	10.2	10.8	11.4	12.0	12.5	13.1
8 min per mile		10.8	11.3	11.9	12.5	13.1	13.6	14.2
7 min per mile		12.2	12.7	13.3	13.9	14.5	15.0	15.6
6 min per mile		13.9	14.4	15.0	15.6	16.2	16.7	17.3
5 min, 30 s per mile		14.5	15.3	16.2	17.1	17.9	18.8	19.7
Scraping paint		3.2	3.3	3.5	3.7	3.9	4.1	4.3
Scrubbing floors (F)		5.5	5.8	6.1	6.4	6.8	7.1	7.4
Scrubbing floors (M)		5.4	5.7	6.0	6.4	6.7	7.0	7.3
Shoe repair, general		2.3	2.4	2.5	2.7	2.8	2.9	3.1
Sitting quietly		1.1	1.1	1.2	1.2	1.3	1.4	1.4
Skiing, hard snow								
level, moderate spped		6.0	6.3	6.7	7.0	7.4	7.7	8.1
level, walking		7.2	7.6	8.0	8.4	8.9	9.3	9.7
uphill, maximum speed		13.7	14.5	15.3	16.2	17.0	17.8	18.6
Skiing, soft snow								
leisure (F)		4.9	5.2	5.5	5.8	6.1	6.4	6.7
leisure (M)		5.6	5.9	6.2	6.5	6.9	7.2	7.5
Skindiving, as frogman								
considerable motion		13.8	14.6	15.5	16.3	17.1	17.9	18.8
moderate motion		10.3	10.9	11.5	12.2	12.8	13.4	14.0
Snowshoeing, soft snow		8.3	8.8	9.3	9.8	10.3	10.8	11.3
Squash		10.6	11.2	11.9	12.5	13.1	13.8	14.4
Standing quietly (F)		1.3	1.3	1.4	1.5	1.6	1.6	1.7
Standing quietly (M)		1.4	1.4	1.5	1.6	1.7	1.8	1.8
Steel mill, working in								
fettling		4.5	4.7	5.0	5.3	5.5	5.8	6.1
forging		5.0	5.3	5.6	5.9	6.2	6.5	6.8
hand rolling		6.9	7.3	7.7	8.1	8.5	8.9	9.3
merchant mill rolling		7.3	7.7	8.1	8.6	9.0	9.4	9.9
removing slag		8.9	9.4	10.0	10.5	11.0	11.6	12.1
tending furnace		6.3	6.7	7.1	7.4	7.8	8.2	8.6
tipping molds		4.6	4.9	5.2	5.4	5.7	6.0	6.3
Stock clerking		2.7	2.9	3.0	3.2	3.3	3.5	3.7
Swimming								
back stroke		8.5	9.0	9.5	10.0	10.5	11.0	11.5
breast stroke		8.1	8.6	9.1	9.6	10.0	10.5	11.0

71 157	74 163	77 170	80 176	83 183	86 190	89 196	92 203	95 209	98 216
2.8	3.0	3.1	3.2	3.3	3.4	3.6	3.7	3.8	3.9
2.2	2.3	2.4	2.5	2.6	2.7	2.8	2.9	2.9	3.0
3.2	3.3	3.5	3.6	3.7	3.9	4.0	4.1	4.3	4.4
2.3	2.4	2.5	2.6	2.7	2.8	2.8	2.9	3.0	3.1
2.4	2.5	2.6	2.7	2.8	2.9	3.0	3.1	3.2	3.3
5.5	5.7	5.9	6.2	6.4	6.6	6.9	7.1	7.3	7.5
5.0	5.2	5.4	5.6	5.8	6.0	6.2	6.4	6.7	6.9
5.5	5.8	6.0	6.2	6.5	6.7	6.9	7.2	7.4	7.6
2.5	2.6	2.7	2.8	2.9	3.0	3.1	3.2	3.3	3.4
12.6	13.2	13.7	14.2	14.8	15.3	15.8	16.4	16.9	17.4
11.6	12.1	12.6	13.0	13.5	14.0	14.5	15.0	15.5	16.0
9.6	10.0	10.5	10.9	11.3	11.7	12.1	12.5	12.9	13.3
13.7	14.3	14.9	15.4	16.0	16.6	17.2	17.8	18.3	18.9
14.8	15.4	16.0	16.5	17.1	17.7	18.3	18.9	19.4	20.0
16.2	16.8	17.4	17.9	18.5	19.1	19.7	20.3	20.8	21.4
17.9	18.5	19.1	19.6	20.2	20.8	21.4	22.0	22.5	23.1
20.5	21.4	22.3	23.1	24.0	24.9	25.7	26.6	27.5	28.3
4.5	4.7	4.9	5.0	5.2	5.4	5.6	5.8	6.0	6.2
7.7	8.1	8.4	8.7	9.0	9.4	9.7	10.0	10.4	10.7
7.7	8.0	8.3	8.6	9.0	9.3	9.6	9.9	10.3	10.6
3.2	3.3	3.5	3.6	3.7	3.9	4.0	4.1	4.3	4.4
1.5	1.6	1.6	1.7	1.7	1.8	1.9	1.9	2.0	2.1
8.4	8.8	9.2	9.5	9.9	10.2	10.6	10.9	11.3	11.7
10.2	10.6	11.0	11.4	11.9	12.3	12.7	13.2	13.6	14.0
19.5	20.3	21.1	21.9	22.7	23.6	24.4	25.2	26.0	26.9
7.0	7.3	7.5	7.8	8.1	8.4	8.7	9.0	9.3	9.6
7.9	8.2	8.5	8.9	9.2	9.5	9.9	10.2	10.5	10.9
19.6	20.4	21.3	22.1	22.9	23.7	24.6	25.4	26.2	27.0
14.6	15.2	15.9	16.5	17.1	17.7	18.3	19.0	19.6	20.2
11.8	12.3	12.8	13.3	13.8	14.3	14.8	15.3	15.8	16.3
15.1	15.7	16.3	17.0	17.6	18.2	18.9	19.5	20.1	20.8
1.8	1.9	1.9	2.0	2.1	2.2	2.2	2.3	2.4	2.5
1.9	2.0	2.1	2.2	2.2	2.3	2.4	2.5	2.6	2.6
6.3	6.6	6.9	7.1	7.4	7.7	7.9	8.2	8.5	8.7
7.1	7.4	7.7	8.0	8.3	8.6	8.9	9.2	9.5	9.8
9.7	10.1	10.6	11.0	11.4	11.8	12.2	12.6	13.0	13.4
10.3	10.7	11.2	11.6	12.0	12.5	12.9	13.3	13.8	14.2
12.6	13.2	13.7	14.2	14.8	15.3	15.8	16.4	16.9	17.4
8.9	9.3	9.7	10.1	10.5	10.8	11.2	11.6	12.0	12.3
6.5	6.8	7.1	7.4	7.6	7.9	8.2	8.5	8.7	9.0
3.8	4.0	4.2	4.3	4.5	4.6	4.8	5.0	5.1	5.3
12.0	12.5	13.0	13.5	14.0	14.5	15.0	15.5	16.1	16.6
11.5	12.0	12.5	13.0	13.4	13.9	14.4	14.9	15.4	15.9

ACTIVITY	KG LB	50 110	53 117	56 123	59 130	62 137	65 143	68 150
Swimming *(continued)*								
crawl, fast		7.8	8.3	8.7	9.2	9.7	10.1	10.6
crawl, slow		6.4	6.8	7.2	7.6	7.9	8.3	8.7
side stroke		6.1	6.5	6.8	7.2	7.6	7.9	8.3
treading, fast		8.5	9.0	9.5	10.0	10.5	11.1	11.6
treading, normal		3.1	3.3	3.5	3.7	3.8	4.0	4.2
Table tennis		3.4	3.6	3.8	4.0	4.2	4.4	4.6
Tailoring								
cutting		2.1	2.2	2.3	2.4	2.5	2.7	2.8
hand-sewing		1.6	1.7	1.8	1.9	2.0	2.1	2.2
machine-sewing		2.3	2.4	2.5	2.7	2.8	2.9	3.1
pressing		3.1	3.3	3.5	3.7	3.8	4.0	4.2
Tennis		5.5	5.8	6.1	6.4	6.8	7.1	7.4
Typing								
electric		1.4	1.4	1.5	1.6	1.7	1.8	1.8
manual		1.6	1.6	1.7	1.8	1.9	2.0	2.1
Volleyball		2.5	2.7	2.8	3.0	3.1	3.3	3.4
Walking, normal pace								
asphalt road		4.0	4.2	4.5	4.7	5.0	5.2	5.4
fields and hillsides		4.1	4.3	4.6	4.8	5.1	5.3	5.6
grass track		4.1	4.3	4.5	4.8	5.0	5.3	5.5
plowed field		3.9	4.1	4.3	4.5	4.8	5.0	5.2
Wallpapering		2.4	2.5	2.7	2.8	3.0	3.1	3.3
Watch repairing		1.3	1.3	1.4	1.5	1.6	1.6	1.7
Window cleaning (F)		3.0	3.1	3.3	3.5	3.7	3.8	4.0
Window cleaning (M)		2.9	3.1	3.2	3.4	3.6	3.8	3.9
Writing (sitting)		1.5	1.5	1.6	1.7	1.8	1.9	2.0

71	74	77	80	83	86	89	92	95	98
157	163	170	176	183	190	196	203	209	216
11.1	11.5	12.0	12.5	12.9	13.4	13.9	14.4	14.8	15.3
9.1	9.5	9.9	10.2	10.6	11.0	11.4	11.8	12.2	12.5
8.7	9.0	9.4	9.8	10.1	10.5	10.9	11.2	11.6	12.0
12.1	12.6	13.1	13.6	14.1	14.6	15.1	15.6	16.2	16.7
4.4	4.6	4.8	5.0	5.1	5.3	5.5	5.7	5.9	6.1
4.8	5.0	5.2	5.4	5.6	5.8	6.1	6.3	6.5	6.7
2.9	3.0	3.2	3.3	3.4	3.5	3.6	3.8	3.9	4.0
2.3	2.4	2.5	2.6	2.7	2.8	2.8	2.9	3.0	3.1
3.2	3.3	3.5	3.6	3.7	3.9	4.0	4.1	4.3	4.4
4.4	4.6	4.8	5.0	5.1	5.3	5.5	5.7	5.9	6.1
7.7	8.1	8.4	8.7	9.0	9.4	9.7	10.0	10.4	10.7
1.9	2.0	2.1	2.2	2.2	2.3	2.4	2.5	2.6	2.6
2.2	2.3	2.4	2.5	2.6	2.7	2.8	2.9	2.9	3.0
3.6	3.7	3.9	4.0	4.2	4.3	4.5	4.6	4.8	4.9
5.7	5.9	6.2	6.4	6.6	6.9	7.1	7.4	7.6	7.8
5.8	6.1	6.3	6.6	6.8	7.1	7.3	7.5	7.8	8.0
5.8	6.0	6.2	6.5	6.7	7.0	7.2	7.5	7.7	7.9
5.5	5.7	5.9	6.2	6.4	6.6	6.9	7.1	7.3	7.5
3.4	3.6	3.7	3.8	4.0	4.1	4.3	4.4	4.6	4.7
1.8	1.9	1.9	2.0	2.1	2.2	2.2	2.3	2.4	2.5
4.2	4.4	4.5	4.7	4.9	5.1	5.3	5.4	5.6	5.8
4.1	4.3	4.5	4.6	4.8	5.0	5.2	5.3	5.5	5.7
2.1	2.1	2.2	2.3	2.4	2.5	2.6	2.7	2.8	2.8

APPENDIX C

EVALUATION OF BODY COMPOSITION

DESCRIPTION OF THE PROCEDURES

In experiments from our laboratories, we have determined the best combination of circumference measures for predicting body fatness in a sample of young adult and older men and women. The younger group ranged in age from 17 to 26 years; the age range of the older subjects was 27 to 50 years. The criterion value for body density and percent body fat were determined in the laboratory by hydrostatic weighing or water displacement methods. The data were analyzed to determine the combination of circumference measures that came closest to predicting actual body fatness as determined by the more sophisticated laboratory techniques. A combination of three circumferences resulted in an accurate prediction of fatness for all subjects. These predicted values for body fat were generally within 2.5 to 4.0% body fat units of values determined in the laboratory. The practical significance of this finding was obvious; percent body fat could be predicted easily from a few simple circumference measurements.

The anatomic landmarks used in taking the various circumference measurements for the young and older women and men are described below and illustrated in the accompanying diagram.

Young women	Older women	Young men	Older men
1. Abdomen	1. Abdomen	1. Right upper arm	1. Buttocks
2. Right thigh	2. Right thigh	2. Abdomen	2. Abdomen
3. Right forearm	3. Right calf	3. Right forearm	3. Right forearm

ANATOMICAL LOCATIONS

Abdomen—one inch above the umbilicus
Buttocks—maximum protrusion with the heels together
Right thigh—upper thigh just below the buttocks
Right upper arm—arm straight, palm up and extended in front of the body (measure at the midpoint between the shoulder and elbow)
Right forearm—maximum circumference with the arm extended in front of the body with palm up
Right calf—widest circumference midway between the ankle and knee

Measurement of circumferences with a tape.

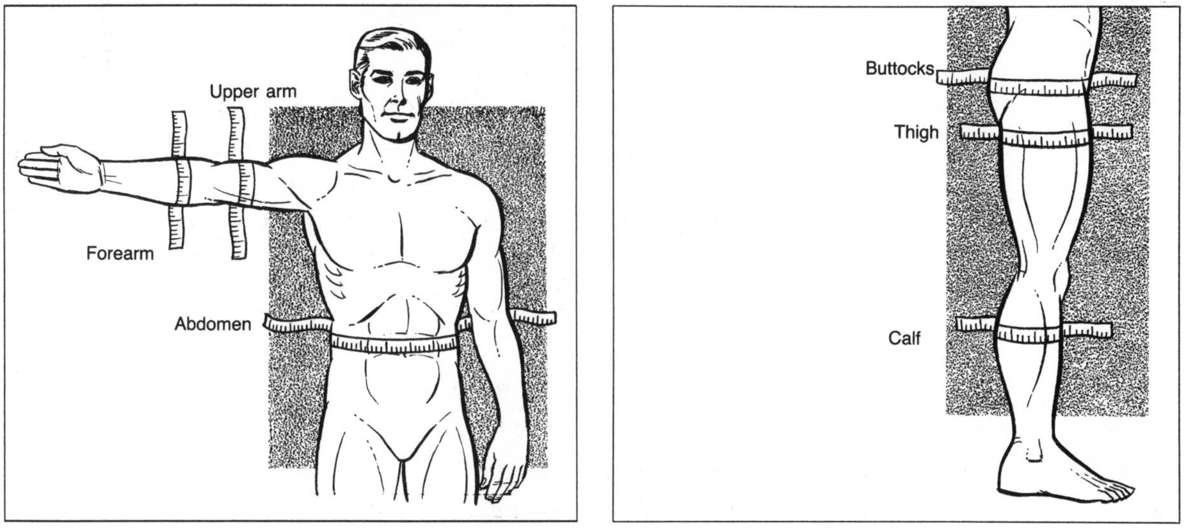
Upper arm
Forearm
Abdomen
Buttocks
Thigh
Calf

HOW TO ESTIMATE PERCENT BODY FAT

You can estimate your percent body fat by using the appropriate table in this section. Table C-1 is for young women (ages 17–26), Table C-2 is for older women (ages 27–50), Table C-3 is for young men (ages 17–26), and Table C-4 is for older men (ages 27–50). Once you have accurate circumference measurements, use the table to determine the value for the corresponding constants A, B, and C. The values corresponding to each constant are substituted in the formula at the bottom of the appropriate table. Percent body fat is obtained after performing the two additions and two subtractions in the formula. It should be emphasized that the equations to predict percent body fat from circumferences may not be valid when applied to athletic young men and women who regularly engage in strenuous physical training, or for large or small individuals who could be visually classified as thin or obese. For physically active individuals (including current athletes), use the adjusted age correction factor listed at the bottom of each table. A further explanation is provided on pages 280–281, Step 3.

EXAMPLE OF CALCULATIONS

The following five-step example illustrates how percent fat, weight of fat, and lean body weight were calculated for a sedentary 24-year-old woman who weighed 125 pounds.

Step 1. The abdomen, right thigh, and right forearm circumference were taken with a cloth tape, and accuracy was to the nearest one-eighth inch. Convert inches to centimeters by multiplying by 2.54 (1 in. = 2.54 cm).
Abdomen = 28.0 in. (71.1 cm)
Right thigh = 20.0 in. (50.8 cm)
Right forearm = 8.0 in. (20.3 cm).

Step 2. The three constants A, B, and C, corresonding to the three circumference measures, were determined from Table C-1.
Constant A, corresponding to 28.0 in. = 37.4
Constant B, corresponding to 20.0 in. = 41.6
Constant C, corresponding to 8.0 in. = 34.5

Step 3. Percent body fat was computed by substituting the appropriate constants in the formula shown at the bottom of Table C-1.

$$\begin{aligned} \text{Percent fat} &= \text{constant A} + \text{constant B} - \text{constant C} - 19.6 \\ &= 37.4 + 41.6 - 34.5 - 19.6 \\ &= 79.0 - 34.5 - 19.6 \\ &= 44.5 - 19.6 \\ &= 24.9\% \end{aligned}$$

Step 4. $\text{Weight of fat} = \dfrac{\text{Percent fat} \times \text{Body weight}}{100}$.

$$\begin{aligned} \text{Weight of fat} &= 24.9/100 \times 125 \text{ lb} \\ &= 0.249 \times 125 \text{ lb} \\ &= 31.1 \text{ lb.} \end{aligned}$$

Step 5. Lean body weight = Body weight − Weight of fat
Lean body weight = 125 pounds − 31.1 pounds
= 93.9 pounds

PERSONAL CALCULATIONS

Use the five step procedure as in the preceding example to calculate your percent body fat, fat weight, and lean body weight.

Step 1. With a tape, measure the three circumferences that correspond to your gender and age group. Record all values in centimeters or to the nearest one-eighth inch.

	Measurement Site	cm	in.
1.	________	______	______
2.	________	______	______
3.	________	______	______

Step 2. Determine the three constants A, B, and C that correspond to the appropriate circumference in Step 1. Use Tables C-1 to C-4 to determine the constants depending on your age and gender.

	cm	Constant
Measurement 1	________	A = ________
Measurement 2	________	B = ________
Measurement 3	________	C = ________

Step 3. Substitute the value for each constant in the equation below. Enter the age constant at the end of the equation depending on your gender and age group; young men = 10.2; older men = 15.0; young women = 19.6; older women = 18.4

If you participate in a regular program of vigorous physical activity a minimum of 240 minutes a week, use the following age-correction factors that incorporate this significantly higher than normal level of physical activity: young men, 14.2; older men, 19.0; young women, 22.6; older women, 21.4.

Percent fat = Constant A + Constant B − Constant C − ______ Age Constant

=

=

=

Percent fat =

Step 4. Weight of fat = percent fat (step 3)/100 × body weight (lb).

Weight of fat = ______ (percent of fat) × ______ (body weight)

=

=

Step 5. Compute lean body weight by subtracting the weight of fat from body weight.

Lean body weight = ______ (body weight, lb) − ______ (weight of fat, lb)

If your value for percent body fat exceeds the guidelines for men (above 20% fat) or women (above 30% fat), compute a value for "desirable" body weight as follows:

$$\text{Desirable body weight} = \frac{\text{current lean body weight}}{1.00 - \text{\% fat desired (expressed as a decimal)}}$$

Desirable body weight = ______________

Desirable body weight =

The total amount of fat weight you should lose to achieve the desired weight (with desired body fat level) is computed simply as your current body weight minus your desirable weight. Suppose your weight is 194 pounds and your desirable weight is 147 pounds. The difference of 47 pounds would be your target weight (fat) loss. This method of computing a target weight loss can be considered a rough approximation toward a realistic goal weight.

CONVERSION CONSTANTS TO PREDICT PERCENT BODY FAT

To use the charts, measure the three girths at the sites indicated on page 279. The specific equation to predict percent body fat with its corresponding constant is presented at the bottom of each chart.

CHART C-1. *Conversion constants to predict percent body fat for* **young women**

ABDOMEN			THIGH			FOREARM		
IN	CM	CONSTANT A	IN	CM	CONSTANT B	IN	CM	CONSTANT C
20.00	50.80	26.74	14.00	35.56	29.13	6.00	15.24	25.86
20.25	51.43	27.07	14.25	36.19	29.65	6.25	15.87	26.94
20.50	52.07	27.41	14.50	36.83	30.17	6.50	16.51	28.02
20.75	52.70	27.74	14.75	37.46	30.69	6.75	17.14	29.10
21.00	53.34	28.07	15.00	38.10	31.21	7.00	17.78	30.17
21.25	53.97	28.41	15.25	38.73	31.73	7.25	18.41	31.25
21.50	54.61	28.74	15.50	39.37	32.25	7.50	19.05	32.33
21.75	55.24	29.08	15.75	40.00	32.77	7.75	19.68	33.41
22.00	55.88	29.41	16.00	40.64	33.29	8.00	20.32	34.48
22.25	56.51	29.74	16.25	41.27	33.81	8.25	20.95	35.56
22.50	57.15	30.08	16.50	41.91	34.33	8.50	21.59	36.64
22.75	57.78	30.41	16.75	42.54	34.85	8.75	22.22	37.72
23.00	58.42	30.75	17.00	43.18	35.37	9.00	22.86	38.79
23.25	59.05	31.08	17.25	43.81	35.89	9.25	23.49	39.87
23.50	59.69	31.42	17.50	44.45	36.41	9.50	24.13	40.95
23.75	60.32	31.75	17.75	45.08	36.93	9.75	24.76	42.03
24.00	60.96	32.08	18.00	45.72	37.45	10.00	25.40	43.10
24.25	61.59	32.42	18.25	46.35	37.97	10.25	26.03	44.18
24.50	62.23	32.75	18.50	46.99	38.49	10.50	26.67	45.26
24.75	62.86	33.09	18.75	47.62	39.01	10.75	27.30	46.34
25.00	63.50	33.42	19.00	48.26	39.53	11.00	27.94	47.41
25.25	64.13	33.76	19.25	48.89	40.05	11.25	28.57	48.49
25.50	64.77	34.09	19.50	49.53	40.57	11.50	29.21	49.57
25.75	65.40	34.42	19.75	50.16	41.09	11.75	29.84	50.65
26.00	66.04	34.76	20.00	50.80	41.61	12.00	30.48	51.73
26.25	66.67	35.09	20.25	51.43	42.13	12.25	31.11	52.80
26.50	67.31	35.43	20.50	52.07	42.65	12.50	31.75	53.88
26.75	67.94	35.76	20.75	52.70	43.17	12.75	32.38	54.96
27.00	68.58	36.10	21.00	53.34	43.69	13.00	33.02	56.04
27.25	69.21	36.43	21.25	53.97	44.21	13.25	33.65	57.11
27.50	69.85	36.76	21.50	54.61	44.73	13.50	34.29	58.19
27.75	70.48	37.10	21.75	55.24	45.25	13.75	34.92	59.27
28.00	71.12	37.43	22.00	55.88	45.77	14.00	35.56	60.35
28.25	71.75	37.77	22.25	56.51	46.29	14.25	36.19	61.42
28.50	72.39	38.10	22.50	57.15	46.81	14.50	36.83	62.50
28.75	73.02	38.43	22.75	57.78	47.33	14.75	37.46	63.58
29.00	73.66	38.77	23.00	58.42	47.85	15.00	38.10	64.66

CHART C-1. *continued*

ABDOMEN			THIGH			FOREARM		
IN	CM	CONSTANT A	IN	CM	CONSTANT B	IN	CM	CONSTANT C
29.25	74.29	39.10	23.25	59.05	48.37	15.25	38.73	65.73
29.50	74.93	39.44	23.50	59.69	48.89	15.50	39.37	66.81
29.75	75.56	39.77	23.75	60.32	49.41	15.75	40.00	67.89
30.00	76.20	40.11	24.00	60.96	49.93	16.00	40.64	68.97
30.25	76.83	40.44	24.25	61.59	50.45	16.25	41.27	70.04
30.50	77.47	40.77	24.50	62.23	50.97	16.50	41.91	71.12
30.75	78.10	41.11	24.75	62.86	51.49	16.75	42.54	72.20
31.00	78.74	41.44	25.00	63.50	52.01	17.00	43.18	73.28
31.25	79.37	41.78	25.25	64.13	52.53	17.25	43.81	74.36
31.50	80.01	42.11	25.50	64.77	53.05	17.50	44.45	75.43
31.75	80.64	42.45	25.75	65.40	53.57	17.75	45.08	76.51
32.00	81.28	42.78	26.00	66.04	54.09	18.00	45.72	77.59
32.25	81.91	43.11	26.25	66.67	54.61	18.25	46.35	78.67
32.50	82.55	43.45	26.50	67.31	55.13	18.50	46.99	79.74
32.75	83.18	43.78	26.75	67.94	55.65	18.75	47.62	80.82
33.00	83.82	44.12	27.00	68.58	56.17	19.00	48.26	81.90
33.25	84.45	44.45	27.25	69.21	56.69	19.25	48.89	82.98
33.50	85.09	44.78	27.50	69.85	57.21	19.50	49.53	84.05
33.75	85.72	45.12	27.75	70.48	57.73	19.75	50.16	85.13
34.00	86.36	45.45	28.00	71.12	58.26	20.00	50.80	86.21
34.25	86.99	45.79	28.25	71.75	58.78			
34.50	87.63	46.12	28.50	72.39	59.30			
34.75	88.26	46.46	38.75	73.02	59.82			
35.00	88.90	46.79	29.00	73.66	60.34			
35.25	89.53	47.12	29.25	74.29	60.86			
35.50	90.17	47.46	29.50	74.93	61.38			
35.75	90.80	47.79	29.75	75.56	61.90			
36.00	91.44	48.13	30.00	76.20	62.42			
36.25	92.07	48.46	30.25	76.83	62.94			
36.50	92.71	48.80	30.50	77.47	63.46			
36.75	93.34	49.13	30.75	78.10	63.98			
37.00	93.98	49.46	31.00	78.74	64.50			
37.25	94.61	49.80	31.25	79.37	65.02			
37.50	95.25	50.13	31.50	80.01	65.54			
37.75	95.88	50.47	31.75	80.64	66.06			
38.00	96.52	50.80	32.00	81.28	66.58			
38.25	97.15	51.13	32.25	81.91	67.10			
38.50	97.79	51.47	32.50	82.55	67.62			
38.75	98.42	51.80	32.75	83.18	68.14			
39.00	99.06	52.14	33.00	83.82	68.66			
39.25	99.69	52.47	33.25	84.45	69.18			
39.50	100.33	52.81	33.50	85.09	69.70			
39.75	100.96	53.14	33.75	85.72	70.22			
40.00	101.60	53.47	34.00	86.36	70.74			

Note: Percent Fat = Constant A + Constant B − Constant C − 19.6

CHART C-2. *Conversion constants to predict body fat for* **older women**

ABDOMEN			THIGH			CALF		
IN	CM	CONSTANT A	IN.	CM	CONSTANT B	IN.	CM	CONSTANT C
25.00	63.50	29.69	14.00	35.56	17.31	10.00	25.40	14.46
25.25	64.13	29.98	14.25	36.19	17.62	10.25	26.03	14.82
25.50	64.77	30.28	14.50	36.83	17.93	10.50	26.67	15.18
25.75	65.40	30.58	14.75	37.46	18.24	10.75	27.30	15.54
26.00	66.04	30.87	15.00	38.10	18.55	11.00	27.94	15.91
26.25	66.67	31.17	15.25	38.73	18.86	11.25	28.57	16.27
26.50	67.31	31.47	15.50	39.37	19.17	11.50	29.21	16.63
26.75	67.94	31.76	15.75	40.00	19.47	11.75	29.84	16.99
27.00	68.58	32.06	16.00	40.64	19.78	12.00	30.48	17.35
27.25	69.21	32.36	16.25	41.27	20.09	12.25	31.11	17.71
27.50	69.85	32.65	16.50	41.91	20.40	12.50	31.75	18.08
27.75	70.48	32.95	16.75	42.54	20.71	12.75	32.38	18.44
28.00	71.12	33.25	17.00	43.18	21.02	13.00	33.02	18.80
28.25	71.75	33.55	17.25	43.81	21.33	13.25	33.65	19.16
28.50	72.39	33.84	17.50	44.45	21.64	13.50	34.29	19.52
28.75	73.02	34.14	17.75	45.08	21.95	13.75	34.92	19.88
29.00	73.66	34.44	18.00	45.72	22.26	14.00	35.56	20.24
29.25	74.29	34.73	18.25	46.35	22.57	14.25	36.19	20.61
29.50	74.93	35.03	18.50	46.99	22.87	14.50	36.83	20.97
29.75	75.56	35.33	18.75	47.62	23.18	14.75	37.46	21.33
30.00	76.20	35.62	19.00	48.26	23.49	15.00	38.10	21.69
30.25	76.83	35.92	19.25	48.89	23.80	15.25	38.73	22.05
30.50	77.47	36.22	19.50	49.53	24.11	15.50	39.37	22.41
30.75	78.10	36.51	19.75	50.16	24.42	15.75	40.00	22.77
31.00	78.74	36.81	20.00	50.80	24.73	16.00	40.64	23.14
31.25	79.37	37.11	20.25	51.43	25.04	16.25	41.27	23.50
31.50	80.01	37.40	20.50	52.07	25.35	16.50	41.91	23.86
31.75	80.64	37.70	20.75	52.70	25.66	16.75	42.54	24.22
32.00	81.28	38.00	21.00	53.34	25.97	17.00	43.18	24.58
32.25	81.91	38.30	21.25	53.97	26.28	17.25	43.81	24.94
32.50	82.55	38.59	21.50	54.61	26.58	17.50	44.45	25.31
32.75	83.18	38.89	21.75	55.24	26.89	17.75	45.08	25.67
33.00	83.82	39.19	22.00	55.88	27.20	18.00	45.72	26.03
33.25	84.45	39.48	22.25	56.51	27.51	18.25	46.35	26.39
33.50	85.09	39.78	22.50	57.15	27.82	18.50	46.99	26.75
33.75	85.72	40.08	22.75	57.78	28.13	18.75	47.62	27.11
34.00	86.36	40.37	23.00	58.42	28.44	19.00	48.26	27.47
34.25	86.99	40.67	23.25	59.05	28.75	19.25	48.89	27.84
34.50	87.63	40.97	23.50	59.69	29.06	19.50	49.53	28.20
34.75	88.26	41.26	23.75	60.32	29.37	19.75	50.16	28.56
35.00	88.90	41.56	24.00	60.96	29.68	20.00	50.80	28.92
35.25	89.53	41.86	24.25	61.59	29.98	20.25	51.43	29.28
35.50	90.17	42.15	24.50	62.23	30.29	20.50	52.07	29.64
35.75	90.80	42.45	24.75	62.86	30.60	20.75	52.70	30.00
36.00	91.44	42.75	25.00	63.50	30.91	21.00	53.34	30.37
36.25	92.07	43.05	25.25	64.13	31.22	21.25	53.97	30.73
36.50	92.71	43.34	25.50	64.77	31.53	21.50	54.61	31.09
36.75	93.35	43.64	25.75	65.40	31.84	21.75	55.24	31.45
37.00	93.98	43.94	26.00	66.04	32.15	22.00	55.88	31.81
37.25	94.62	44.23	26.25	66.67	32.46	22.25	56.51	32.17
37.50	95.25	44.53	26.50	67.31	32.77	22.50	57.15	32.54
37.75	95.89	44.83	26.75	67.94	33.08	22.75	57.78	32.90
38.00	96.52	45.12	27.00	68.58	33.38	23.00	58.42	33.26
38.25	97.16	45.42	27.25	69.21	33.69	23.25	59.05	33.62
38.50	97.79	45.72	27.50	69.85	34.00	23.50	59.69	33.98

CHART C-2. *Continued*

ABDOMEN			THIGH			CALF		
IN	CM	CONSTANT A	IN	CM	CONSTANT B	IN	CM	CONSTANT C
38.75	98.43	46.01	27.75	70.48	34.31	23.75	60.32	34.34
39.00	99.06	46.31	28.00	71.12	34.62	24.00	60.96	34.70
39.25	99.70	46.61	28.25	71.75	34.93	24.25	61.59	35.07
39.50	100.33	46.90	28.50	72.39	35.24	24.50	62.23	35.43
39.75	100.97	47.20	28.75	73.02	35.55	24.75	62.86	35.79
40.00	101.60	47.50	29.00	73.66	35.86	25.00	63.50	36.15
40.25	101.24	47.79	29.25	74.29	36.17			
40.50	102.87	48.09	29.50	74.93	36.48			
40.75	103.51	48.39	29.75	75.56	36.79			
41.00	104.14	48.69	30.00	76.20	37.09			
41.25	104.78	48.98	30.25	76.83	37.40			
41.50	105.41	49.28	30.50	77.47	37.71			
41.75	106.05	49.58	30.75	78.10	38.02			
42.00	106.68	49.87	31.00	78.74	38.33			
42.25	107.32	50.17	31.25	79.37	38.64			
42.50	107.95	50.47	31.50	80.01	38.95			
42.75	108.59	50.76	31.75	80.64	39.26			
43.00	109.22	51.06	32.00	81.28	39.57			
43.25	109.86	51.36	32.25	81.91	39.88			
43.50	110.49	51.65	32.50	82.55	40.19			
43.75	111.13	51.95	32.75	83.18	40.49			
44.00	111.76	52.25	33.00	83.82	40.80			
44.25	112.40	52.54	33.25	84.45	41.11			
44.50	113.03	52.84	33.50	85.09	41.42			
44.75	113.67	53.14	33.75	85.72	41.73			
45.00	114.30	53.44	34.00	86.36	42.04			

Note: Percent Fat = Constant A + Constant B − Constant C − 18.4

CHART C-3. *Conversion constants to predict percent body fat for* **young men**

UPPER ARM			ABDOMEN			FOREARM		
IN	CM	CONSTANT A	IN	CM	CONSTANT B	IN	CM	CONSTANT C
7.00	17.78	25.91	21.00	53.34	27.56	7.00	17.78	38.01
7.25	18.41	26.83	21.25	53.97	27.88	7.25	18.41	39.37
7.50	19.05	27.76	21.50	54.61	28.21	7.50	19.05	40.72
7.75	19.68	28.68	21.75	55.24	28.54	7.75	19.68	42.08
8.00	20.32	29.61	22.00	55.88	28.87	8.00	20.32	43.44
8.25	20.95	30.53	22.25	56.51	29.20	8.25	20.95	44.80
8.50	21.59	31.46	22.50	57.15	29.52	8.50	21.59	46.15
8.75	22.22	32.38	22.75	57.78	29.85	8.75	22.22	47.51

CHART C-3. *Continued*

UPPER ARM			ABDOMEN			FOREARM		
IN	CM	CONSTANT A	IN	CM	CONSTANT B	IN	CM	CONSTANT C
9.00	22.86	33.31	23.00	58.42	30.18	9.00	22.86	48.87
9.25	23.49	34.24	23.25	59.05	30.51	9.25	23.49	50.23
9.50	24.13	35.16	23.50	59.69	30.84	9.50	24.13	51.58
9.75	24.76	36.09	23.75	60.32	31.16	9.75	24.76	52.94
10.00	25.40	37.01	24.00	60.96	31.49	10.00	25.40	54.30
10.25	26.03	37.94	24.25	61.59	31.82	10.25	26.03	55.65
10.50	26.67	38.86	24.50	62.23	32.15	10.50	26.67	57.01
10.75	27.30	39.79	24.75	62.86	32.48	10.75	27.30	58.37
11.00	27.94	40.71	25.00	63.50	32.80	11.00	27.94	59.73
11.25	28.57	41.64	25.25	64.13	33.13	11.25	28.57	61.08
11.50	29.21	42.56	25.50	64.77	33.46	11.50	29.21	62.44
11.75	29.84	43.49	25.75	65.40	33.79	11.75	29.84	63.80
12.00	30.48	44.41	26.00	66.04	34.12	12.00	30.48	65.16
12.25	31.11	45.34	26.25	66.67	34.44	12.25	31.11	66.51
12.50	31.75	46.26	26.50	67.31	34.77	12.50	31.75	67.87
12.75	32.38	47.19	26.75	67.94	35.10	12.75	32.38	69.23
13.00	33.02	48.11	27.00	68.58	35.43	13.00	33.02	70.59
13.25	33.65	49.04	27.25	69.21	35.76	13.25	33.65	71.94
13.50	34.29	49.96	27.50	69.85	36.09	13.50	34.29	73.30
13.75	34.92	50.89	27.75	70.48	36.41	13.75	34.92	74.66
14.00	35.56	51.82	28.00	71.12	36.74	14.00	35.56	76.02
14.25	36.19	52.74	28.25	71.75	37.07	14.25	36.19	77.37
14.50	36.83	53.67	28.50	72.39	37.40	14.50	36.83	78.73
14.75	37.46	54.59	28.75	73.02	37.73	14.75	37.46	80.09
15.00	38.10	55.52	29.00	73.66	38.05	15.00	38.10	81.45
15.25	38.73	56.44	29.25	74.29	38.38	15.25	38.73	82.80
15.50	39.37	57.37	29.50	74.93	38.71	15.50	39.37	84.16
15.75	40.00	58.29	29.75	75.56	39.04	15.75	40.00	85.52
16.00	40.64	59.22	30.00	76.20	39.37	16.00	40.64	86.88
16.25	41.27	60.14	30.25	76.83	39.69	16.25	41.27	88.23
16.50	41.91	61.07	30.50	77.47	40.02	16.50	41.91	89.59
16.75	42.54	61.99	30.75	78.10	40.35	16.75	42.54	90.95
17.00	43.18	62.92	31.00	78.74	40.68	17.00	43.18	92.31
17.25	43.81	63.84	31.25	79.37	41.01	17.25	43.81	93.66
17.50	44.45	64.77	31.50	80.01	41.33	17.50	44.45	95.02
17.75	45.08	65.69	31.75	80.64	41.66	17.75	45.08	96.38
18.00	45.72	66.62	32.00	81.28	41.99	18.00	45.72	97.74
18.25	46.35	67.54	32.25	81.91	42.32	18.25	46.35	99.09
18.50	46.99	68.47	32.50	82.55	42.65	18.50	46.99	100.45
18.75	47.62	69.40	32.75	83.18	42.97	18.75	47.62	101.81
19.00	48.26	70.32	33.00	83.82	43.30	19.00	48.26	103.17
19.25	48.89	71.25	33.25	84.45	43.63	19.25	48.89	104.52
19.50	49.53	72.17	33.50	85.09	43.96	19.50	49.53	105.88
19.75	50.16	73.10	33.75	85.72	44.29	19.75	50.16	107.24
20.00	50.80	74.02	34.00	86.36	44.61	20.00	50.80	108.60
20.25	51.43	74.95	34.25	86.99	44.94	20.25	51.43	109.95
20.50	52.07	75.87	34.50	87.63	45.27	20.50	52.07	111.31
20.75	52.70	76.80	34.75	88.26	45.60	20.75	52.70	112.67
21.00	53.34	77.72	35.00	88.90	45.93	21.00	53.34	114.02
21.25	53.97	78.65	35.25	89.53	46.25	21.25	53.97	115.38
21.50	54.61	79.57	35.50	90.17	46.58	21.50	54.61	116.74
21.75	55.24	80.50	35.75	90.80	46.91	21.75	55.24	118.10
22.00	55.88	81.42	36.00	91.44	47.24	22.00	55.88	119.45
			36.25	92.07	47.57			
			36.50	92.71	47.89			

CHART C-3. *Continued*

UPPER ARM			ABDOMEN			FOREARM		
IN	CM	CONSTANT A	IN	CM	CONSTANT B	IN	CM	CONSTANT C
			36.75	93.34	48.22			
			37.00	93.98	48.55			
			37.25	94.61	48.88			
			37.50	95.25	49.21			
			37.75	95.88	49.54			
			38.00	96.52	49.86			
			38.25	97.15	50.19			
			38.50	97.79	50.52			
			38.75	98.42	50.85			
			39.00	99.06	51.18			
			39.25	99.69	51.50			
			39.50	100.33	51.83			
			39.75	100.96	52.16			
			40.00	101.60	52.49			
			40.25	102.23	52.82			
			40.50	102.87	53.14			
			40.75	103.50	53.47			
			41.00	104.14	53.80			
			41.25	104.77	54.13			
			41.50	105.41	54.46			
			41.75	106.04	54.78			
			42.00	106.68	55.11			

Note: Percent Fat = Constant A + Constant B − Constant C − 10.2

CHART C-4. *Conversion constants to predict percent body fat for* **older men**

BUTTOCKS			ABDOMEN			FOREARM		
IN	CM	CONSTANT A	IN	CM	CONSTANT B	IN	CM	CONSTANT C
28.00	71.12	29.34	25.50	64.77	22.84	7.00	17.78	21.01
28.25	71.75	29.60	25.75	65.40	23.06	7.25	18.41	21.76
28.50	72.39	29.87	26.00	66.04	23.29	7.50	19.05	22.52
28.75	73.02	30.13	26.25	66.67	23.51	7.75	19.68	23.26
29.00	73.66	30.39	26.50	67.31	23.73	8.00	20.32	24.02
29.25	74.29	30.65	26.75	67.94	23.96	8.25	20.95	24.76
29.50	74.93	30.92	27.00	68.58	24.18	8.50	21.59	25.52
29.75	75.56	31.18	27.25	69.21	24.40	8.75	22.22	26.26
30.00	76.20	31.44	27.50	69.85	24.63	9.00	22.86	27.02
30.25	76.83	31.70	27.75	70.48	24.85	9.25	23.49	27.76
30.50	77.47	31.96	28.00	71.12	25.08	9.50	24.13	28.52
30.75	78.10	32.22	28.25	71.75	25.29	9.75	24.76	29.26
31.00	78.74	32.49	28.50	72.39	25.52	10.00	25.40	30.02
31.25	79.37	32.75	28.75	73.02	25.75	10.25	26.03	30.76
31.50	80.01	33.01	29.00	73.66	25.97	10.50	26.67	31.52
31.75	80.64	33.27	29.25	74.29	26.19	10.75	27.30	32.27
32.00	81.28	33.54	29.50	74.93	26.42	11.00	27.94	33.02
32.25	81.91	33.80	29.75	75.56	26.64	11.25	28.57	33.77
32.50	82.55	34.06	30.00	76.20	26.87	11.50	29.21	34.52
32.75	83.18	34.32	30.25	76.83	27.09	11.75	29.84	35.27
33.00	83.82	34.58	30.50	77.47	27.32	12.00	30.48	36.02
33.25	84.45	34.84	30.75	78.10	27.54	12.25	31.11	36.77

CHART C-4. *Continued*

BUTTOCKS			ABDOMEN			FOREARM		
IN	CM	CONSTANT A	IN	CM	CONSTANT B	IN	CM	CONSTANT C
33.50	85.09	35.11	31.00	78.74	27.76	12.50	31.75	37.53
33.75	85.72	35.37	31.25	79.37	27.98	12.75	32.38	38.27
34.00	86.36	35.63	31.50	80.01	28.21	13.00	33.02	39.03
34.25	86.99	35.89	31.75	80.64	28.43	13.25	33.65	39.77
34.50	87.63	36.16	32.00	81.28	28.66	13.50	34.29	40.53
34.75	88.26	36.42	32.25	81.91	28.88	13.75	34.92	41.27
35.00	88.90	36.68	32.50	82.55	29.11	14.00	35.56	42.03
35.25	89.53	36.94	32.75	83.18	29.33	14.25	36.19	42.77
35.50	90.17	37.20	33.00	83.82	29.55	14.50	36.83	43.53
35.75	90.80	37.46	33.25	84.45	29.78	14.75	37.46	44.27
36.00	91.44	37.73	33.50	85.09	30.00	15.00	38.10	45.03
36.25	92.07	37.99	33.75	85.72	30.22	15.25	38.73	45.77
36.50	92.71	38.25	34.00	86.36	30.45	15.50	39.37	46.53
36.75	93.34	38.51	34.25	86.99	30.67	15.75	40.00	47.28
37.00	93.98	38.78	34.50	87.63	30.89	16.00	40.64	48.03
37.25	94.61	39.04	34.75	88.26	31.12	16.25	41.27	48.78
37.50	95.25	39.30	35.00	88.90	31.35	16.50	41.91	49.53
37.75	95.88	39.56	35.25	89.53	31.57	16.75	42.54	50.28
38.00	96.52	39.82	35.50	90.17	31.79	17.00	43.18	51.03
38.25	97.15	40.08	35.75	90.80	32.02	17.25	43.81	51.78
38.50	97.79	40.35	36.00	91.44	32.24	17.50	44.45	52.54
38.75	98.42	40.61	36.25	92.07	32.46	17.75	45.08	53.28
39.00	99.06	40.87	36.50	92.71	32.69	18.00	45.72	54.04
39.25	99.69	41.13	36.75	93.34	32.91	18.25	46.35	54.78
39.50	100.33	41.39	37.00	93.98	33.14			
39.75	100.96	41.66	37.25	94.61	33.36			
40.00	101.60	41.92	37.50	95.25	33.58			
40.25	102.23	42.18	37.75	95.88	33.81			
40.50	102.87	42.44	38.00	96.52	34.03			
40.75	103.50	42.70	38.25	97.15	34.26			
41.00	104.14	42.97	38.50	97.79	34.48			
42.25	104.77	43.23	38.75	98.42	34.70			
41.50	105.41	43.49	39.00	99.06	34.93			
41.75	106.04	43.75	39.25	99.69	35.15			
42.00	106.68	44.02	39.50	100.33	35.38			
42.25	107.31	44.28	39.75	100.96	35.59			
42.50	107.95	44.54	40.00	101.60	35.82			
42.75	108.58	44.80	40.25	102.23	36.05			
43.00	109.22	45.06	40.50	102.87	36.27			
43.25	109.85	45.32	40.75	103.50	36.49			
43.50	110.49	45.59	41.00	104.14	36.72			
43.75	111.12	45.85	41.25	104.77	36.94			
44.00	111.76	46.12	41.50	105.41	37.17			
44.25	112.39	46.37	41.75	106.04	37.39			
44.50	113.03	46.64	42.00	106.68	37.62			
44.75	113.66	46.89	42.25	107.31	37.87			
45.00	114.30	47.16	42.50	107.95	38.06			
42.25	114.93	47.42	42.75	108.58	38.28			
45.50	115.57	47.68	43.00	109.22	38.51			
45.75	116.20	47.94	43.25	109.85	38.73			
46.00	116.84	48.21	43.50	110.49	38.96			
46.25	117.47	48.47	43.75	111.12	39.18			
46.50	118.11	48.73	44.00	111.76	39.41			
46.75	118.74	48.99	44.25	112.39	39.63			
47.00	119.38	49.26	44.50	113.03	39.85			

CHART C-4. *Continued*

BUTTOCKS			ABDOMEN			FOREARM		
IN	CM	CONSTANT A	IN	CM	CONSTANT B	IN	CM	CONSTANT C
47.25	120.01	49.52	44.75	113.66	40.08			
47.50	120.65	49.78	45.00	114.30	40.30			
47.75	121.28	50.04						
48.00	121.92	50.30						
48.25	122.55	50.56						
48.50	123.19	50.83						
48.75	123.82	51.09						
49.00	124.46	51.35						

Note: Percent Fat = Constant A + Constant B − Constant C − 15.0

Comment on "computerized fat machines"

Since the publication of the second edition of *Nutrition, Weight Control, and Exercise,* considerable research has been devoted to the evaluation of body composition. Published studies have verified the accuracy of the girth equations in men and women. We have been encouraged by such findings because the use of the girth equations permits application to various nonlaboratory settings (health clubs, spas, fitness and sports medicine centers, hospitals) without a need to invest in expensive equipment and electronic instrumentation. What is somewhat disturbing, however, are the overzealous claims and pronouncements by some manufacturers that their "computerized fat machines" provide a more valid approach to the assessment of body composition in people who vary widely in body size, body build, and fitness status. The manufacturers argue forcibly in their advertising that a $2500–$4500 device (with computer and printer) can essentially substitute for the densitometric procedure (or be used in lieu of other more standard laboratory techniques such as girths, fatfolds, or ultrasound. It is noteworthy that detailed experiments, which involved hundreds of male and female children, adults, and athletes and were carried out in our labs and throughout the United States and Canada, confirm that such "fat machines" (i.e. those that require the attachment of electrodes to the hands and feet, using the procedure of *bioelectrical impedance*) are unable to provide the necessary degree of accuracy to estimate an individual's body fat and lean body weight. Although a few reports do show that the impedance method does correlate highly with established criterion methods such as densitometry and total body water, the majority of research published or presented at national scientific meetings in 1985, 1986, and 1987, indicates that the bioelectrical impedance procedure to estimate percent body fat is not as valid as claimed. The "fat machines" should probably not be used in a general way for application in the overall population, or to document changes that occur with dietary or exercise intervention.

APPENDIX **D**

Nutritive Value of Commonly Used Foods*

Explanation of the nutrient sources listed in Appendix D

The foods have been arranged in alphabetical order. The weight of the food is given in grams (g) as well as in ounces (oz), followed by the approximate measure of the food and its description. The next columns present the caloric value of the food (kcal); the number of grams of protein, fat, and carbohydrates; and the number of milligrams of calcium, iron, ascorbic acid, thiamin, riboflavin, and vitamin-A activity expressed in international units (IU). Page 316 lists the caloric value of alcoholic beverages, and pages 316 to 327 list the caloric value of specialty items purchased at selected fast-food chain stores. The abbreviation *tr* indicates that only a trace of food nutrient is present.

Equivalents by Weight

1 pound (16 ounces)	= 454 grams
1 ounce	= 28.4 grams
3½ ounces	= 100 grams

Equivalents by Volume

1 quart	= 4 cups
1 cup	= 8 fluid ounces
	= ½ pint
	= 16 tablespoons
2 tablespoons	= 1 fluid ounce
1 tablespoon	= 3 teaspoons
1 pound regular margarine or butter	= 4 sticks
	= 2 cups
1 pound whipped butter or margarine	= 6 sticks
	= two 8-ounce containers

* Data from Watt, B.K., and Merrill, A.L.: *Composition of Foods—Raw, Processed and Prepared.* U.S. Department of Agriculture, Washington, D.C., 1963; *Nutritive Value of Foods.* Home and Garden Bulletin no. 72, rev. U.S. Department of Agriculture, Washington, D.C., 1971; Adams, C. *Nutritive Value of American Foods.* In common units. Agricultural Handbook no. 456. U.S. Department of Agriculture, Washington, D.C., 1975.

Conversions

To convert	*into*	*multiply by*
gallons	liters	3.785
milligrams	grams	0.001
quarts (liquid)	liters	0.9463
ounces	pounds	0.0625
ounces (fluid)	liters	0.02957
grams	kilograms	0.001

Other Conversions

Units of Length

METRIC UNIT	EQUIVALENT METRIC UNIT	EQUIVALENT ENGLISH UNIT
meter (m)	100 cm 1000 mm	39.37 in. (3.28 ft; 1.09 yd)
centimeter (cm)	0.01 m 10 mm	0.3937 in.
millimeter (mm)	0.001 m 0.1 cm	0.03937 in.

Units of Weight

METRIC UNIT	EQUIVALENT METRIC UNIT	EQUIVALENT ENGLISH UNIT
kilogram (kg)	1000 g 1,000,000 mg	35.3 oz (2.2046 lb)
gram (g)	0.001 kg 1000 mg	0.0353 oz
milligram (mg)	0.000001 kg 0.001 g	0.0000353 oz

Units of Volume

METRIC UNIT	EQUIVALENT METRIC UNIT	EQUIVALENT ENGLISH UNIT
liter (l)	1000 ml	1.057 qt
milliliter (ml) or cubic centimeter (cc)	0.001 l	0.001057 qt

Common Expressions of Work, Energy, and Power

WATTS	KILOCALORIES (KCAL)	FOOT-POUNDS (FT-LB)
1 watt = 0.73756 ft-lb · s^{-1}	1 kcal = 3086 ft-lb	1 ft-lb = 3.2389 × 10^{-3} kcal
1 watt = 0.01433 kcal · min^{-1}	1 kcal = 426.8 kg-m	1 ft-lb = 0.13825 kg-m
1 watt = 1.341 × 10^{-3} hp or 0.0013 hp	1 kcal = 3087.4 ft-lb	1 ft-lb = 5.050 × 10^{-3} hp · h^{-1}
1 watt = 6.12 kg-m · min^{-1}	1 kcal = 1.5593 × 10^{-3} hp · h^{-1}	

FOOD	WEIGHT G	WEIGHT OZ	APPROXIMATE MEASURE AND DESCRIPTION	KCAL
Alcoholic beverages (*see* p. 316)				
Apples, raw	150	5.3	1 apple, about 3 per lb.	70
Apple, baked	130	4.6	1 medium apple, 2½ in. dia.	120
Apple brown betty	115	4.0	½ cup	175
Apple juice (sweet cider)	124	4.3	½ cup, bottled or canned	60
Apple pie (*see* pies)				
Applesauce, canned sweetened	128	4.5	½ cup	115
Apricots, fresh, raw (as purchased)	114	4.0	3 apricots, about 12 per lb.	55
Apricots, canned	130	4.6	½ cup or 4 medium halves, 2 tbsp. juice (syrup pack)	110
Apricots, dried, stewed	108	3.8	½ cup (scant) or 8 halves, 2 tbsp. juice, sweetened	135
Apricot nectar (peach and pear nectar have similar values)	125	4.4	½ cup	70
Asparagus, cooked, green	73	2.6	½ cup, 1½- to 2-in. lengths	15
Avocado, raw (as purchased)	142	5.0	½ avocado, 3⅛ in. dia., pitted and peeled	185
Bacon, broiled or fried	15	0.5	2 slices, cooked crisp (20 slices per lb., raw)	90
Bacon, Canadian, cooked	43	1.5	3 slices, cooked crisp	100
Bananas, raw (as purchased)	175	6.1	1 medium banana	100
Bavarian cream, orange	99	3.5	½ cup	210
Bean sprouts, mung, cooked	63	2.2	½ cup, drained	18
Beans, green snap, cooked	63	2.2	½ cup	15
Beans, dry, green lima, cooked	144	5.0	¾ cup	195
Beans, immature, green lima, cooked	85	2.8	½ cup	95
Beans, dry, red kidney, canned	191	6.7	¾ cup	173
Beans, dry, white, canned with tomato sauce, without pork	196	6.9	¾ cup	233
Beans, dry, white, canned with tomato sauce and pork	191	6.7	¾ cup	233
Beef, corned, canned	85	3.0	3 slices, 3 × 2 × ¼ in.	185
Beef, corned hash, canned	85	3.0	½ cup (approx.)	155
Beef, dried or chipped	57	2.0	4 thin slices, 4 × 5 in.	115
Beef, hamburger, broiled	85	3.0	1 patty, 3 in. dia. (regular ground beef)	245
Beef, heart, braised	85	3.0	2 round slices, 2½ in. dia., ½ in. thick	160

PROTEIN G	FAT G	CARBOHYDRATE G	CALCIUM MG	IRON MG	VITAMIN-A ACTIVITY IU	ASCORBIC ACID MG	THIAMIN MG	RIBOFLAVIN MG
tr	tr	18	8	0.4	50	3	0.04	0.02
tr	tr	30	8	0.4	50	3	0.04	0.02
2	4	34	21	0.7	115	2	0.07	0.05
tr	tr	15	8	0.8	—	1	0.01	0.03
tr	tr	31	5	0.7	50	2	0.03	0.02
1	tr	14	18	0.5	2890	10	0.03	0.04
1	tr	29	14	0.4	2255	5	0.03	0.03
2	tr	34	26	1.5	2287	3	tr	0.04
1	tr	19	12	0.3	1190	4	0.02	0.02
2	tr	3	15	0.5	655	19	0.12	0.13
3	19	7	11	0.7	315	15	0.12	0.22
5	8	1	2	0.5	0	—	0.08	0.05
18	12	tr	13	2.2	0	0	0.62	0.12
1	tr	26	10	0.8	230	12	0.06	0.07
2	10	30	27	0.1	627	54	0.10	0.05
2	tr	4	11	0.6	15	4	0.06	0.07
1	tr	4	32	0.4	340	8	0.05	0.06
12	1	37	41	4.2	—	—	0.19	0.08
7	1	17	40	2.2	240	15	0.16	0.09
11	1	32	56	3.5	8	—	0.10	0.08
12	1	45	133	3.9	120	4	0.14	0.07
12	5	37	104	3.5	248	4	0.15	0.06
22	10	0	17	3.7	20	—	0.01	0.20
7	10	9	11	1.7	—	—	0.01	0.08
19	4	0	11	2.9	—	—	0.04	0.18
21	17	0	9	2.7	30	—	0.07	0.18
27	5	1	5	5.0	20	1	0.21	1.04

FOOD	WEIGHT G	WEIGHT OZ	APPROXIMATE MEASURE AND DESCRIPTION	KCAL
Beef liver (*see* liver)				
Beef loaf (*see* meat loaf)				
Beef potpie, baked	227	7.9	1 pie, $4\frac{1}{4}$ in. dia.	560
Beef, pot roast, cooked	85	3.0	1 piece, $4 \times 3\frac{3}{4} \times \frac{1}{2}$ in.	245
Beef roast, oven-cooked	85	3.0	2 slices, $6 \times 3\frac{1}{4} \times \frac{1}{8}$ in., relatively lean	165
Beef steak, broiled	85	3.0	1 piece, $3\frac{1}{2} \times 2 \times \frac{3}{4}$ in., relatively fat, no bone	330
Beef stroganoff, cooked	130	4.6	$\frac{1}{2}$ cup	250
Beef tongue, braised	85	3.0	7 slices, $2\frac{1}{4} \times 2\frac{1}{4} \times \frac{1}{8}$ in.	210
Beets, cooked	85	3.0	$\frac{1}{2}$ cup, diced	28
Beverages, alcoholic (*see* p. 316)				
Beverages, cola-type	185	6.5	about $\frac{3}{4}$ cup	75
Beverages, ginger ale	240	8.4	1 cup	75
Biscuits, baking powder	28	1.0	1 biscuit, 2 in. dia. (enriched flour)	105
Blackberries, raw	72	2.5	$\frac{1}{2}$ cup	45
Blueberries, raw	70	2.5	$\frac{1}{2}$ cup	45
Bluefish, cooked	85	3.0	1 piece, $3\frac{1}{2} \times 2 \times \frac{1}{2}$ in.	135
Bologna (*see* sausage)				
Bouillon cubes	4	0.1	1 cube, $\frac{5}{8}$ in.	5
Bran flakes	26	0.9	$\frac{3}{4}$ cup, 40% bran, (thiamin and iron added)	80
Bread, Boston brown	48	1.7	1 slice, $3 \times \frac{3}{4}$ in.	100
Bread, cracked wheat	25	0.9	1 slice, 18 slices per lb. loaf	65
Bread, French or Vienna	20	0.7	1 slice, $3\frac{1}{4} \times 2 \times 1$ in. (enriched flour)	60
Bread, Italian	20	0.7	1 slice, $3\frac{1}{4} \times 2 \times 1$ in. (enriched flour)	55
Bread, light rye	25	0.9	1 slice, 18 slices per lb. loaf ($\frac{1}{3}$ rye, $\frac{2}{3}$ wheat)	60
Bread, pumpernickel	34	1.2	1 slice, $3\frac{1}{4} \times 2 \times 1$ in. (dark rye flour)	85
Bread, raisin	25	0.9	1 slice, 18 slices per lb. loaf	65
Bread, white firm crumb (enriched)	23	0.8	1 slice, 20 slices per lb. loaf	65
Bread, white soft crumb (enriched)	25	0.9	1 slice, 18 slices per lb loaf	70
Bread, white soft crumb (enriched), toasted	22	0.8	1 slice, 18 slices per lb loaf	70
Bread, white soft crumb (unenriched)	25	0.9	1 slice, 18 slices per lb loaf	70
Bread, whole wheat firm crumb	25	0.9	1 slice, 18 slices per lb loaf	60
Bread crumbs	25	0.9	$\frac{1}{4}$ cup, dry grated	98

PROTEIN G	FAT G	CARBOHYDRATE G	CALCIUM MG	IRON MG	VITAMIN-A ACTIVITY IU	ASCORBIC ACID MG	THIAMIN MG	RIBOFLAVIN MG
23	33	43	32	4.1	1860	7	0.25	0.27
23	16	0	10	2.9	30	—	0.04	0.18
25	7	0	11	3.2	10	—	0.06	0.19
20	27	0	9	2.5	50	—	0.05	0.16
17	18	6	41	2.6	395	2	0.12	0.29
18	14	tr	6	1.9	—	—	0.04	0.25
1	tr	6	12	0.5	15	5	0.03	0.04
0	0	19	—	—	0	0	0	0
0	0	19	—	—	0	0	0	0
2	5	13	34	0.4	tr	tr	0.06	0.06
1	1	10	23	0.7	145	15	0.03	0.03
1	1	11	11	0.7	70	10	0.02	0.04
22	4	0	25	0.6	40	—	0.09	0.08
1	tr	tr	—	—	—	—	—	—
3	1	21	19	9.3	0	0	0.11	0.05
3	1	22	43	0.9	0	0	0.05	0.03
2	1	13	22	0.3	tr	tr	0.03	0.02
2	1	11	9	0.4	tr	tr	0.06	0.04
2	tr	11	3	0.4	0	0	0.06	0.04
2	tr	13	19	0.4	0	0	0.05	0.02
3	0	19	30	0.8	0	0	0.08	0.05
2	1	13	18	0.3	tr	tr	0.01	0.02
2	1	12	22	0.6	tr	tr	0.06	0.05
2	1	13	21	0.6	tr	tr	0.06	0.05
2	1	13	21	0.6	tr	tr	0.05	0.05
2	1	13	21	0.2	tr	tr	0.02	0.02
3	1	12	25	0.8	tr	tr	0.06	0.03
3	1	18	31	0.9	tr	tr	0.06	0.08

FOOD	WEIGHT G	WEIGHT OZ	APPROXIMATE MEASURE AND DESCRIPTION	KCAL
Broccoli, cooked	78	2.7	½ cup, stalks cut into ½-in. pieces	20
Brussels sprouts, cooked	78	2.7	½ cup or 5 medium sprouts	28
Buns (*see* rolls)				
Butter	14	0.5	1 tbsp or ⅛ stick	100
Cabbage, cooked	73	2.6	½ cup, cooked short time in little water	15
Cabbage, raw	45	1.6	½ cup, finely shredded	10
Cabbage, raw, Chinese	38	1.3	½ cup, 1-in. pieces	5
Cake, angel food (from mix)	53	1.9	1 piece, $\frac{1}{12}$ of 10-in.-dia. cake	135
Cake, Boston cream pie	69	2.4	1 piece, $\frac{1}{12}$ of 8-in.-dia. pie (unenriched flour)	210
Cake, plain chocolate-iced cupcake (from mix)	36	1.3	1 cupcake, 2½ in. dia.	130
Cake, plain uniced cupcakes (from mix)	25	0.9	1 cupcake, 2½ in. dia.	90
Cake, 2-layer devil's food with chocolate icing (from mix)	69	2.4	1 piece (mix), $\frac{1}{16}$ of 9-in.-dia. cake	235
Cake, fruit, dark	15	0.5	1 slice, $\frac{1}{30}$ of 8-in.-long loaf (enriched flour)	55
Cake, pound	30	1.1	1 slice, 2¾ × 3 × ⅝ in. (unenriched flour)	140
Cake, sponge	66	1.4	1 piece, $\frac{1}{12}$ of 10-in.-dia. cake (unenriched)	195
Cake, 2-layer white with chocolate icing	71	2.5	1 piece, $\frac{1}{16}$ of 9-in.-dia. cake	250
Candy, caramels	28	1.0	4 small	115
Candy, plain chocolate	28	1.0	1 bar, 3¾ × 1½ × ¼ in.	145
Candy, chocolate with almonds	51	1.8	1 bar, 5⅓ × 1⅞ × ⅓ in.	265
Candy, chocolate creams	28	1.0	2 pieces, 1¼ in. dia. (base), ⅝ in. thick	110
Candy, chocolate fudge	28	1.0	1 piece, 1¼ × 1¼ × 1 in.	115
Candy, hard	28	1.0	6 pieces, 1 in. dia., ¼ in. thick	110
Candy, peanut brittle	28	1.0	1 piece, 3¼ × 2½ × ¼ in.	125
Cantaloupes	385	13.5	½ melon, 5 in. dia.	60
Carrots, raw grated	55	1.9	½ cup grated	23
Carrots, raw whole or strips	50	1.8	1 carrot, 5½ in. long, or 25 thin strips	20
Carrots, cooked	73	2.6	½ cup diced	23
Catsup, tomato (*see* tomato)				
Cauliflower, cooked	60	2.1	½ cup flowerets	13
Celery, raw diced	50	1.8	½ cup	8
Celery, raw whole	40	1.4	1 stalk, large outer, 8 in. long	5
Cheese, blue (Roquefort type)	28	1.0	¾-in. sector or 3 tbsp	105

PROTEIN G	FAT G	CARBOHYDRATE G	CALCIUM MG	IRON MG	VITAMIN-A ACTIVITY IU	ASCORBIC ACID MG	THIAMIN MG	RIBOFLAVIN MG
3	1	4	68	0.6	1940	70	0.07	0.16
4	1	5	25	0.9	405	68	0.06	0.11
tr	12	tr	3	0	470	0	—	—
1	tr	3	32	0.2	95	24	0.03	0.03
1	tr	3	22	0.2	60	21	0.03	0.03
1	tr	1	16	0.3	55	10	0.02	0.02
3	tr	32	50	0.2	0	0	tr	0.06
4	6	34	46	0.3	140	tr	0.02	0.08
2	5	21	47	0.3	60	tr	0.01	0.04
1	3	14	40	0.1	40	tr	0.01	0.03
3	9	40	41	0.6	100	tr	0.02	0.06
1	2	9	11	0.4	20	tr	0.02	0.02
2	9	14	6	0.2	80	0	0.01	0.03
5	4	36	20	0.8	300	tr	0.03	0.09
3	8	45	70	0.4	40	tr	0.01	0.06
1	3	22	42	0.4	tr	tr	0.01	0.05
2	9	16	65	0.3	80	tr	0.02	0.10
4	19	25	102	1.4	70	0	0.07	0.25
1	4	20	—	—	—	0	—	—
1	4	21	22	0.3	tr	tr	0.01	0.03
0	tr	28	6	0.5	0	0	0	0
2	4	21	11	0.6	10	0	0.03	0.01
1	tr	14	27	0.8	6540	63	0.08	0.06
1	tr	6	21	0.4	6050	5	0.03	0.03
1	tr	5	18	0.4	5500	4	0.03	0.03
1	tr	5	24	0.5	7610	5	0.04	0.04
2	tr	3	13	0.4	35	33	0.06	0.05
1	tr	2	20	0.2	120	5	0.02	0.02
tr	tr	2	16	0.1	100	4	0.01	0.01
6	9	1	89	0.1	350	0	0.01	0.17

FOOD	WEIGHT G	WEIGHT OZ	APPROXIMATE MEASURE AND DESCRIPTION	KCAL
Cheese, cheddar (American), cubed	28	1.0	1 cube, 1⅛ in.	115
Cheese, cheddar (American), grated	7	0.3	1 tbsp	30
Cheese, creamed cottage	61	2.1	¼ cup (made from skim milk)	65
Cheese, uncreamed cottage	28	1.0	2 tbsp (made from skim milk)	25
Cheese, cream	16	0.5	1 tbsp	60
Cheese, Swiss (domestic)	28	1.0	1 slice, 7 × 4 × ⅛ in.	105
Cheese foods, cheddar	28	1.0	2 round slices, 1⅝ in. dia., ¼ in. thick or 2 tbsp	90
Cheese sauce	60	2.1	¼ cup	110
Cheese soufflé	79	2.8	¾ cup	200
Cheesecake	162	5.7	1/10 of 9-in.-dia. cake	400
Cherries, raw sweet	130	4.6	1 cup with stems	80
Cherries, raw West Indian (acerola)	11	0.4	2 medium cherries	3
Chick peas, dry raw (garbanzos)	105	3.7	½ cup	380
Chicken, broiled	85	3.0	3 slices, flesh only	115
Chicken, canned	85	3.0	⅓ cup boned meat	170
Chicken, creamed	99	3.5	½ cup	222
Chicken breast, fried	94	3.3	½ breast with bone	155
Chicken drumstick, fried	59	2.1	1 drumstick with bone	90
Chicken pie (*see* poultry potpie)				
Chili con carne with beans, canned	188	6.5	¾ cup	250
Chili con carne without beans, canned	191	6.7	¾ cup	383
Chili powder	15	0.5	1 tbsp hot red peppers, dried and ground	50
Chili sauce	17	0.6	1 tbsp, mainly tomatoes	20
Chocolate, bitter (baking chocolate)	28	1.0	1 square	145
Chocolate candy (*see* candy)				
Chocolate-flavored milk drink	250	8.8	1 cup (made with skim milk)	190
Chocolate morsels	15	0.5	30 morsels or 1½ tbsp	80
Chocolate syrup	40	1.4	2 tbsp	80
Chop suey, cooked	122	4.3	¾ cup	325
Clams, canned	85	3.0	½ cup or 3 medium clams	45
Cocoa, beverage	182	6.3	¾ cup (made with milk)	176
Coconut, dried shredded, sweetened	16	0.6	¼ cup	85
Coconut, fresh shredded	33	1.2	¼ cup	113
Codfish, dried	51	1.8	½ cup	190
Coffee cake, frosted	79	2.8	1 piece, 3 × 3 × 1¼ in.	260
Cole slaw	60	2.1	½ cup	50
Cookies, brownies	26	0.9	1 piece, 1⅞ × 1⅞ × ⅝ in.	145
Cookies, chocolate chip	11	0.4	1 cookie, 2¼ in. dia.	60
Cookies, coconut bar chews	11	0.4	1 cookie, 3 × ⅞ × ⅓ in.	55
Cookies, oatmeal with raisins and nuts	11	0.4	1 cookie, 2⅛ in. dia.	65

PROTEIN G	FAT G	CARBOHYDRATE G	CALCIUM MG	IRON MG	VITAMIN-A ACTIVITY IU	ASCORBIC ACID MG	THIAMIN MG	RIBOFLAVIN MG
6	10	2	206	0.3	368	0	0.02	0.13
2	2	tr	52	0.1	90	0	tr	0.03
8	3	2	58	0.2	105	0	0.02	0.15
5	tr	1	26	0.1	tr	0	0.01	0.08
1	6	tr	10	tr	250	0	tr	0.04
8	8	1	262	0.3	320	0	tr	0.11
6	6	2	160	0.2	280	0	tr	0.16
5	9	4	156	0.1	337	1	0.02	0.14
10	16	7	210	1.0	826	1	0.08	0.23
15	23	35	128	0.8	958	1	0.08	0.33
2	tr	20	26	0.5	130	12	0.06	0.07
—	—	1	1	—	—	100	—	0.01
22	5	64	97	7.5	tr	2	0.58	0.19
20	2	0	8	1.4	80	—	0.05	0.16
18	10	0	18	1.3	200	3	0.03	0.11
20	12	6	84	1.1	445	1	0.04	0.20
25	5	1	9	1.3	70	—	0.04	0.17
12	4	tr	6	0.9	50	—	0.03	0.15
14	11	23	60	3.2	113	—	0.06	0.14
20	29	11	73	2.7	285	—	0.04	0.23
2	2	8	40	2.3	9750	2	0.03	0.17
tr	tr	4	3	0.1	240	3	0.02	0.01
3	15	8	22	1.9	20	0	0.01	0.07
8	6	27	270	0.5	210	3	0.10	0.40
1	4	10	5	0.3	tr	0	tr	tr
tr	tr	22	6	0.6	—	—	—	—
19	20	16	43	2.9	85	17	0.11	0.13
7	1	2	47	3.5	—	—	0.01	0.09
7	8	20	215	0.7	293	2	0.07	0.34
1	6	8	3	0.3	0	0	0.01	0.01
1	12	3	4	0.6	0	1	0.02	0.01
41	2	0	25	1.8	0	0	0.04	0.23
4	11	37	25	1.0	477	0	0.12	0.13
1	4	5	24	0.3	40	25	0.03	0.03
2	9	17	12	0.5	231	—	0.03	0.04
1	3	7	4	0.2	81	—	0.01	0.01
tr	2	9	7	0.3	76	0	0.01	0.01
1	4	6	5	0.3	18	tr	0.04	0.02

FOOD	WEIGHT G	WEIGHT OZ	APPROXIMATE MEASURE AND DESCRIPTION	KCAL
Cookies, sugar, plain	9	0.3	1 cookie, 2½ in. dia.	40
Corn, sweet, cooked	140	4.9	1 ear, 5 in. long	70
Corn, sweet, canned	128	4.5	½ cup, solids and liquid	85
Corn grits, cooked	163	5.7	⅔ cup, enriched and degermed	85
Corn muffins	40	1.4	1 muffin, 2⅜ in. dia., enriched flour and enriched degermed meal	125
Corned beef (*see* beef)				
Corned beef hash (*see* beef)				
Cornflakes	33	1.2	1⅓ cup (added nutrients)	133
Cornmeal, dry	138	4.8	1 cup, white or yellow, enriched and degermed	500
Cow peas (*see* peas)				
Crabmeat, canned	85	3.0	½ cup flakes	85
Crackers, graham, plain	14	0.6	2 medium or 4 small	55
Crackers, saltines	8	0.3	2 crackers, 2 in. square	35
Cranberry juice, canned	125	4.4	½ cup or 1 small glass, ascorbic acid added	85
Cranberry sauce, canned	69	2.4	¼ cup, strained and sweetened	85
Cream, coffee (light cream)	15	0.5	1 tbsp	30
Cream, half-and-half	15	0.5	1 tbsp	20
Cream, heavy, whipping	15	0.5	1 tbsp, unwhipped (volume doubled when whipped)	55
Creamer, coffee (imitation cream)	2	—	1 tsp powder	10
Cucumber, raw	50	1.8	6 slices, pared, ⅛ in. thick	5
Custard, baked	124	4.3	½ cup	143
Dates, pitted	45	1.6	¼ cup or 8 dates	123
Dessert topping, whipped	11	0.4	2 tbsp (low-calorie, with nonfat dry milk)	17
Doughnuts, cake-type	32	1.1	1 (enriched flour)	125
Egg, raw, boiled, or poached	50	1.8	1 whole egg	80
Egg white, raw	33	1.2	1 egg white	15
Egg yolk, raw	17	0.6	1 egg yolk	60
Eggs, creamed	113	4.0	½ cup (1 egg in ¼ cup white sauce)	190
Eggs, fried	54	1.9	1 egg, cooked in 1 tsp fat	115
Eggs, scrambled	64	2.2	1 egg, with milk and fat	110
Endive, curly, raw	57	2.0	3 leaves (includes escarole)	10
Farina, cooked	163	5.7	⅔ cup (quick, enriched)	70
Fats, cooking, lard	13	0.5	1 tbsp solid fat	115
Fats, cooking, vegetable	13	0.5	1 tbsp solid fat	110
Figs, dried	21	0.7	1 large fig, 1 × 2 in.	60
Figs, fresh raw	114	4.0	3 small, 1½ in. dia.	90
Fish (*see* various kinds of fish)				

PROTEIN G	FAT G	CARBOHYDRATE G	CALCIUM MG	IRON MG	VITAMIN-A ACTIVITY IU	ASCORBIC ACID MG	THIAMIN MG	RIBOFLAVIN MG
1	2	6	2	0.1	64	0	0.02	0.01
3	1	16	2	0.5	310	7	0.09	0.08
3	1	20	5	0.5	345	7	0.04	0.06
2	tr	18	1	0.5	100	0	0.07	0.05
3	4	19	42	0.7	120	tr	0.08	0.09
3	tr	28	5	0.5	0	0	0.15	0.03
11	2	108	8	4.0	610	0	0.61	0.36
15	2	1	38	0.7	—	—	0.07	0.07
1	1	10	6	0.2	0	0	0.01	0.03
1	1	6	2	0.1	0	0	tr	tr
tr	tr	21	7	0.4	tr	20	0.02	0.02
tr	tr	21	4	0.1	13	1	0.01	0.01
1	3	1	15	tr	130	tr	tr	0.02
1	2	1	16	tr	70	tr	tr	0.02
tr	6	1	11	tr	230	tr	tr	0.02
tr	1	1	1	tr	tr	—	—	—
tr	tr	2	8	0.2	tr	6	0.02	0.02
7	7	14	139	0.5	435	1	0.05	0.24
1	tr	33	26	1.3	23	0	0.04	0.04
1	—	3	29	—	1	1	0.01	0.04
1	6	16	13	0.4	30	tr	0.05	0.05
6	6	tr	27	1.1	590	0	0.05	0.15
4	tr	tr	3	tr	0	0	tr	0.09
3	5	tr	24	0.9	580	0	0.04	0.07
9	14	7	103	1.2	928	tr	0.07	0.25
6	10	tr	28	1.1	590	0	0.05	0.15
7	8	1	51	1.1	690	0	0.05	0.18
1	tr	2	46	1.0	1870	6	0.04	0.08
2	tr	14	98	0.5	0	0	0.08	0.05
0	13	0	0	0	0	0	0	0
0	13	0	0	0	—	0	0	0
1	tr	15	26	0.6	20	0	0.02	0.02
1	tr	23	40	0.7	90	2	0.07	0.06

FOOD	WEIGHT G	WEIGHT OZ	APPROXIMATE MEASURE AND DESCRIPTION	KCAL
Fish, creamed (tuna, salmon, or other, in white sauce)	136	4.8	½ cup	220
Fish sticks, breaded, cooked	114	4.0	5 sticks, each 3.8 × 1.0 × 0.5 in.	200
Frankfurter, heated	56	2.0	1 frankfurter	170
French toast, fried	79	2.8	1 slice (enriched bread)	180
Fruit balls, raw (dried apricots, dates, nuts)	11	0.4	1 ball, 1 in. dia.	45
Fruit cocktail, canned	128	4.5	½ cup, with heavy syrup	98
Gelatin, plain, dry	7	0.3	1 tbsp (1 envelope)	25
Gelatin dessert, plain	120	4.2	½ cup, ready to eat	70
Gingerbread	63	2.2	1 piece (mix), $\frac{1}{9}$ of 8-in.-square cake	175
Grapefruit, white, raw (as purchased)	241	8.4	½ medium, 3¾ in. dia.	45
Grapefruit, white, canned	125	4.4	½ cup, syrup pack	88
Grapefruit juice, canned	124	4.3	½ cup, unsweetened	50
Grapefruit juice, dehydrated crystals	124	4.3	½ cup or 1 small glass, prepared, ready to serve	50
Grapes, raw American-type	153	5.4	1 cup or 1 medium bunch (slip skin, as Concord)	65
Grapes, raw European-type	160	5.6	1 cup or 40 grapes (adherent skin, as Tokay)	95
Grape juice, canned	127	4.4	½ cup	83
Greens, collards, cooked	95	3.3	½ cup	28
Greens, dandelion, cooked	90	3.2	½ cup	30
Greens, kale, cooked	55	1.9	½ cup, leaves and stems	15
Greens, mustard, cooked	70	2.5	½ cup	18
Greens, spinach, cooked	90	3.2	½ cup	20
Greens, turnip, cooked	73	2.6	½ cup	15
Guavas, raw	82	2.8	1 guava	50
Haddock, fried	85	3.0	1 fillet, 4 × 2½ × ½ in.	140
Ham, boiled	57	2.0	1 slice, 6¼ × 3¾ × ⅛ in.	135
Ham, cured, roasted	85	3.0	2 slices, 5½ × 3¾ × ⅛ in.	245
Ham, luncheon, canned	57	2.0	2 tbsp, spiced or unspiced	165
Hamburger (*see* beef, hamburger)				
Honey, strained	21	0.7	1 tbsp	65
Hot dog (*see* frankfurter)				
Ice cream, plain	50	1.8	1 container, 3 fluid oz (factory packed)	95
Ice cream, plain brick	71	2.5	1 slice, ⅛ of qt brick	145
Ice milk	66	2.3	½ cup	100

PROTEIN G	FAT G	CARBOHYDRATE G	CALCIUM MG	IRON MG	VITAMIN-A ACTIVITY IU	ASCORBIC ACID MG	THIAMIN MG	RIBOFLAVIN MG
20	13	8	81	0.9	385	tr	0.05	0.18
19	10	8	13	0.5	—	—	0.05	0.08
7	15	1	3	0.8	—	—	0.08	0.11
6	12	14	78	1.0	568	tr	0.09	0.17
1	1	8	10	0.4	285	tr	0.02	0.02
1	tr	25	12	0.5	180	3	0.03	0.02
6	tr	0	—	—	—	—	—	—
2	0	17	—	—	—	—	—	—
2	4	32	57	1.0	tr	tr	0.02	0.06
1	tr	12	19	0.5	10	44	0.05	0.02
1	tr	22	16	0.4	10	38	0.04	0.02
1	tr	12	10	0.5	10	42	0.04	0.02
1	tr	12	11	0.1	10	46	0.05	0.03
1	1	15	15	0.4	100	3	0.05	0.03
1	tr	25	17	0.6	140	6	0.07	0.04
1	tr	21	14	0.4	—	tr	0.05	0.03
3	1	5	145	0.6	5130	44	0.14	0.19
2	1	6	126	1.6	10,530	16	0.12	0.15
2	1	2	74	0.7	4070	34	—	—
2	1	3	97	1.3	4060	34	0.06	0.10
3	1	3	84	2.0	7290	25	0.07	0.13
2	tr	3	126	0.8	4135	34	0.08	0.17
1	tr	12	21	0.5	180	212	0.05	0.03
17	5	5	34	1.0	—	2	0.03	0.06
11	10	0	6	1.6	0	—	0.25	0.09
18	19	0	8	2.2	0	—	0.40	0.16
8	14	1	5	1.2	0	—	0.18	0.12
tr	0	17	1	0.1	0	tr	tr	0.01
2	5	10	73	0.2	220	1	0.02	0.11
3	9	15	87	0.1	370	1	0.03	0.13
3	4	15	102	0.1	140	1	0.04	0.15

FOOD	WEIGHT G	OZ	APPROXIMATE MEASURE AND DESCRIPTION	KCAL
Jams, jellies, preserves	20	0.7	1 tbsp	55
Kale (*see* greens)				
Lamb chop, cooked	137	4.8	1 thick chop with bone	400
Lamb, leg, roasted	85	3.0	2 slices, 3 × 3¼ × ⅛ in., lean and fat, no bone	235
Lard (*see* fats, cooking)				
Lemon juice, fresh	15	0.5	1 tbsp	5
Lemonade	248	8.7	1 cup (made from frozen, sweetened concentrate)	110
Lentils, dry, cooked	100	3.5	½ cup	120
Lettuce, headed, raw	454	16.0	1 head (compact, as iceberg), 4¾ in. dia.	60
Lettuce, loose leaf, raw	50	1.8	2 large leaves or 4 small leaves	10
Lime juice, canned	62	2.2	¼ cup	15
Liver, beef, fried	57	2.0	1 slice, 5 × 2 × ⅓ in.	130
Liver, calf, fried	74	2.6	1 slice, 5 × 2 × ½ in.	230
Liver, chicken, fried	85	3.0	3 medium livers	235
Liver, pork, fried	70	2.5	1 slice, 3¾ × 1¾ × ½ in.	225
Macaroni, cooked	105	3.7	¾ cup (enriched)	115
Macaroni and cheese, baked	150	5.3	¾ cup (enriched macaroni)	325
Mackerel, broiled	85	3.0	1 piece	200
Mangoes, raw	198	7.0	1 medium mango	90
Margarine	14	0.5	1 tbsp or ⅛ stick (fortified with vitamin A)	100
Marshmallows	9	0.3	1, 1¼ in. dia.	25
Meat loaf, beef, baked	77	2.7	1 slice, 3¾ × 2¼ × ¾ in.	240
Milk, dry skim (nonfat)	17	0.6	¼ cup powder, instant	61
Milk, dry whole	26	0.9	¼ cup powder	129
Milk, evaporated, canned	126	4.4	½ cup, undiluted and unsweetened	173
Milk, fluid, skim or buttermilk	245	8.6	1 cup (½ pt)	90
Milk, fluid, whole	244	8.5	1 cup (½ pt), 3.5% fat	160
Milk, malted, plain	353	12.4	1 fountain size glass (about 1½ cup)	368
Milkshake, chocolate	342	12.0	1 fountain size glass	420
Molasses, cane, blackstrap	20	0.7	1 tbsp, 3rd extraction	45
Molasses, cane, light	20	0.7	1 tbsp, 1st extraction	50
Muffins, plain	40	1.4	1 muffin, 2¾ in. dia. (enriched white flour)	120
Mushrooms, canned	122	4.3	½ cup, solids and liquid	20
Noodles, egg, cooked	120	4.2	¾ cup (enriched)	150
Nuts, almonds	36	1.3	¼ cup shelled	213
Nuts, cashew, roasted	35	1.2	¼ cup	196
Nuts, peanuts (*see* peanuts, roasted)				
Nuts, pecan halves	27	0.9	¼ cup	185
Nuts, walnut halves	25	0.9	¼ cup, English or Persian	163

PROTEIN G	FAT G	CARBOHYDRATE G	CALCIUM MG	IRON MG	VITAMIN-A ACTIVITY IU	ASCORBIC ACID MG	THIAMIN MG	RIBOFLAVIN MG
tr	tr	14	4	0.2	tr	tr	tr	0.01
25	33	0	10	1.5	—	—	0.14	0.25
22	16	0	9	1.4	—	—	0.13	0.23
tr	tr	1	1	tr	tr	7	tr	tr
tr	tr	28	2	tr	tr	17	tr	0.02
9	tr	22	12	2.5	200	0	0.20	0.09
4	tr	13	91	2.3	1500	29	0.29	0.27
1	tr	2	34	0.7	950	9	0.03	0.04
tr	tr	6	6	0.1	5	13	0.01	0.01
15	6	3	6	5.0	30,280	15	0.15	2.37
15	15	4	5	9.0	19,130	30	0.18	2.65
20	15	5	15	6.4	27,370	17	0.19	2.11
17	15	3	8	15.3	12,070	19	0.34	2.53
4	1	24	6	1.0	0	0	0.15	0.08
13	17	30	272	1.4	645	tr	0.15	0.30
19	13	0	5	1.0	450	—	0.13	0.23
1	—	23	12	0.3	8380	55	0.08	0.07
tr	12	tr	3	0	470	0	—	—
tr	0	8	2	0.2	0	0	0	tr
19	17	3	34	2.9	138	—	0.10	0.21
6	tr	9	220	0.1	5	1	0.06	0.30
7	7	10	234	0.1	290	2	0.08	0.38
9	10	12	318	0.2	405	2	0.05	0.43
9	tr	12	296	0.1	10	2	0.09	0.44
9	9	12	288	0.1	350	2	0.07	0.41
17	15	42	476	1.1	885	3	0.21	0.74
11	18	58	363	0.9	687	4	0.12	0.55
—	—	11	137	3.2	—	—	0.02	0.04
—	—	13	33	0.9	—	—	0.01	0.01
3	4	17	42	0.6	40	tr	0.07	0.09
3	tr	3	8	0.6	tr	2	0.02	0.30
5	2	28	12	1.1	83	0	0.17	0.11
7	19	7	83	1.7	0	tr	0.09	0.33
6	16	10	13	1.3	35	—	0.15	0.09
3	19	4	20	0.7	35	1	0.23	0.04
4	16	4	25	0.8	8	1	0.08	0.03

FOOD	WEIGHT G	WEIGHT OZ	APPROXIMATE MEASURE AND DESCRIPTION	KCAL
Oatmeal or rolled oats, cooked	160	5.6	$\frac{2}{3}$ cup (regular or quick-cooking)	87
Oils, salad or cooking	14	0.5	1 tbsp	125
Okra, cooked	43	1.5	4 pods, 3 × $\frac{5}{8}$ in.	13
Olives, green	16	0.6	4 medium or 3 large	15
Olives, ripe	10	0.4	3 small or 2 large	15
Onions, raw	110	3.9	1 onion, 2$\frac{1}{2}$ in. dia.	40
Onions, cooked	105	3.7	$\frac{1}{2}$ cup or 5 onions, 1$\frac{1}{4}$ in. dia.	30
Onions, young green	50	1.8	6 small, without tops	20
Oranges	180	6.3	1 orange, 2$\frac{5}{8}$ in. dia. (all commercial varieties)	65
Orange juice, canned unsweetened	125	4.4	$\frac{1}{2}$ cup or 1 small glass	60
Orange juice, dehydrated crystals	124	4.3	$\frac{1}{2}$ cup or 1 small glass, prepared, ready to serve	60
Orange juice, fresh	124	4.3	$\frac{1}{2}$ cup or 1 small glass (all varieties)	55
Orange juice, frozen concentrate	125	4.4	$\frac{1}{2}$ cup or 1 small glass, diluted, ready to serve	60
Oysters, raw	120	4.2	$\frac{1}{2}$ cup or 8–10 oysters	80
Oyster stew, milk	230	8.1	1 cup with 3–4 oysters	200
Pancakes, wheat	27	0.9	1 griddle cake, 4 in. dia. (enriched flour)	60
Papayas, raw	91	3.2	$\frac{1}{2}$ cup in $\frac{1}{2}$-in. cubes	35
Parsley, raw	4	0.1	1 tbsp chopped	tr
Parsnips, cooked	77	2.7	$\frac{1}{2}$ cup	50
Peaches, canned halves or slices	129	4.5	$\frac{1}{2}$ cup, solids and liquid, syrup-pack	100
Peaches, canned whole	123	4.3	$\frac{1}{2}$ cup, solids liquid (water pack)	38
Peaches, raw sliced	84	2.9	$\frac{1}{2}$ cup fresh or frozen	33
Peaches, raw whole	114	4.0	1 peach, 2 in. dia.	35
Peanuts, roasted	36	1.3	$\frac{1}{4}$ cup halves, salted	210
Peanut butter	32	1.1	2 tbsp	190
Pears, canned	117	4.1	2 medium halves with 2 tbsp juice (syrup pack)	90
Pears, raw (as purchased)	182	6.3	1 pear, 3 × 2$\frac{1}{2}$ in. dia.	100
Peas, cowpeas, dry, cooked (blackeye peas or frijoles)	124	4.3	$\frac{1}{2}$ cup	95
Peas, green, cooked	80	2.8	$\frac{1}{2}$ cup	58
Peas, pigeon, dry raw (gandules)	99	3.5	6 tbsp	310
Peas, split, dry cooked	125	4.4	$\frac{1}{2}$ cup	145
Peppers, green, stuffed	113	4.0	1 medium pepper, cooked with meat stuffing	200
Peppers, hot red (*see* chili powder)				
Peppers, pimientos, canned	38	1.3	1 medium pod	10
Peppers, raw sweet green	74	2.6	1 medium pod without stem and seeds, 5 pods per lb	15

PROTEIN G	FAT G	CARBOHYDRATE G	CALCIUM MG	IRON MG	VITAMIN-A ACTIVITY IU	ASCORBIC ACID MG	THIAMIN MG	RIBOFLAVIN MG
3	1	15	15	0.9	0	0	0.13	0.03
0	14	0	0	0	—	0	0	0
1	tr	3	39	0.2	210	9	0.06	0.08
tr	2	tr	8	0.2	40	—	—	—
tr	2	tr	9	0.1	10	—	tr	tr
2	tr	10	30	0.6	40	11	0.04	0.04
2	tr	7	25	0.4	40	7	0.03	0.03
1	tr	5	20	0.3	tr	12	0.02	0.02
1	tr	16	54	0.5	260	66	0.13	0.05
1	1	13	14	0.3	250	62	0.11	0.04
1	tr	14	13	0.5	250	50	0.09	0.03
1	tr	15	13	0.1	275	60	0.11	0.01
1	tr	14	13	0.3	250	55	0.10	0.04
10	2	4	113	6.6	370	—	0.17	0.22
11	12	11	269	3.3	640	—	0.13	0.41
2	2	9	27	0.4	30	tr	0.05	0.06
1	tr	9	18	0.3	1595	51	0.04	0.04
tr	tr	tr	8	0.2	340	7	tr	0.01
1	1	12	35	0.5	25	8	0.06	0.07
1	tr	26	5	0.4	550	4	0.01	0.03
1	tr	10	5	0.4	550	4	0.01	0.03
1	tr	8	8	0.4	1115	6	0.02	0.04
1	tr	10	9	0.5	1320	7	0.02	0.05
9	18	7	27	0.8	—	0	0.12	0.05
8	16	6	18	0.6	—	0	0.04	0.04
tr	tr	23	6	0.2	tr	2	0.01	0.02
1	1	25	13	0.5	30	7	0.04	0.07
7	1	17	21	1.6	10	tr	0.21	0.06
5	1	10	19	1.5	430	17	0.22	0.09
22	2	50	140	4.0	169	0	0.45	0.34
10	1	26	14	2.1	50	—	0.19	0.11
12	14	12	31	1.9	637	64	0.09	0.14
tr	tr	2	3	0.6	870	36	0.01	0.02
1	tr	4	7	0.5	310	94	0.06	0.06

FOOD	WEIGHT G	WEIGHT OZ	APPROXIMATE MEASURE AND DESCRIPTION	KCAL
Peppers, raw sweet red	60	2.1	1 medium pod without stem and seeds	20
Perch, ocean, fried	85	3.0	1 piece, 4 × 3 × ½ in.	195
Persimmons, raw (Japanese)	125	4.4	1 fruit, 2½ in. dia.	75
Pickle relish	15	0.5	1 tbsp	20
Pickles, cucumber, bread and butter	42	1.5	6 slices, ¼ × 1½ in. dia.	30
Pickles, cucumber, dill	65	2.3	1 large pickel, 3¾ × 1¼ in.	10
Pickles, cucumber, sweet	15	0.5	1 pickle, 2½ × ¾ in. dia.	20
Pie, apple	135	4.7	4-in. sector or ⅐ of 9-in.-dia. pie (unenriched flour)	350
Pie, cherry	135	4.7	4-in. sector or ⅐ of 9-in.-dia. pie (unenriched flour)	350
Pie, custard	130	4.6	4-in. sector or ⅐ of 9-in.-dia. pie (unenriched flour)	285
Pie, lemon meringue	120	4.2	4-in. sector or ⅐ of 9-in.-dia. pie (unenriched flour)	305
Pie, mince	135	4.7	4-in. sector or ⅐ of 9-in.-dia. pie (unenriched flour)	365
Pie, pumpkin	130	4.6	4-in. sector or ⅐ of 9-in.-dia. pie (unenriched flour)	275
Pineapple, canned crushed	130	4.6	½ cup (syrup pack)	100
Pineapple, canned slices	122	4.3	1 large or 2 small slices, 2 tbsp juice (syrup pack)	90
Pineapple, raw	70	2.5	½ cup, diced	38
Pineapple juice, canned	125	4.4	½ cup or 1 small glass	68
Pizza (cheese)	75	2.6	5½-in. sector or ⅛ of 14-in.-dia. pie	185
Plantain, raw, green	100	3.5	1 baking banana, 6 in.	135
Plums, canned	128	4.5	½ cup or 3 plums with 2 tbsp juice (syrup pack)	100
Plums, raw	60	2.1	1 plum, 2 in. diameter	25
Popcorn, popped	9	0.3	1 cup (oil and salt) added	40
Pork chop, cooked	99	3.5	1 thick chop, trimmed, with bone	260
Pork roast, cooked	85	3.0	2 slices, 5 × 4 × ⅛ in.	310
Potato chips	20	0.7	10 medium chips, 2 in. dia.	115
Potatoes, baked	99	3.5	1 medium potato, about 3 per pound raw	90
Potatoes, boiled	122	4.3	1 potato, peeled before boiling	80
Potatoes, French fried	57	2.0	10 pieces, 2 × ½ × ½ in., cooked in deep fat	155
Potatoes, mashed	98	3.4	½ cup (milk and butter added)	95
Poultry (chicken or turkey) potpie	227	7.9	1 indiv. pie, 4¼ in. dia.	535
Pretzels	3	0.1	5, 3⅛-in. sticks	10
Prunes, dried, cooked	105	3.7	5 medium prunes with 2 tbsp juice, sweetened	160
Prune juice, canned	128	4.5	½ cup or 1 small glass	100
Pudding, chocolate blanc mange	130	4.6	½ cup	190

PROTEIN G	FAT G	CARBOHYDRATE G	CALCIUM MG	IRON MG	VITAMIN-A ACTIVITY IU	ASCORBIC ACID MG	THIAMIN MG	RIBOFLAVIN MG
1	tr	4	8	0.4	2670	122	0.05	0.05
16	11	6	1.1	1.1	—	—	0.08	0.09
1	tr	20	6	0.4	2740	11	0.03	0.02
tr	tr	5	3	0.1	—	—	—	—
tr	tr	7	13	0.8	80	4	0.01	0.02
1	tr	1	17	0.7	70	4	tr	0.01
tr	tr	6	2	0.2	10	1	tr	tr
3	15	51	11	0.4	40	1	0.03	0.03
4	15	52	19	0.4	590	tr	0.03	0.03
8	14	30	125	0.8	300	0	0.07	0.21
4	12	45	17	0.6	200	4	0.04	0.10
3	16	56	38	1.4	tr	1	0.09	0.05
5	15	32	66	0.7	3210	tr	0.04	0.13
1	tr	25	15	0.4	60	9	0.10	0.03
tr	tr	24	13	0.4	50	8	0.09	0.03
1	tr	10	12	0.4	50	12	0.06	0.02
1	tr	17	19	0.4	60	11	0.06	0.02
7	6	27	107	0.7	290	4	0.04	0.12
1	—	32	8	0.8	380	28	0.07	0.04
1	tr	27	11	1.1	1485	2	0.03	0.03
tr	tr	7	7	0.3	140	3	0.02	0.02
1	2	5	1	0.2	—	0	—	0.01
16	21	0	8	2.2	0	—	0.63	0.18
21	24	0	9	2.7	0	—	0.78	0.22
1	8	10	8	0.4	tr	3	0.04	0.01
3	tr	21	9	0.7	tr	20	0.10	0.04
2	tr	18	7	0.6	tr	20	0.11	0.04
2	7	20	9	0.7	tr	12	0.07	0.04
2	4	12	24	0.4	165	9	0.08	0.05
23	31	42	68	3.0	3020	5	0.25	0.26
tr	tr	2	1	tr	0	0	tr	tr
1	tr	42	21	1.5	733	1	0.03	0.06
1	tr	25	18	5.3	—	3	0.02	0.02
6	8	26	158	0.9	211	1	0.06	0.27

FOOD	WEIGHT G	WEIGHT OZ	APPROXIMATE MEASURE AND DESCRIPTION	KCAL
Pudding, cornstarch (plain blanc mange)	124	4.3	½ cup	140
Pudding, rice with raisins (old-fashioned)	136	4.8	½ cup	300
Pudding, tapioca	74	2.6	½ cup	140
Radishes, raw	40	1.4	4 small	5
Raisins, seedless	10	0.4	1 tbsp pressed down	30
Raspberries, raw, red	62	2.2	½ cup	35
Rhubarb, cooked	136	4.8	½ cup (sugar added)	190
Rice, parboiled, cooked	131	4.6	¾ cup (enriched)	140
Rice, puffed	15	0.5	1 cup (nutrients added)	60
Rice flakes	30	1.1	1 cup (nutrients added)	115
Rolls, bagel (egg)	55	1.9	1 roll, 3 in. dia.	165
Rolls, barbecue bun	40	1.3	1 bun, 3½ in. dia. (enriched)	120
Rolls, hard	52	1.8	1 round roll	160
Rolls, plain, white	28	1.0	1 commercial pan roll (enriched flour)	85
Rolls, sweet, pan	43	1.5	1 roll	135
Rutabagas, cooked	77	2.7	½ cup	25
Salad, chicken	125	4.4	½ cup, with mayonnaise	280
Salad, egg	128	4.5	½ cup, with mayonnaise	190
Salad, fresh fruit (orange, apple, banana, grapes)	125	4.4	½ cup, with French dressing	130
Salad, jellied, vegetable	122	4.3	½ cup, no dressing	70
Salad, lettuce	130	4.6	¼ solid head, with French dressing	80
Salad, potato	139	4.9	½ cup, with mayonnaise	185
Salad, tomato aspic	119	4.2	½ cup, no dressing	45
Salad, tuna fish	102	3.6	½ cup, with mayonnaise	250
Salad dressing, blue cheese	15	0.5	1 tbsp	75
Salad dressing, boiled	16	0.6	1 tbsp, home-made	25
Salad dressing, commercial	15	0.5	1 tbsp, mayonnaise-type	65
Salad dressing, French	16	0.6	1 tbsp	65
Salad dressing, low-calorie	26	0.9	2 tbsp (cottage cheese, nonfat dry milk, no oil)	17
Salad dressing, mayonnaise	14	0.5	1 tbsp	100
Salad dressing, Thousand Island	16	0.6	1 tbsp	80
Salmon, boiled or baked	119	4.2	1 steak, 4 × 3 × ½ in.	200
Salmon, pink, canned	85	3.0	½ cup	120
Salmon loaf	113	4.0	½ cup or 1 slice, 4 × 1¼ × 1¼ in.	235
Sardines, canned oil	57	2.0	5 small fish, 3 × 1 × ¼ in.	120
Sauce, chocolate	40	1.4	2 tbsp	75
Sauce, custard	31	1.1	2 tbsp (low calorie, with nonfat dry milk)	45
Sauce, hard	17	0.6	1 tbsp	90

PROTEIN G	FAT G	CARBOHYDRATE G	CALCIUM MG	IRON MG	VITAMIN-A ACTIVITY IU	ASCORBIC ACID MG	THIAMIN MG	RIBOFLAVIN MG
5	5	20	145	0.1	195	1	0.04	0.20
8	8	52	243	0.8	313	3	0.10	0.35
5	5	12	104	0.4	327	1	0.04	0.19
tr	tr	1	12	0.4	tr	10	0.01	0.01
tr	tr	8	7	0.4	2	tr	0.01	0.01
1	1	9	14	0.6	80	16	0.02	0.06
1	tr	50	106	0.8	110	9	0.03	0.08
3	tr	31	25	1.1	0	0	0.14	0.02
1	tr	13	3	0.3	0	0	0.07	0.01
2	tr	26	9	0.5	0	0	0.10	0.02
6	2	28	9	1.2	30	0	0.14	0.10
3	2	21	30	0.8	tr	tr	0.11	0.07
5	2	31	24	0.4	tr	tr	0.03	0.05
2	2	15	21	0.5	tr	tr	0.08	0.05
4	4	21	37	0.3	30	tr	0.03	0.06
1	tr	6	43	0.3	270	18	0.04	0.06
25	19	1	20	1.7	200	1	0.04	0.15
6	18	1	35	1.3	630	1	0.06	0.16
—	6	21	25	0.6	154	22	0.06	0.05
3	—	16	14	0.2	25	20	0.03	0.02
1	6	5	28	0.7	618	9	0.05	0.10
2	12	17	21	0.8	40	17	0.11	0.05
5	0	7	12	0.5	1441	22	0.07	0.05
21	18	1	14	1.2	98	1	0.04	0.09
1	8	1	12	tr	30	tr	tr	0.02
1	2	2	14	0.1	80	tr	0.01	0.03
tr	6	2	2	tr	30	—	tr	tr
tr	6	3	2	0.1	—	—	—	—
2	0	2	31	0	18	1	0.01	0.06
tr	11	tr	3	0.1	40	—	tr	0.01
tr	8	3	2	0.1	50	tr	tr	tr
34	7	tr	—	1.4	—	—	0.12	0.33
17	5	0	167	0.7	60	—	0.03	0.16
29	10	5	43	1.8	332	2	0.08	0.20
13	6	0	248	1.7	127	—	0.01	0.11
1	4	9	32	0.2	87	—	0.01	0.05
2	1	7	56	0.2	89	—	0.02	0.09
—	6	11	1	0	231	0	0	0

FOOD	WEIGHT G	WEIGHT OZ	APPROXIMATE MEASURE AND DESCRIPTION	KCAL
Sauce, hollandaise (mock)	26	0.9	2 tbsp	75
Sauce, lemon	28	1.0	2 tbsp	40
Sauerkraut, canned	118	4.1	½ cup, solids and liquid	25
Sausage, bologna	57	2.0	2 slices, 4.1 × 0.1 in.	173
Sausage, frankfurters (*see* frankfurters)				
Sausage, liverwurst	57	2.0	3 slices, 2½ in. dia. ¼ in. thick	150
Sausage, pork, cooked	26	0.9	2 small patties or links	125
Sausage, Vienna	16	0.6	1 canned sausage, about 2 in. long	40
Shad, baked	85	3.0	1 piece, 4 × 3 × ½ in.	170
Sherbet, orange	97	3.4	½ cup	130
Shrimp, canned	85	3.0	½ cup, meat only	100
Syrup, table blends	21	0.7	1 tbsp, light and dark	60
Soup, bean with pork, canned	250	8.8	1 cup, ready to serve	170
Soup, beef broth, bouillon, consommé, canned	240	8.4	1 cup, ready to serve	30
Soup, chicken noodle, canned	250	8.8	1 cup, ready to serve	65
Soup, clam chowder, canned	255	8.9	1 cup, ready to serve	85
Soup, cream of vegetable (e.g., tomato, mushroom), canned	240	8.4	1 cup, ready to serve	135
Soup, minestrone, canned	245	8.6	1 cup, ready to serve	105
Soup, tomato, canned	245	8.6	1 cup, ready to serve	90
Soup, vegetable, canned	250	8.8	1 cup, ready to serve	80
Spaghetti, cooked	105	3.7	¾ cup (enriched)	115
Spaghetti, in tomato sauce, with cheese	188	6.5	¾ cup	200
Spaghetti, in tomato sauce, with meat balls	186	6.5	¾ cup	250
Spinach (*see* greens)				
Squash, summer, cooked	105	3.7	½ cup, diced	15
Squash, winter, baked	103	3.6	½ cup, mashed	65
Stew, beef and vegetable	176	6.2	¾ cup	160
Strawberries, raw	75	2.6	½ cup, capped	30
Sugar, brown	14	0.5	1 tbsp firmly packed	50
Sugar, granulated	11	0.4	1 tbsp (beet or cane)	40
Sugar, lump	6	0.2	1 domino, 1⅛ × ¾ × ⅜ in.	25
Sugar, powdered	8	0.3	1 tbsp	30
Sweet potatoes, baked	110	3.9	1 medium potato, about 6 oz raw	155
Sweet potatoes, candied	175	6.1	1 potato, 3½ × 2¼ in.	295
Tangerine	116	4.1	1 medium tangerine, 2⅜ in. dia.	40

PROTEIN G	FAT G	CARBOHYDRATE G	CALCIUM MG	IRON MG	VITAMIN-A ACTIVITY IU	ASCORBIC ACID MG	THIAMIN MG	RIBOFLAVIN MG
2	7	3	36	0.2	353	1	0.02	0.06
0	1	8	—	—	34	2	—	—
1	tr	5	43	0.6	60	17	0.04	0.05
7	16	1	4	1.0	—	—	0.09	0.12
10	12	1	5	3.1	3260	0	0.10	0.63
5	11	tr	2	0.6	0	—	0.21	0.09
2	3	tr	1	0.3	—	—	0.01	0.02
20	10	0	20	0.5	20	—	0.11	0.22
1	1	30	16	tr	60	2	0.01	0.03
21	1	1	98	2.6	50	—	0.01	0.03
0	0	15	9	0.8	0	0	0	0
8	6	22	63	2.3	650	3	0.13	0.08
5	0	3	tr	0.5	tr	—	tr	0.02
4	2	8	10	0.5	50	tr	0.02	0.02
2	3	13	36	1.0	920	—	0.03	0.03
2	10	10	41	0.5	70	tr	0.02	0.12
5	3	14	37	1.0	2350	—	0.07	0.05
2	3	16	15	0.7	1000	12	0.05	0.05
3	2	14	20	0.8	3250	—	0.05	0.02
4	1	24	8	1.0	0	0	0.15	0.08
7	7	28	60	1.7	810	10	0.18	0.14
15	9	30	93	2.8	1193	17	0.20	0.23
1	tr	4	26	0.4	410	11	0.05	0.08
2	1	16	29	0.8	4305	14	0.05	0.14
11	8	11	21	2.1	1733	11	0.10	0.13
1	1	7	16	0.8	45	44	0.02	0.05
0	0	13	12	0.5	0	0	tr	tr
0	0	11	0	tr	0	0	0	0
0	0	6	0	tr	0	0	0	0
0	0	8	0	tr	0	0	0	0
2	1	36	44	1.0	8910	24	0.10	0.07
2	6	60	65	1.6	11,030	17	0.10	0.08
1	tr	10	34	0.3	360	27	0.05	0.02

FOOD	WEIGHT G	WEIGHT OZ	APPROXIMATE MEASURE AND DESCRIPTION	KCAL
Tartar sauce (*see* salad dressing, mayonnaise)				
Toast, melba	6	0.2	1 slice, $3\frac{3}{4} \times 1\frac{3}{4}$ in.	20
Tomato catsup	15	0.5	1 tbsp	15
Tomato juice, canned	122	4.3	½ cup or 1 small glass	23
Tomatoes, canned	121	4.2	½ cup	25
Tomatoes, raw	200	7.0	1 tomato, about 3 in. dia., $2\frac{1}{8}$ in. high	40
Topping, whipped	4	0.1	1 tbsp, pressurized	10
Tortillas	20	0.7	1 tortilla, 5 in. dia.	50
Tuna fish, canned in oil	85	3.0	½ cup, drained solids	170
Tuna salad (*see* salad, tuna fish)				
Turnip greens (*see* greens)				
Turnips, cooked	78	2.7	½ cup, diced	18
Veal cutlet, breaded (wiener schnitzel)	136	4.8	2 slices, $2\frac{1}{2} \times 2\frac{1}{2} \times \frac{3}{4}$ in.	315
Veal cutlet, broiled	85	3.0	1 cutlet, $3\frac{3}{4} \times 3 \times \frac{1}{2}$ in.	185
Veal roast, cooked	85	3.0	2 slices, $3 \times 2\frac{1}{2} \times \frac{1}{4}$ in.	230
Vinegar	15	0.5	1 tbsp	2
Waffles	75	2.6	1 waffle, 7 in. dia. (enriched flour)	210
Watermelon, raw	925	32.4	1 wedge, 4 × 8 in., with rind	115
Welsh rarebit	125	4.4	½ cup	330
Wheat flour, white enriched	115	4.0	1 cup, sifted	420
Wheat flour, white unenriched	110	3.9	1 cup, sifted	400
Wheat flour, whole wheat	120	4.2	1 cup, hard wheat	400
Wheat germ	9	0.3	2 tbsp	30
Wheat flakes	30	1.1	1 cup (nutrients added)	105
Wheat, shredded	25	0.9	1 biscuit, $4 \times 2\frac{1}{4}$ in.	90
White sauce (medium)	65	2.3	¼ cup	110
Yeast, brewers, dry	8	0.3	1 tbsp	25
Yeast, compressed	28	1.0	one 1-oz cake	25
Yeast, dry active	28	1.0	four ¼-oz packages	80
Yogurt, plain	245	8.6	1 cup (made from partially skimmed milk)	125

PROTEIN G	FAT G	CARBOHYDRATE G	CALCIUM MG	IRON MG	VITAMIN-A ACTIVITY IU	ASCORBIC ACID MG	THIAMIN MG	RIBOFLAVIN MG
1	tr	4	5	0.1	0	0	0.01	0.01
tr	tr	4	3	0.1	210	2	0.01	0.01
1	tr	5	9	1.1	970	20	0.06	0.04
1	1	5	7	0.6	1085	21	0.06	0.04
2	tr	9	24	0.9	1640	42	0.11	0.07
tr	1	tr	tr	—	20	—	—	0
1	1	10	22	0.4	40	—	0.04	0.01
24	7	0	7	1.6	70	—	0.04	0.10
1	tr	4	27	0.3	tr	17	0.03	0.04
26	21	5	37	4.2	295	—	0.22	0.41
23	9	—	9	2.7	—	—	0.06	0.21
23	14	0	10	2.9	—	—	0.11	0.26
0	—	1	1	0.1	—	—	—	—
7	7	28	85	1.3	250	tr	0.13	0.19
2	1	27	30	2.1	2510	30	0.13	0.13
19	26	6	534	0.7	1118	—	0.04	0.40
12	1	88	18	3.3	0	0	0.51	0.30
12	1	84	18	0.9	0	0	0.07	0.05
16	2	85	49	4.0	0	0	0.66	0.14
2	1	4	6	0.8	0	0	0.17	0.06
3	tr	24	12	1.3	0	0	0.19	0.04
2	1	20	11	0.9	0	0	0.06	0.03
3	8	6	76	0.1	305	tr	0.03	0.11
3	tr	3	17	1.4	tr	tr	1.25	0.34
3	tr	3	4	1.4	tr	tr	0.20	0.47
12	tr	12	12	4.4	tr	tr	0.69	1.52
8	4	13	294	0.1	170	2	0.10	0.44

Alcoholic Beverages

BEVERAGE		NUMBER OF CALORIES
Beer	8-oz glass	100
Eggnog, holiday variety, made with whiskey and rum	½ cup	225
Whiskey, gin, rum, and vodka		
100 proof	1 jigger (1½ oz)	125
90 proof	1 jigger (1½ oz)	110
86 proof	1 jigger (1½ oz)	105
80 proof	1 jigger (1½ oz)	100
70 proof	1 jigger (1½ oz)	85
Wines		
table wines (such as chablis, claret, Rhine wine, and sauterne)	1 wine glass (about 3 oz)	75
dessert wines (such as muscatel, port, sherry, or Tokay)	1 wine glass (about 3 oz)	125

Specialty and Fast Food Items (Dashes indicate information not provided by sources.)

	WT (G)	KCAL	P G	F G	CAR G	CAL G	IRON G	VITA IU	ASCOR-BIC MG	THIA-MIN MG	RIBO MG
ARBY'S											
Bac'n Cheddar Deluxe	225	561	28	34	78	—	—	—	—	—	—
Baked Potato											
Plain	312	290	8	0.5	0	—	—	—	—	—	—
Beef 'n Cheddar	190	490	24	21	51	—	—	—	—	—	—
Chicken Breast Sandwich	210	592	28	27	57	—	—	—	—	—	—
Chocolate Shake	300	384	9	11	32	—	—	—	—	—	—
French Fries	71	211	2	8	6	—	—	—	—	—	—
Hot Ham 'n Cheese Sandwich	161	353	26	13	50	—	—	—	—	—	—
Jamocha Shake	305	424	8	10	31	—	—	—	—	—	—
Junior Roast Beef	86	218	12	8	22	—	—	—	—	—	—
King Roast Beef	192	467	27	19	49	—	—	—	—	—	—
Potato Cakes	85	201	2	14	13	—	—	—	—	—	—
Regular Roast Beef	147	353	22	15	32	—	—	—	—	—	—
Super Roast Beef	234	501	25	22	40	—	—	—	—	—	—
Superstuffed Potato											
Broccoli and Cheddar	340	541	13	22	24	—	—	—	—	—	—
Superstuffed Potato											
Deluxe	312	648	18	38	72	—	—	—	—	—	—
Superstuffed Potato											
Mushroom and Cheese	300	506	16	22	21	—	—	—	—	—	—
Superstuffed Potato											
Taco	425	619	23	27	145	—	—	—	—	—	—
Turkey Deluxe	197	375	24	17	39	—	—	—	—	—	—
Vanilla Shake	250	295	8	10	30	—	—	—	—	—	—

Source: Arby's Inc. Nutritional information provided by Consumer Affairs, Arby's Inc. Atlanta, GA., 1986.

	WT (G)	KCAL	P G	F G	CAR G	CAL G	IRON G	VITA IU	ASCOR-BIC MG	THIA-MIN MG	RIBO MG
ARTHUR TREACHER'S											
Chicken	136	369	27.1	21.6	16.5	11.2	0.799	102	1.5	0.07	0.148
Chicken Sandwich	156	41.3	16.2	19.2	44.0	58.8	1.70	117	19.2	0.17	0.240
Chips	113	276	4.0	13.2	34.9	12.4	0.473	85	5.9	0.17	0.035
Chowder	170	112	4.6	5.4	11.2	61.4	0.092	340	1.7	0.07	0.14
Cole Slaw	85	123	1.0	8.2	11.1	24.0	0.185	170	59.1	0.026	0.025
Fish	147	355	19.2	19.8	25.4	14.9	0.566	111	1.5	0.1	0.075
Fish Sandwich	156	440	16.4	24.0	39.4	88.9	1.49	117	1.6	0.27	0.215
Krunch Pups	57	203	5.4	14.8	12.0	7.99	0.601	43	3.5	0.05	0.052
Lemon Luvs	85	276	2.6	13.9	35.1	9.87	0.851	64	0.94	0.18	0.0885
Shrimp	115	381	13.1	24.4	27.2	56.7	0.638	86	1.3	0.08	0.051

Source: Arthur Treacher's Inc., Youngstown, OH. All sampling and analysis was conducted by Warf Institute, Inc., Madison, WI. July, 1977.

	WT (G)	KCAL	P G	F G	CAR G	CAL G	IRON G	VITA IU	ASCOR-BIC MG	THIA-MIN MG	RIBO MG
BURGER CHEF											
Big Chef	186	542	23	34	35	189	3.4	282	2	0.34	0.35
Cheeseburger	104	304	14	17	24	156	2.0	266	1	0.22	0.23
Double Cheeseburger	145	434	24	26	24	246	3.1	430	1	0.25	0.34
French Fries	68	187	3	9	25	10	0.9	tr	14	0.09	0.05
Hamburger, Regular	91	258	11	13	24	69	1.9	114	1	0.22	0.18
Mariner Platter	373	680	32	24	85	137	4.7	448	24	0.37	0.40
Rancher Platter	316	640	30	38	44	57	5.1	367	24	0.30	0.37
Shake	305	326	11	11	47	411	0.2	10	2	0.11	0.57
Skipper's Treat	179	604	21	37	47	201	2.5	303	1	0.29	0.30
Super Shef	252	600	29	37	39	240	4.2	763	9	0.37	0.43

Source: Burger King Corporation, Miami, FL.

	WT (G)	KCAL	P G	F G	CAR G	CAL G	IRON G	VITA IU	ASCOR-BIC MG	THIA-MIN MG	RIBO MG
BURGER KING											
Bacon Double Cheeseburger	159	510	31.92	31	27	167.79	3.80	383.68	—	0.31	0.42
Breakfast Croissan'wich Bacon, Egg, Cheese	119	355	14.55	24	20	135.70	2.01	426.11	—	0.32	0.30
Breakfast Croissan'wich Ham, Egg, Cheese	145	386	17.53	20	20	136.46	2.16	426.11	—	0.49	0.32
Breakfast Croissan'wich Sausage, Egg, Cheese	163	538	19.36	41	20	145.22	2.89	426.11	—	0.36	0.32
Cheeseburger	120	317	17.26	15	30	102.17	2.74	341.40	3.09	0.23	0.29
Chicken Sandwich	230	688	26.03	40	56	78.51	3.30	126.13	—	0.45	0.31
Chicken Tenders	95	204	20.24	10	10	18.29	0.67	95.26	—	0.08	0.08
Coffee, Reg.	244	2	0	0	0	—	—	—	—	—	—
Double Beef Whopper	351	—	46.36	—	—	91.31	7.31	617.34	13.88	0.34	0.56
Double Beef Whopper w/Cheese	374	—	50.82	—	—	221.95	7.34	1000.64	13.88	0.35	0.63
French Fries, Reg.	74	227	3	13	24	—	0.52	—	—	0.10	0.30
French Toast Platter w/Bacon	117	469	11.02	30	41	59.09	2.72	—	—	0.24	0.24
French Toast Platter w/Sausage	158	635	16.08	46	41	69.92	3.71	—	—	0.29	0.29
Ham and Cheese	230	471	23.74	23	44	194.90	3.19	725.02	7.37	0.87	0.42

	WT (G)	KCAL	P G	F G	CAR G	CAL G	IRON G	VITA IU	ASCOR-BIC MG	THIA-MIN MG	RIBO MG
BURGER KING *(continued)*											
Hamburger	109	275	15.03	12	29	36.86	2.73	149.76	3.09	0.23	0.25
Hot Chocolate	244	131	1.34	4	22	26.71	0.71	—	—	—	—
Hot Dog	—	291	11	17	23	40	2.0	0	0	0.04	0.02
Milk 2% lowfat	244	121	8.13	5	12	296.70	—	500.20	2.32	0.10	0.40
Milk Whole	244	157	8.00	9	11	290.36	—	336.72	3.59	0.09	0.39
Onion Rings, Reg.	79	274	3.64	16	28	124.01	0.80	—	—	—	—
Orange Juice	183	82	1	0	20	—	—	142.74	71.19	0.14	—
Pies Apple	125	305	3.12	12	44	—	1.18	—	4.99	0.27	0.16
Pies Cherry	128	357	3.57	13	55	—	1.12	370.04	7.66	0.24	0.16
Pies Pecan	113	459	4.99	20	64	23.81	1.13	—	—	0.28	0.18
Salad w/1000 Island	176	145	2.46	12	9	42.38	1.44	1659.13	42.55	0.06	0.13
Salad w/Bleu Cheese	176	184	3.43	16	7	66.19	1.33	1638.16	41.70	0.06	0.15
Salad w/Creamy Italian	176	NA	NA	NA	NA	NA	NA	NA	NA	NA	NA
Salad w/French	176	152	2.29	11	13	40.40	1.35	1688.62	43.26	0.06	0.12
Salad w/Golden Italian	176	162	2.24	14	7	39.83	1.26	1597.90	42.32	0.05	0.12
Salad w/House	176	159	2.92	13	8	44.36	1.31	1604.42	41.84	0.06	0.15
Salad w/Reduced Calorie Italian	176	42	2.21	1	7	40.40	1.35	1591.38	42.04	0.05	0.12
Salad—Plain	148	28	2.16	0	5	36.71	1.24	1582.60	41.67	0.06	0.12
Salad Dressings 1000 Island	—	117	—	12	4	—	—	—	—	—	—
Salad Dressings Bleu Cheese	—	156	—	16	2	—	—	—	—	—	—
Salad Dressings Creamy Italian	—	NA	—	NA	NA	—	—	—	—	—	—
Salad Dressings French	—	123	—	11	8	—	—	—	—	—	—
Salad Dressings Golden Italian	—	134	—	14	2	—	—	—	—	—	—
Salad Dressings House	—	130	—	13	3	—	—	—	—	—	—
Salad Dressings Reduced Calorie Italian	—	14	—	0	2	—	—	—	—	—	—
Scrambled Egg Platter	195	—	14.24	—	—	101.45	2.69	374.90	2.62	0.31	0.35
Scrambled Egg Platter w/Bacon	206	536	18.02	36	33	102.84	2.82	374.90	2.62	0.39	0.38
Scrambled Egg Platter w/Sausage	247	702	21.88	52	33	112.04	3.66	375.01	2.62	0.42	0.40
Shakes, Med. Chocolate	273	320	8.02	12	46	259.88	1.61	—	—	0.13	0.55
Shakes, Med. Chocolate (added syrup)	284	374	8.33	11	60—	247.58	1.55	—	—	0.12	0.51
Shakes, Med. Vanilla	273	321	8.73	10	49	294.52	—	—	—	0.11	0.57
Shakes, Med. Vanilla (added syrup)	284	334	9	10	51	NA	NA	NA	NA	NA	NA
Soft Drinks, Med. 7-Up	366	144	0	0	38	—	—	—	—	—	—
Soft Drinks, Med. Diet Pepsi	366	1	0	0	0	—	—	—	—	—	—
Soft Drinks, Med. Dr. Pepper	366	155	0	0	40	—	—	—	—	—	—
Soft Drinks, Med. Mountain Dew	366	158	0	0	42	—	—	—	—	—	—
Soft Drinks, Med. Pepsi Cola	366	159	0	0	40	—	—	—	—	—	—
Whaler Sandwich	189	488	18.64	27	45	46.46	2.22	35.54	—	0.28	0.21
Whaler w/Cheese	201	530	20.86	30	46	111.78	2.24	227.19	—	0.27	0.24
Whopper Jr. Sandwich	136	322	15.19	17	30	39.97	2.81	296.38	6.24	0.23	0.25
Whopper Jr. w/Cheese	147	364	17.42	20	31	105.29	2.82	488.02	6.24	0.23	0.29
Whopper Sandwich	265	640	26.94	41	42	79.79	4.88	617.57	13.88	0.33	0.41
Whopper w/Cheese	289	723	31.39	48	43	210.40	4.91	1000.64	13.88	0.34	0.48

Source: Burger Chef Systems, Inc., Indianapolis, Ind., 1978 (Analyses obtained from USDA Handbook No. 8).

	WT (G)	DESCRIPTION	KCAL	P G	F G	CAR G	CAL G	IRON G	VITA IU	ASCORBIC MG	THIAMIN MG	RIBO MG
CHURCH'S FRIED CHICKEN												
Catfish	21		66.7	3.9	4.0	3.8	—	—	—	—	—	
Corn	168	1 ear with Butter Oil	236.5	4.2	9.3	32.9	—	—	—	—	—	
French Fries	85	1 reg. w/100 mg. salt added	138	2.1	5.5	20.1	—	—	—	—	—	—
Fried Chicken	—		—	—	—	—	—	—	—	—	—	—
Fried Chicken Breast	93		278	21.3	17.3	9.4	—	—	—	—	—	—
Fried Chicken Leg	56		147.1	12.9	8.6	4.5	—	—	—	—	—	—
Fried Chicken Thigh	93		305.8	18.5	21.6	9.2	—	—	—	—	—	—
Fried Chicken Wing-Breast	97		—	—	—	—	—	—	—	—	—	—
Hushpuppy	23	1	78.0	1.3	2.9	11.6	—	—	—	—	—	—
Nuggets Regular	18		55.1	3.0	3.1	3.7	—	—	—	—	—	—
Nuggets Spicy	18		51.8	3.1	2.9	3.4	—	—	—	—	—	—

Source: Church's Fried Chicken, Inc., San Antonio, TX. Nutritional information based on Texas Testing Laboratories, Inc., May, 1985., Pioneer Flour Mills, Inc., August, 1985, and Bowes & Church's Food Values of Portions Commonly Used—Pennington & Church, 14th Edition, 1985.

	WT (G)	DESCRIPTION	KCAL	P G	F G	CAR G	CAL G	IRON G	VITA IU	ASCORBIC MG	THIAMIN MG	RIBO MG
DAIRY QUEEN												
Banana Split	383		540	9	11	103	—	—	—	—	—	—
Big Brazier Deluxe	213		470	28	24	36	111	5.2	—	<2.5	0.34	0.37
Big Brazier Regular	184		184	27	23	37	113	5.2	—	<2.0	0.37	0.39
Big Brazier w/Cheese	213		553	32	30	38	268	5.2	495	<2.3	0.34	0.53
Blizzard Banana Split	—	regular	763	—	—	—	—	—	—	—	—	—
Blizzard Banana Split	—	large	1333	—	—	—	—	—	—	—	—	—
Blizzard Chocolate Sandwich Cookies	—	regular	600	—	—	—	—	—	—	—	—	—
Blizzard Chocolate Sandwich Cookies	—	large	1050	—	—	—	—	—	—	—	—	—
Blizzard German Chocolate	—	regular	794	—	—	—	—	—	—	—	—	—
Blizzard German Chocolate	—	large	1460	—	—	—	—	—	—	—	—	—
Blizzard Heath	—	regular	824	—	—	—	—	—	—	—	—	—
Blizzard Heath	—	large	1212	—	—	—	—	—	—	—	—	—
Blizzard M&M	—	regular	766	—	—	—	—	—	—	—	—	—
Blizzard M&M	—	large	1154	—	—	—	—	—	—	—	—	—
Brazier Cheese Dog	113		330	15	19	24	168	1.6	—	—	—	0.18
Brazier Chili Dog	128		330	13	20	25	86	2.0	—	11.0	0.15	0.23
Brazier Dog	99		273	11	15	23	75	1.5	—	11.0	0.12	0.15
Brazier French Fries	71		200	2	10	25	tr	0.4	tr	3.6	0.06	tr
Brazier French Fries	113		320	3	16	40	tr	0.4	tr	4.8	0.09	0.03
Brazier Onion Rings	85		300	6	17	33	20	0.4	tr	2.4	0.09	tr
Brazier Regular	106		260	13	9	28	70	3.5	—	<1.0	0.28	0.26
Brazier w/Cheese	121		318	18	14	30	163	3.5	—	<1.2	0.29	0.29
Buster Bar	149		460	10	29	41	—	—	—	—	—	—
Chicken Sandwich	220		670	29	41	46	—	—	—	—	—	—
Cone large	213		340	9	10	57	—	—	—	—	—	—
Cone regular	142		240	6	7	38	—	—	—	—	—	—
Cone small	85		140	3	4	22	—	—	—	—	—	—
Dairy Queen Parfait	284		460	10	11	81	300	1.8	400	tr	0.12	0.43
Dilly Bar	85		240	4	15	22	100	0.4	100	tr	0.06	0.17

	WT (G)	DESCRIPTION	KCAL	P G	F G	CAR G	CAL G	IRON G	VITA IU	ASCORBIC MG	THIAMIN MG	RIBO MG
DAIRY QUEEN *(continued)*												
Dilly Bar	85		210	3	13	21	—	—	—	—	—	—
Dipped Cone large	234		510	9	24	64	—	—	—	—	—	—
Dipped Cone regular	156		340	6	16	42	—	—	—	—	—	—
Dipped Cone small	92		190	3	9	25	—	—	—	—	—	—
Double Delight	255		490	9	20	69	—	—	—	—	—	—
Double Hamburger	210		530	36	28	33	—	—	—	—	—	—
Double w/Cheese	239		650	43	37	34	—	—	—	—	—	—
Chocolate Dipped Cone	234	large	450	10	20	58	300	0.4	400	tr	0.12	0.51
Chocolate Dipped Cone	156	medium	300	7	13	40	200	0.4	300	tr	0.09	0.34
Chocolate Dipped Cone	78	small	150	3	7	20	100	tr	100	tr	0.03	0.17
Chocolate Malt	588	large	840	22	28	125	600	5.4	750	6.0	0.15	0.85
Chocolate Malt	418	medium	600	15	20	89	500	3.6	750	3.6	0.12	0.60
Chocolate Malt	241	small	340	10	11	51	300	1.8	400	2.4	0.06	0.34
Chocolate Sundae	248	large	400	9	9	71	300	1.8	400	tr	0.09	0.43
Chocolate Sundae	184	medium	300	6	7	53	200	1.1	300	tr	0.06	0.26
Chocolate Sundae	106	small	170	4	4	30	100	0.7	100	tr	0.03	0.17
Cone	213	large	340	10	10	52	300	tr	400	tr	0.15	0.43
Cone	142	medium	230	6	7	35	200	tr	300	tr	0.09	0.26
Cone	71	small	110	3	3	18	100	tr	100	tr	0.03	0.14
Float	397		330	6	8	59	200	tr	100	tr	0.12	0.17
Freeze	397		520	11	13	89	300	tr	200	tr	0.15	0.34
Sandwich	60		140	3	4	24	60	0.4	100	tr	0.03	0.14
Fiesta Sundae	269		570	9	22	84	200	tr	200	tr	0.23	0.26
Fish Sandwich	170		400	20	17	41	60	1.1	tr	tr	0.15	0.26
Fish Sandwich w/cheese	177		440	24	21	39	150	0.4	100	tr	0.15	0.26
Float	397		410	5	7	82	—	—	—	—	—	—
Freeze	397		500	9	12	89	—	—	—	—	—	—
French Fries	71		200	2	10	25	—	—	—	—	—	—
French Fries	113	large	320	3	16	40	—	—	—	—	—	—
Frozen Dessert	113		180	4	6	27	—	—	—	—	—	—
Hot Dog	100		280	11	16	21	—	—	—	—	—	—
Hot Dog w/Cheese	114		330	15	21	21	—	—	—	—	—	—
Hot Dog w/Chili	128		320	13	20	23	—	—	—	—	—	—
Hot Fudge Brownie Delight	266		600	9	25	85	—	—	—	—	—	—
Malt large	588		1060	20	25	187	—	—	—	—	—	—
Malt regular	418		760	14	18	134	—	—	—	—	—	—
Malt small	291		520	10	13	91	—	—	—	—	—	—
Mr. Misty	439	large	340	0	0	84	—	—	—	—	—	—
Mr. Misty	330	regular	250	0	0	63	—	—	—	—	—	—
Mr. Misty	248	small	190	0	0	48	—	—	—	—	—	—
Mr. Misty Float	404		440	6	8	85	200	tr	120	tr	0.12	0.17
Mr. Misty Float	411		390	5	7	74	—	—	—	—	—	—
Mr. Misty Freeze	411		500	9	12	91	—	—	—	—	—	—
Mr. Misty Kiss	89		70	0	0	17	—	—	—	—	—	—
Onion Rings	85		280	4	16	31	—	—	—	—	—	—
Parfait	283		430	8	8	76	—	—	—	—	—	—
Peanut Buster Parfait	305		740	16	34	94	—	—	—	—	—	—
Shake large	588		990	19	26	168	—	—	—	—	—	—
Shake regular	418		710	14	19	120	—	—	—	—	—	—
Shake small	291		490	10	13	82	—	—	—	—	—	—
Single Hamburger	148		360	21	16	33	—	—	—	—	—	—
Single w/Cheese	162		410	24	20	33	—	—	—	—	—	—
Strawberry Shortcake	312		540	10	11	100	—	—	—	—	—	—
Sundae large	248		440	8	10	78	—	—	—	—	—	—
Sundae regular	177		310	5	8	56	—	—	—	—	—	—
Sundae small	106		190	3	4	33	—	—	—	—	—	—
Super Brazier	298		783	53	48	35	282	7.3	—	<3.2	0.39	0.69
Super Brazier Chili Dog	210		555	23	33	42	158	4.0	—	18.0	0.42	0.48

	WT (G)	DESCRIPTION	KCAL	P G	F G	CAR G	CAL G	IRON G	VITA IU	ASCOR-BIC MG	THIA-MIN MG	RIBO MG
DAIRY QUEEN *(continued)*												
Super Brazier Dog	182		518	20	30	41	158	4.3	tr	14.0	0.42	0.44
Super Brazier Dog w/Cheese	203		593	26	36	43	297	4.4	—	14.0	0.43	0.48
Super Hot Dog	175		520	17	27	44	—	—	—	—	—	—
Super Hot Dog w/Cheese	196		580	22	34	45	—	—	—	—	—	—
Super Hot Dog w/Chili	218		570	21	32	47	—	—	—	—	—	—
Triple Hamburger	272		710	51	45	33	—	—	—	—	—	—
Triple w/Cheese	301		820	58	50	34	—	—	—	—	—	—

Source: International Dairy Queen, Inc., Minneapolis, MN, 1982. Nutritional information reviewed and edited by Dr. David J. Aulik in cooperation with Raltech Scientific Services.

	WT (G)	DESCRIPTION	KCAL	P G	F G	CAR G	CAL G	IRON G	VITA IU	ASCOR-BIC MG	THIA-MIN MG	RIBO MG
JACK IN THE BOX												
1000 Island Dressing	—		250	0	24	9	—	—	—	—	—	—
Apple Turnover	—		410	4	24	45	—	—	—	—	—	—
Bacon	—	2 slices	70	3	6	0	—	—	—	—	—	—
Bacon Cheeseburger Supreme	—		724	34	46	44	—	—	—	—	—	—
Bleu Cheese Dressing	—		210	0	18	11	—	—	—	—	—	—
Breakfast Jack	—		307	18	13	30	—	—	—	—	—	—
Buttermilk House Dressing	—		290	0	29	6	—	—	—	—	—	—
Canadian Crescent	—		451.7	18.6	31.0	24.6	—	—	—	—	—	—
Cheese Nachos	—		571	15	35	49	—	—	—	—	—	—
Cheeseburger	—		323	16	15	32	—	—	—	—	—	—
Chicken Strips Dinner	—		689	40	30	65	—	—	—	—	—	—
Chicken Supreme	—		601	31	36	39	—	—	—	—	—	—
Chocolate Shake	—		330	11	7	55	—	—	—	—	—	—
Club Pita	—		284	22	8	30	—	—	—	—	—	—
Grape Jelly	—		38	0	0	9	—	—	—	—	—	—
Ham & Swiss Burger	—		638	35.6	38.5	37.3	—	—	—	—	—	—
Hamburger	—		276	13	12	30	—	—	—	—	—	—
Jumbo Jack	—		485	26	26	38	—	—	—	—	—	—
Jumbo Jack w/Cheese	—		630	32	35	45	—	—	—	—	—	—
Ketchup	—		10	0	2	0	—	—	—	—	—	—
Milk	—		137	10	5	14	—	—	—	—	—	—
Moby Jack	—		444	16	25	39	—	—	—	—	—	—
Mushroom Burger	—		477	27.7	27.2	30.4	—	—	—	—	—	—
Onion Rings	—		382	5	23	39	—	—	—	—	—	—
Orange Juice	—		80	1	0	20	—	—	—	—	—	—
Pancake Breakfast	—		630	16	27	79	—	—	—	—	—	—
Pasta Seafood Salad	—		394	15.0	22.0	32.0	—	—	—	—	—	—
Regular French Fries	—		221	2	12	27	—	—	—	—	—	—
Regular Taco	—		191	8	11	16	—	—	—	—	—	—
Sausage Crescent	—		584	22	43	28	—	—	—	—	—	—
Scrambled Eggs Breakfast	—		720	26	44	55	—	—	—	—	—	—
Shrimp Dinner	—		731	22	37	77	—	—	—	—	—	—
Sirloin Steak Dinner	—		699	38	27	75	—	—	—	—	—	—
Strawberry Shake	—		320	10	7	55	—	—	—	—	—	—
Super Taco	—		288	12	17	21	—	—	—	—	—	—
Supreme Crescent	—		547	20	40	27	—	—	—	—	—	—
Supreme Nachos	—		718	23	40	66	—	—	—	—	—	—
Swiss & Bacon Burger	—		643	33	43	31	—	—	—	—	—	—
Taco Salad	—		377	31	24	10	—	—	—	—	—	—
Vanilla Shake	—		320	10	6	57	—	—	—	—	—	—

Source: Jack In The Box; nutritional information provided by Foodmaker, Inc., San Diego, CA.

	WT (G)	KCAL	P G	F G	CAR G	CAL G	IRON G	VITA IU	ASCOR-BIC MG	THIA-MIN MG	RIBO MG
KENTUCKY FRIED CHICKEN											
9 Pieces	652	1892	152	116	59	—	8.8	—	—	0.49	1.27
Drumstick	54	136	14	8	2	20	0.9	30	0.6	0.04	0.12
Extra Crispy Dinner	437	950	52	54	63	150	3.6	750	27.0	0.38	0.56
Keel	96	283	25	13	6	—	0.9	50	1.2	0.07	0.13
Original Recipe Dinner	425	830	52	46	56	150	4.5	750	27.0	0.38	0.56
Rib	82	241	19	15	8	55	1.0	58	<1.0	0.06	0.14
Thigh	97	276	20	19	12	39	1.4	74	<1.0	0.08	0.24
Wing	45	151	11	10	4	—	0.6	—	<1.0	0.03	0.07

Source: Nutritional Content of Average Serving, Heublein Food Service and Franchising Group, June 1976.

	WT G	DESCRIPTION	KCAL	P G	F G	CAR G	CAL G	IRON G	VITA IU	ASCOR-BIC MG	THIA-MIN MG	RIBO MG
LONG JOHN SILVER'S												
3 Pc. Nugget Dinner	—	6 chicken nuggets, Fryes, slaw	699	23	45	54	—	—	—	—	—	—
Apple Pie	113		280	2	11	43	—	—	—	—	—	—
Barbecue Sauce	34		45	0	0	11	—	—	—	—	—	—
Battered Shrimp Dinner	—	6 battered shrimp, Fryes, slaw	711	17	45	60	—	—	—	—	—	—
Bleu Cheese Dressing	45		225	4	23	3	—	—	—	—	—	—
Breaded Clams	—		465	13	25	46	—	—	—	—	—	—
Breaded Fish Sandwich Platter	—	Fish sandwich, Fryes, slaw	835	30	42	84	—	—	—	—	—	—
Breaded Oysters	—	6 pc.	460	14	19	58	—	—	—	—	—	—
Breaded Shrimp Platter	—	Breaded shrimp, Fryes, slaw, 2 hush puppies	962	20	57	93	—	—	—	—	—	—
Cherry Pie	113		294	3	11	46	—	—	—	—	—	—
Chicken Planks	—	4 pc.	458	27	23	35	—	—	—	—	—	—
Clam Chowder	187		128	7	5	15	—	—	—	—	—	—
Clam Dinner	—	Clams, Fryes, slaw	955	22	58	100	—	—	—	—	—	—
Cole Slaw	—		138	1	8	16	—	—	—	—	—	—
Cole Slaw, drained on fork	98		182	1	15	11	—	—	—	—	—	—
Combo Salad	—	4.25 oz, seafood salad, 2 oz. salad shrimp, 6 oz. lettuce 2.4 oz. tomato, 1 pkg. crackers	397	27	29	21	—	—	—	—	—	—
Corn on Cob	—	1 pc.	174	5	4	29	—	—	—	—	—	—
Corn on the Cob	150	1 ear	176	5	4	29	—	—	—	—	—	—
Fish & Chicken	—	1 fish, 2 Tender Chicken Planks, Fryes, slaw	935	36	55	73	—	—	—	—	—	—
Fish & Fryes	—	3 fish, fryes	853	43	48	64	—	—	—	—	—	—
Fish & Fryes	—	2 pc. fish, fryes	651	30	36	53	—	—	—	—	—	—
Fish & More	—	2 fish, Fryes, slaw, 2 hush puppies	978	34	58	92	—	—	—	—	—	—
Fish w/Batter	—	2 pc.	319	19	19	19	—	—	—	—	—	—
Fish w/Batter	—	3 pc.	477	28	28	28	—	—	—	—	—	—
Four Nuggets and Fryes	—		427	16	24	39	—	—	—	—	—	—
Fryes	85		247	4	12	31	—	—	—	—	—	—
Fryes	—		275	4	15	32	—	—	—	—	—	—
Honey-Mustard Sauce	35		56	—	—	14	—	—	—	—	—	—
Hush Puppies	47	2 pieces	145	3	7	18	—	—	—	—	—	—

	WT G	DESCRIPTION	KCAL	P G	F G	CAR G	CAL G	IRON G	VITA IU	ASCOR-BIC MG	THIA-MIN MG	RIBO MG
LONG JOHN SILVER'S *(continued)*												
Hush Puppies	—	3 pc.	158	1	7	20	—	—	—	—	—	—
Kitchen-Breaded Fish (Three Piece Dinner)	—	3 kitchen breaded fish, Fryes, slaw, 2 hush puppies	940	35	52	84	—	—	—	—	—	—
Kitchen-Breaded Fish (Two Piece Dinner)	—	2 kitchen-breaded fish, Fryes, slaw, 2 hush puppies	818	26	46	76	—	—	—	—	—	—
Lemon Meringue Pie	99		200	2	6	37	—	—	—	—	—	—
Ocean Chef Salad	—	6 oz. lettuce, 1.25 oz. shrimp, 2 oz. seafood blend, 2 tomato wedges, ¾ oz. cheese	229	27	8	13	—	—	—	—	—	—
Ocean Scallops	—	6 pc.	257	10	12	27	—	—	—	—	—	—
One Fish and Fryes	—		449	16	24	42	—	—	—	—	—	—
One Fish, Two Nuggets, and Fryes	—		539	23	30	46	—	—	—	—	—	—
Oyster Dinner	—	6 oysters, Fryes, slaw	789	17	45	78	—	—	—	—	—	—
Pecan Pie	113		446	5	22	59	—	—	—	—	—	—
Peg Leg w/Batter	—	5 pc.	514	25	33	30	—	—	—	—	—	—
Pumpkin Pie	113		251	4	11	34	—	—	—	—	—	—
Reduced Calorie Italian Dressing	49		20	0	1	3	—	—	—	—	—	—
Scallop Dinner	—	6 scallops, Fryes, slaw	747	17	45	66	—	—	—	—	—	—
Sea Salad Dressing	45		220	4	21	5	—	—	—	—	—	—
Seafood Platter	—	1 fish, 2 battered shrimp, 2 scallops, Fryes, slaw	976	29	58	85	—	—	—	—	—	—
Seafood Salad	—	5.6 oz. seafood salad, 6 oz. lettuce, 2.4 oz. tomato	426	19	30	22	—	—	—	—	—	—
Shrimp & Fish Dinner	—	1 fish, 3 battered shrimp, Fryes, slaw, 2 hush puppies	917	27	55	80	—	—	—	—	—	—
Shrimp Salad	—	4.5 oz. salad shrimp, 6 oz. lettuce, 2.4 oz. tomato	203	28	3	16	—	—	—	—	—	—
Shrimp w/Batter	—	5 pc.	269	9	13	31	—	—	—	—	—	—
Sweet-n-Sour Sauce	30		—	—	—	—	—	—	—	—	—	—
Tartar Sauce	30		117	—	11	5	—	—	—	—	—	—
Tender Chicken Plank Dinner	—	3 Chicken Planks, Fryes, slaw	885	32	51	72	—	—	—	—	—	—
Tender Chicken Plank Dinner	—	4 Chicken Planks, Fryes, slaw	1037	41	59	82	—	—	—	—	—	—
Thousand Island Dressing	48		223	—	22	8	—	—	—	—	—	—
Three Piece Fish Dinner	—	3 fish, Fryes, slaw, 2 hush puppies	1180	47	70	93	—	—	—	—	—	—
Treasure Chest	—	2 pc. Fish, 2 Peg Legs	467	25	29	27	—	—	—	—	—	—
Two Planks and Fryes	—		551	22	28	51	—	—	—	—	—	—

Source: Long John Silver's Seafood Shoppes, sampling and nutrient analysis conducted independently by the Department of Nutrition and Food Science, University of Kentucky, April 10, 1986.

	WT G	DESCRIP-TION	KCAL	P G	F G	CAR G	CAL G	IRON G	VITA IU	ASCOR-BIC MG	THIA-MIN MG	RIBO MG
MCDONALD'S												
Apple Pie	85		253	1.87	14.3	29.3	14	0.62	<34	<0.85	0.02	0.02
Barbeque Sauce	32		60	0.4	0.4	13.7	4	0.12	45	<0.64	0.01	0.01
Big Mac	200		570	24.6	35	39.2	203	4.90	380	3	0.48	0.38
Biscuit with Bacon, Egg and Cheese	145		483	16.5	31.6	33.2	2	2.57	653	1.60	0.30	0.43
Biscuit with Sausage	121		467	12.1	30.9	35.3	82	2.05	61	<1.2	0.56	0.22
Biscuit with Sausage and Egg	175		585	19.8	39.9	36.4	119	3.43	420	<1.75	0.53	0.49
Biscuit, plain	85		330	4.9	18.2	36.6	74	1.30	179	<0.85	0.21	0.15
Cake Cones	115		185	4.3	5.2	30.2	20	<2	4	—	4	20
Carmel Sundae	165		361	7.2	10	608	200	0.23	279	3.61	0.07	0.31
Cheeseburger	114		318	15	16	28.5	169	2.84	353	2.05	0.30	0.24
Cherry Pie	88		260	2	13.6	32.1	12	0.59	114	<0.88	0.03	0.02
Chocolate Milk Shake	291		383	9.9	9	65.5	320	0.84	349	<2.91	0.12	0.44
Chocolaty Chip Cookies	69		342	4.2	16.3	44.8	29	1.56	75.9	1.04	0.12	0.21
Cones	115		185	4.3	5.2	30.2	183	0.12	218	<1.15	0.06	0.36
Egg McMuffin	138		340	18.5	15.8	31	226	2.93	591	<1.38	0.47	0.44
English Muffin w/Butter	63		186	5	5.3	29.5	117	1.51	164	0.82	0.28	0.49
Filet-O-Fish	143		435	14.7	25.7	35.9	133	2.47	186	<2.15	0.36	0.23
French Fries	68		220	3	11.5	26.1	9	0.61	<17	12.53	0.12	0.02
Hamburger	100		263	12.4	11.3	28.3	84	2.85	100	1.79	0.31	0.22
Hash Brown Potatoes	55		125	1.5	7	14	5.33	0.40	<13.75	4.14	0.06	<0.01
Honey	14		50	0.04	0.04	12.4	1	0.02	<14.2	<0.15	0.002	0.003
Hot Fudge Sundae	164		357	7	10.8	58	215	0.61	230	2.46	0.07	0.31
Hot Mustard Sauce	30		63	0.6	2.1	10.5	8	0.17	9	<0.3	0.01	0.003
Hotcakes w/Butter & Syrup	214		500	7.9	10.3	93.9	103	2.23	257	4.71	0.26	0.36
McD.L.T.	254		680	30	44	40	230	6.6	508	8	0.56	0.46
McDonaldLand Cookies	67		308	4.2	10.8	48.7	12	1.47	<26.8	<0.94	0.23	0.23
McNuggets	109	6 pc.	323	19.1	21.3	13.7	11	1.25	<109	2.07	0.16	0.14
Quarter Pounder	160		427	24.6	23.5	29.3	98	4.3	128	2.56	0.35	0.32
Quarter Pounder w/Cheese	186		525	29.6	31.6	30.5	255	4.84	614	2.79	0.37	0.41
Sausage	53		210	9.8	18.6	.6	16	0.82	<31.8	<0.53	0.27	0.11
Sausage McMuffin with Egg	165		517	22.9	32.9	32.2	196	3.47	660	1.65	0.84	0.50
Scrambled Eggs	98		180	13.2	13	2.5	61	2.53	652	1.18	0.08	0.47
Strawberry Milk Shake	290		362	9	8.7	62.1	30	<2	377	4.06	0.12	0.44
Strawberry Sundae	164		320	6	8.7	54	174	0.38	230	2.79	0.07	0.30
Sweet & Sour Sauce	32		64	0.2	0.3	15	2	0.08	200	<0.3	0.01	<0.01
Vanilla Milk Shake	291		352	9.3	8.4	59.6	329	0.18	349	3.2	0.12	0.70

Source: McDonald's Corporation. Nutritional analysis reported by Hazleton Laboratories, Inc., 1986.

	WT G	KCAL	P G	F G	CAR G	CAL G	IRON G	VITA IU	ASCOR-BIC MG	THIA-MIN MG	RIBO MG
PIZZA HUT											
Thick 'N' Chewy, Beef	—	620	38	20	73	400	7.2	750	<1.2	0.68	0.60
Thick 'N' Chewy, Cheese	—	560	34	14	71	500	5.4	1000	<1.2	0.68	0.68
Thick 'N' Chewy, Pepperoni	—	560	31	18	68	400	5.4	1250	3.6	0.68	0.68
Thick 'N' Chewy, Pork	—	640	36	23	71	400	7.2	750	1.2	0.90	0.77
Thick 'N' Chewy, Supreme	—	640	36	22	74	400	7.2	1000	9.0	0.75	0.85
Thin 'N' Crispy, Beef	—	490	29	19	51	350	6.3	750	<1.2	0.30	0.60
Thin 'N' Crispy, Cheese	—	450	25	15	54	450	4.5	750	<1.2	0.30	0.51
Thin 'N' Crispy, Pepperoni	—	430	23	17	45	300	4.5	1000	<1.2	0.30	0.51
Thin 'N' Crispy, Pork	—	520	27	23	51	350	6.3	1000	<1.2	0.38	0.68
Thin 'N' Crispy, Supreme	—	510	27	21	51	350	7.2	1250	2.4	0.38	0.68

Source: Research 900 and Pizza Hut, Inc., Wichita, Kan.

	WT G	DESCRIPTION	KCAL	P G	F G	CAR G	CAL G	IRON G	VITA IU	ASCOR-BIC MG	THIA-MIN MG	RIBO MG
ROY ROGERS												
Apple Danish	71		249	4.5	11.6	31.6	—	—	—	—	—	—
Bacon Cheeseburger	180		581	32.3	39.2	25.0	—	—	—	—	—	—
Biscuit	63		231	4.4	12.1	26.2	—	—	—	—	—	—
Breakfast Crescent Sandwich	127		401	13.3	27.3	25.3	—	—	—	—	—	—
Breakfast Crescent Sandwich w/bacon	133		431	15.4	29.7	25.5	—	—	—	—	—	—
Breakfast Crescent Sandwich w/ham	165		557	19.8	41.7	25.3	—	—	—	—	—	—
Breakfast Crescent Sandwich w/sausage	162		449	19.9	29.4	25.9	—	—	—	—	—	—
Breast & Wing	196		604	43.5	36.5	25.4	—	—	—	—	—	—
Brownie	64		264	3.3	11.4	37.3	—	—	—	—	—	—
Caramel Sundae	145		293	7.0	8.5	51.5	—	—	—	—	—	—
Cheese Danish	71		254	4.9	12.2	31.4	—	—	—	—	—	—
Cheeseburger	173		563	29.5	37.3	27.4	—	—	—	—	—	—
Cherry Danish	71		271	4.4	14.4	31.7	—	—	—	—	—	—
Chicken Breast	144		412	33.0	23.7	16.9	—	—	—	—	—	—
Chocolate Shake	319		358	7.9	10.2	61.3	—	—	—	—	—	—
Cole Slaw	99		110	1.0	6.9	11.0	—	—	—	—	—	—
Crescent Roll	70		287	4.7	17.7	27.2	—	—	—	—	—	—
Egg and Biscuit Platter	165		394	16.9	26.5	21.9	—	—	—	—	—	—
Egg and Biscuit Platter w/bacon	173		435	19.7	29.6	22.1	—	—	—	—	—	—
Egg and Biscuit Platter w/ham	200		442	23.5	28.6	22.5	—	—	—	—	—	—
Egg and Biscuit Platter w/sausage	203		550	23.4	40.9	21.9	—	—	—	—	—	—
French Fries	85		268	3.9	13.5	32.0	—	—	—	—	—	—
Hamburger	143		456	23.8	28.3	65.6	—	—	—	—	—	—
Hot Chocolate	—		123	3.0	2.0	22.0	—	—	—	—	—	—
Hot Fudge Sundae	151		337	6.5	12.5	53.3	—	—	—	—	—	—
Hot Topped Potato plain	227		211	5.9	.2	47.9	—	—	—	—	—	—
Hot Topped Potato w/bacon 'n cheese	248		397	17.1	21.7	33.3	—	—	—	—	—	—
Hot Topped Potato w/broccoli 'n cheese	312		376	13.7	18.1	39.6	—	—	—	—	—	—
Hot Topped Potato w/oleo	236		274	5.9	7.3	47.9	—	—	—	—	—	—
Hot Topped Potato w/sour cream 'n chives	297		408	7.3	20.9	47.6	—	—	—	—	—	—
Hot Topped Potato w/taco beef 'n cheese	359		463	21.8	21.8	45.0	—	—	—	—	—	—
Large Fries	113		357	5.3	18.4	42.7	—	—	—	—	—	—
Large Roast Beef	182		360	33.9	11.9	29.6	—	—	—	—	—	—
Large Roast Beef w/Cheese	211		467	39.6	20.9	30.3	—	—	—	—	—	—
Leg	53		140	11.5	8.0	5.5	—	—	—	—	—	—
Macaroni	100		186	3.1	10.7	19.4	—	—	—	—	—	—
Milk	—		150	8.0	8.2	11.4	—	—	—	—	—	—
Orange Juice	—		99	1.5	.2	22.8	—	—	—	—	—	—
Orange Juice	—		136	2.0	.3	31.3	—	—	—	—	—	—
Pancake Platter (w.syrup, butter)	165		452	7.7	15.2	71.8	—	—	—	—	—	—
Pancake Platter (w.syrup, butter) w/bacon	173		493	10.4	18.3	72.0	—	—	—	—	—	—
Pancake Platter (w.syrup, butter) w/ham	200		506	14.3	17.3	72.4	—	—	—	—	—	—
Pancake Platter (w.syrup, butter) w/sausage	203		608	14.2	29.6	71.8	—	—	—	—	—	—
Potato Salad	100		107	2.0	6.1	10.9	—	—	—	—	—	—
Roast Beef Sandwich	154		317	27.2	10.2	29.1	—	—	—	—	—	—
Roast Beef Sandwich w/Cheese	182		424	32.9	19.2	29.9	—	—	—	—	—	—
RR Bar Burger	208		611	36.1	39.4	28.0	—	—	—	—	—	—

	WT G	DESCRIPTION	KCAL	P G	F G	CAR G	CAL G	IRON G	VITA IU	ASCORBIC MG	THIAMIN MG	RIBO MG
ROY ROGERS *(continued)*												
Salad Bar 1,000 Island	—	2 T	160	—	16.0	4.0	—	—	—	—	—	—
Salad Bar Bacon 'n Tomato	—	2 T	136	—	12.0	6.0	—	—	—	—	—	—
Salad Bar Bacon Bits	—	1 T	24	4.0	1.0	38.0	—	—	—	—	—	—
Salad Bar Blue Cheese Dressing	—	2 T	150	2.0	16.0	2.0	—	—	—	—	—	—
Salad Bar Cheddar Cheese	—	¼ cup	112	5.8	9.0	.8	—	—	—	—	—	—
Salad Bar Chinese Noodles	—	¼ cup	55	1.5	2.8	6.5	—	—	—	—	—	—
Salad Bar Chopped Eggs	—	2 T	55	4.0	4.0	.7	—	—	—	—	—	—
Salad Bar Croutons	—	2 T	132	5.5	0	31.0	—	—	—	—	—	—
Salad Bar Cucumbers	—	5-6 slices	4	—	0	1.0	—	—	—	—	—	—
Salad Bar Green Peas	—	¼ cup	7	.5	0	1.2	—	—	—	—	—	—
Salad Bar Green Peppers	—	2 T	4	.3	0	1.0	—	—	—	—	—	—
Salad Bar Lettuce	—	1 cup	10	—	0	4.0	—	—	—	—	—	—
Salad Bar Lo-cal Italian	—	2 T	70	—	6.0	2.0	—	—	—	—	—	—
Salad Bar Macaroni Salad	—	2 T	60	1.0	3.6	6.2	—	—	—	—	—	—
Salad Bar Mushrooms	—	¼ cup	5	.5	0	.7	—	—	—	—	—	—
Salad Bar Potato Salad	—	2 T	50	1.0	3.0	5.5	—	—	—	—	—	—
Salad Bar Ranch	—	2 T	155	—	14.0	4.0	—	—	—	—	—	—
Salad Bar Shredded Carrots	—	¼ cup	12	.6	0	24.0	—	—	—	—	—	—
Salad Bar Sliced Beets	—	¼ cup	16	.5	0	3.8	—	—	—	—	—	—
Salad Bar Sunflower Seeds	—	2 T	101	4.0	9.0	5.0	—	—	—	—	—	—
Salad Bar Tomatoes	—	3 slices	20	.8	0	4.8	—	—	—	—	—	—
Strawberry Shake	312		315	7.6	10.2	49.4	—	—	—	—	—	—
Strawberry Shortcake	205		447	10.1	19.2	59.3	—	—	—	—	—	—
Strawberry Sundae	142		216	5.7	7.1	33.1	—	—	—	—	—	—
Thigh	98		296	18.4	19.5	11.7	—	—	—	—	—	—
Thigh & Leg	151		436	29.9	27.5	17.2	—	—	—	—	—	—
Vanilla Shake	306		306	8.0	10.7	45.0	—	—	—	—	—	—
Wing	52		192	10.5	12.8	8.5	—	—	—	—	—	—

Source: Roy Rogers Restaurants, Marriott Corporation, Washington, DC. Nutritional data furnished by Lancaster Laboratories, 1985.

	WT G	KCAL	P G	F G	CAR G	CAL G	IRON G	VITA IU	ASCORBIC MG	THIAMIN MG	RIBO MG
TACO BELL											
Bean Burrito	166	343	11	12	48	98	2.8	1657	15.2	0.37	0.22
Beef Burrito	184	466	30	21	37	83	4.6	1675	15.2	0.30	0.39
Beefy Tostada	184	291	19	15	21	208	3.4	3450	12.7	0.16	0.27
Bellbeefer	123	221	15	7	23	40	2.6	2961	10.0	0.15	0.20
Bellbeefer w/Cheese	137	278	19	12	23	147	2.7	3146	10.0	0.16	0.27
Burrito Supreme	225	457	21	22	43	121	3.8	3462	16.0	0.33	0.35
Combination Burrito	175	404	21	16	43	91	3.7	1666	15.2	0.34	0.31
Enchirito	207	454	25	21	42	259	3.8	1178	9.5	0.31	0.37
Pintos 'N' Cheese	158	168	11	5	21	150	2.3	3123	9.3	0.26	0.16
Taco	83	186	15	8	14	120	2.5	120	0.2	0.09	0.16
Tostada	138	179	9	6	25	191	2.3	3152	9.7	0.18	0.15

Sources: Menu Item Portions, July 1976. Taco Bell Co., San Antonio, Tex.
Adams CF: *Nutritive Value of American Foods in Common Units.* USDA Agricultural Research Service, Agricultural Handbook No. 456, November 1975.
Church CF, Church HN: *Food Values of Portions Commonly Used,* ed 12. Philadelphia, J. B. Lippincott Co., 1975.
Valley Baptist Medical Center, Food Service Department: Descriptions of Mexican-American Foods, NASCO. Fort Atkinson, Wisc.

	WT G	DESCRIPTION	KCAL	P G	F G	CAR G	CAL G	IRON G	VITA IU	ASCOR-BIC MG	THIA-MIN MG	RIBO MG
WENDY'S												
Bacon	18	2 strips	110	5	10	—	—	—	—	—	—	—
Bacon Cheeseburger on white bun	147		460	29	28	23	—	—	—	—	—	—
Breakfast Sandwich	129		370	17	19	33	—	—	—	—	—	—
Chicken Sandwich on multi-grain wheat bun	128		320	25	10	31	—	—	—	—	—	—
Chili	256		260	21	8	26	—	—	—	—	—	—
Danish	85	1 pc.	360	6	18	44	—	—	—	—	—	—
Double Hamburger on white bun	197		560	41	34	24	—	—	—	—	—	—
French Fries (salted) (reg)	98		280	4	14	35	—	—	—	—	—	—
French Toast	135	2 slices	400	11	19	45	—	—	—	—	—	—
Frosty Dairy Desert	243		400	8	14	59	—	—	—	—	—	—
Home Fries	103		360	4	22	37	—	—	—	—	—	—
Hot Stuffed Baked Potatoes Bacon & Cheese	350		570	19	30	57	—	—	—	—	—	—
Hot Stuffed Baked Potatoes Broccoli & Cheese	365		500	13	25	54	—	—	—	—	—	—
Hot Stuffed Baked Potatoes Cheese	350		590	17	34	55	—	—	—	—	—	—
Hot Stuffed Baked Potatoes Chili & Cheese	400		510	22	20	63	—	—	—	—	—	—
Hot Stuffed Baked Potatoes Plain	250		250	6	2	52	—	—	—	—	—	—
Hot Stuffed Baked Potatoes Sour Cream & Chives	310		460	6	24	53	—	—	—	—	—	—
KIDS' MEAL Hamburger	75		220	13	8	11	—	—	—	—	—	—
Multi-grain Wheat Bun	48		135	5	3	23	—	—	—	—	—	—
Omelet #1 Ham & Cheese	114		250	18	17	6	—	—	—	—	—	—
Omelet #2 Ham, Cheese & Mushroom	118		290	18	21	7	—	—	—	—	—	—
Omelet #3 Ham, Cheese, Onion, Green Pepper	128		280	19	19	7	—	—	—	—	—	—
Omelet #4 Mushroom, Onion, Green Pepper	114		210	14	15	7	—	—	—	—	—	—
Orange Juice	180		80	1	—	17	—	—	—	—	—	—
Pick-Up Window Salad	510		110	8	6	5	—	—	—	—	—	—
Sausage	45	1 patty	200	9	18	—	—	—	—	—	—	—
Scrambled Eggs	91		190	14	12	7	—	—	—	—	—	—
Single Hamburger on multi-grain wheat bun	119		340	25	17	20	—	—	—	—	—	—
Single Hamburger on white bun	117		350	21	18	27	—	—	—	—	—	—
Taco Salad	357		390	23	18	36	—	—	—	—	—	—
Toast with Margarine	69	2 slices	250	6	9	35	—	—	—	—	—	—
White Bun	52		160	5	3	28	—	—	—	—	—	—

Source: Wendy's International, Inc., Dublin, OH., 1985. Nutritional information provided by Hazelton Laboratories America, Inc., and U.S. Department of Agriculture Handbook #8.

APPENDIX E

Basic Free Weight Resistance Exercises for the Neck, Arms, Shoulders, Chest, Abdomen, Back, and Legs

Group A. Exercises to strengthen the neck, arms, and shoulders*

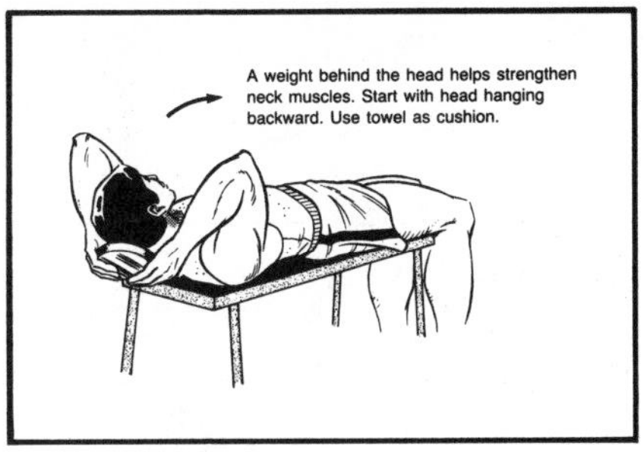

A weight behind the head helps strengthen neck muscles. Start with head hanging backward. Use towel as cushion.

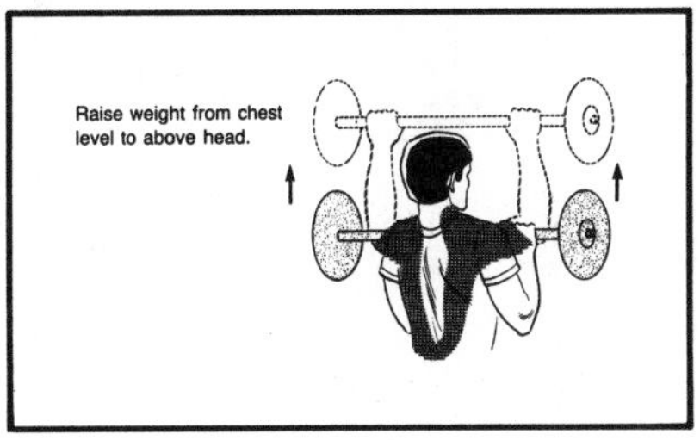

Raise weight from chest level to above head.

Bend at hips, keep arms straight, raise and lower as shown.

Start with arms straight down, lift weight toward shoulders. Place feet shoulder width apart, keep hips steady.

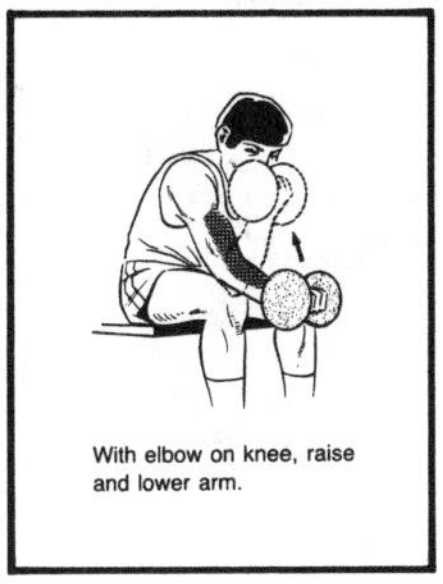

With elbow on knee, raise and lower arm.

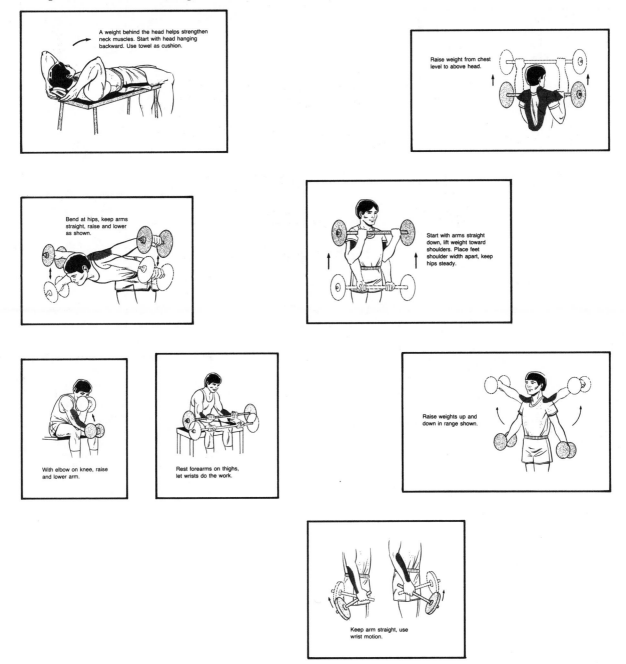

Rest forearms on thighs, let wrists do the work.

Raise weights up and down in range shown.

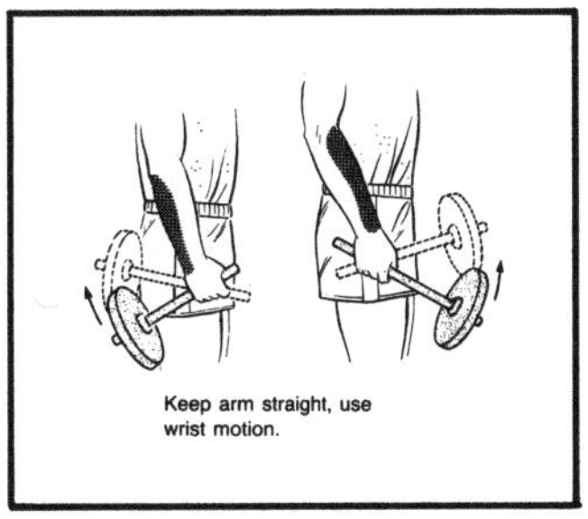

Keep arm straight, use wrist motion.

*–Shaded areas represent primary muscle groups exercised.

Group B. Exercises to strengthen the chest, abdomen, and back*

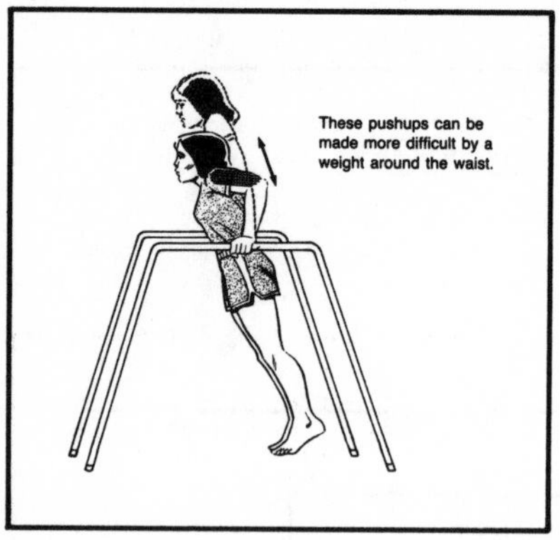
These pushups can be made more difficult by a weight around the waist.

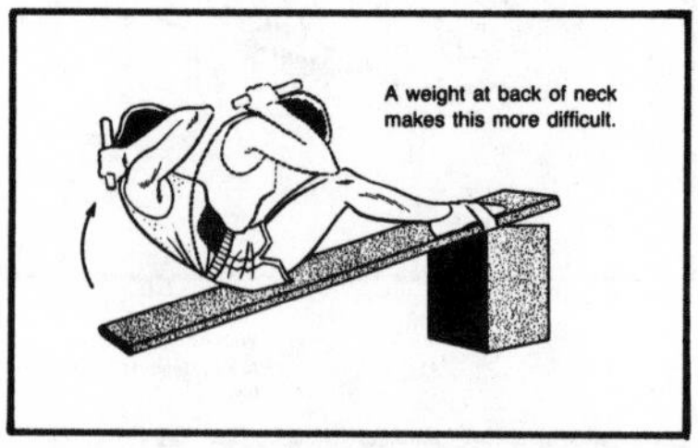
A weight at back of neck makes this more difficult.

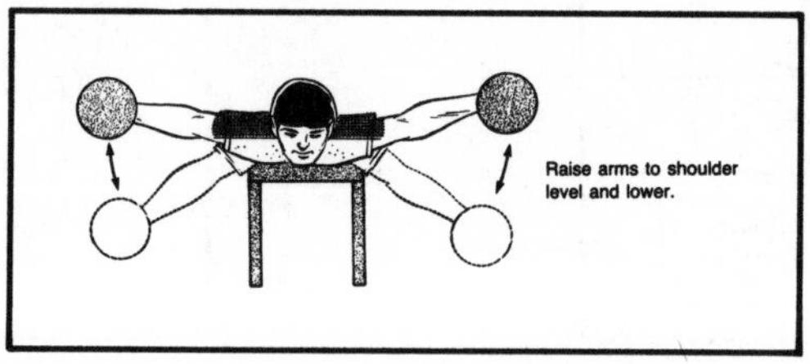
Raise arms to shoulder level and lower.

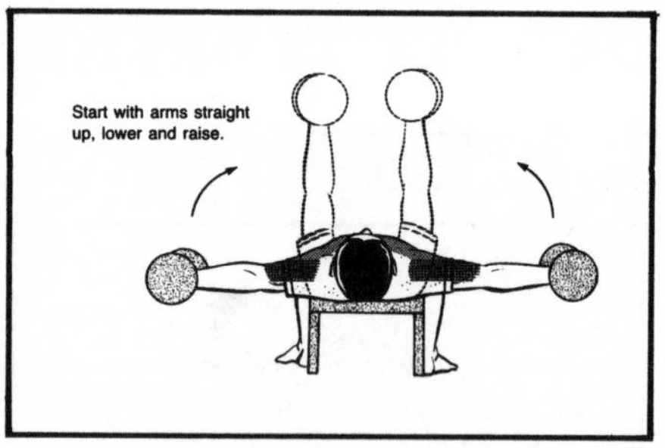
Start with arms straight up, lower and raise.

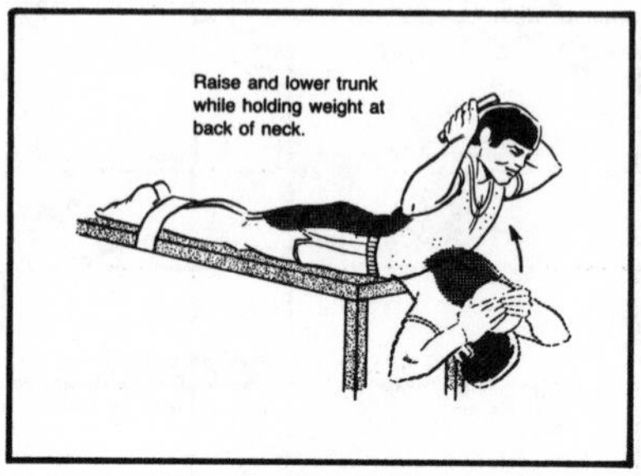
Raise and lower trunk while holding weight at back of neck.

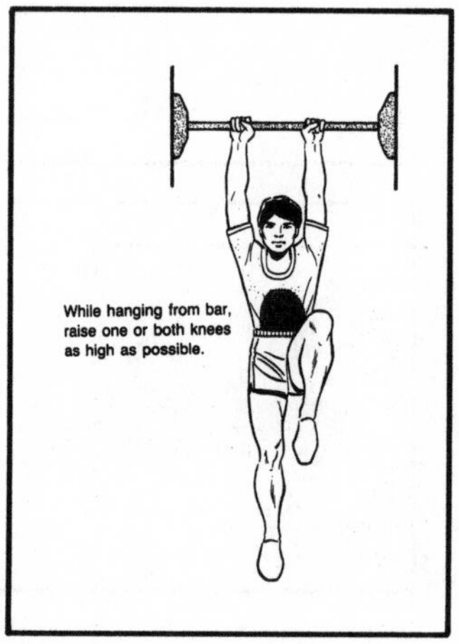
While hanging from bar, raise one or both knees as high as possible.

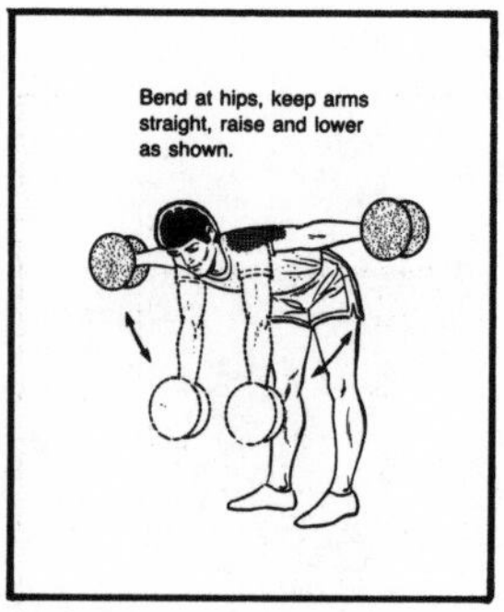
Bend at hips, keep arms straight, raise and lower as shown.

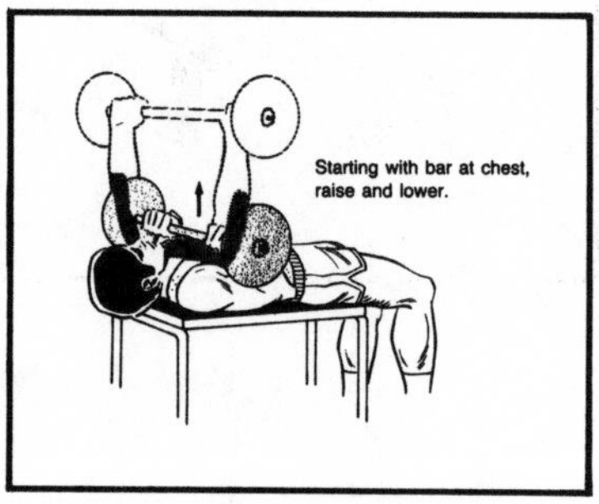
Starting with bar at chest, raise and lower.

*–Shaded areas represent primary muscle groups exercised.

Group C. Exercises to strengthen the buttocks and legs*

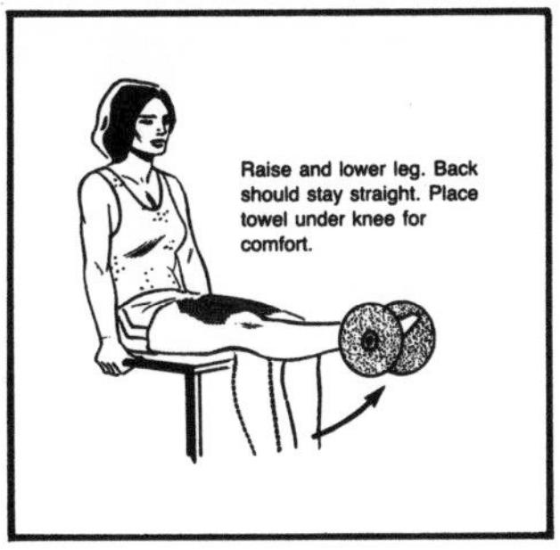
Raise and lower leg. Back should stay straight. Place towel under knee for comfort.

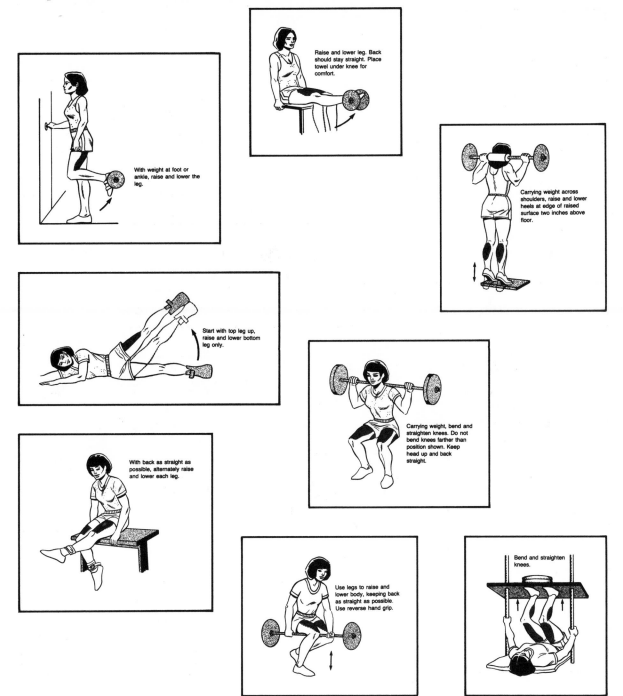

With weight at foot or ankle, raise and lower the leg.

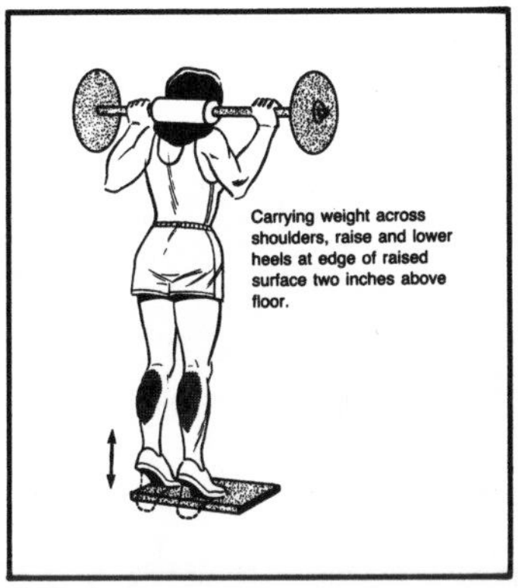
Carrying weight across shoulders, raise and lower heels at edge of raised surface two inches above floor.

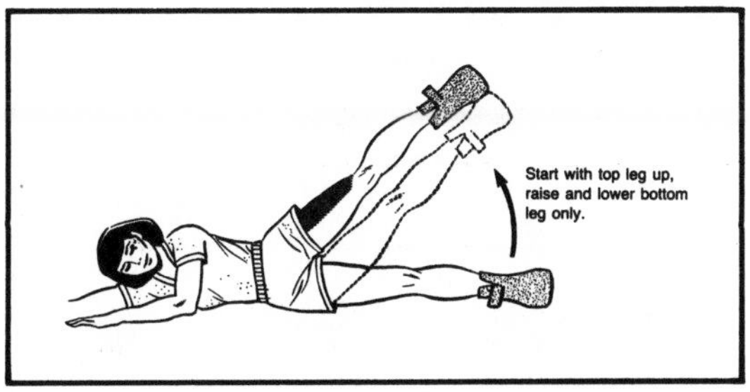
Start with top leg up, raise and lower bottom leg only.

Carrying weight, bend and straighten knees. Do not bend knees farther than position shown. Keep head up and back straight.

With back as straight as possible, alternately raise and lower each leg.

Use legs to raise and lower body, keeping back as straight as possible. Use reverse hand grip.

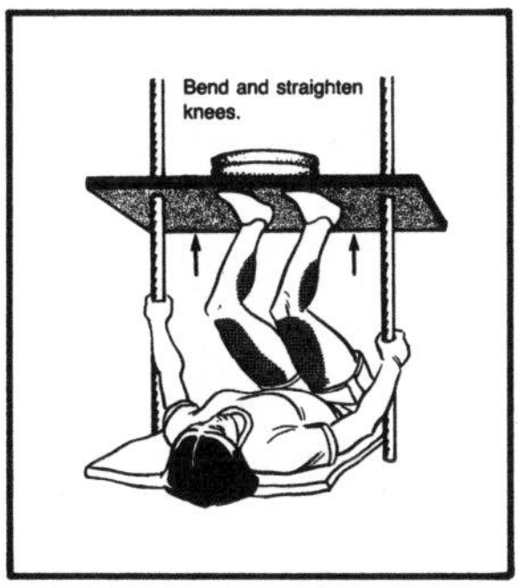
Bend and straighten knees.

*–Shaded areas represent primary muscle groups exercised.

Index

Page numbers followed by "f" indicate figures; page numbers followed by "t" indicate tables.

Abdomen, strengthening exercises, 330
Acetyl Co-A, in aerobic glucose metabolism, 59, 60
Adenosine, 54. *See also* ADP; ATP
Adipose tissue. *See also* Fat cells; Fatness; Obesity
  development of cellularity, 144–147, 146–147f
  early childhood nutrition effects on, 147–148
  exercise effects on, 148–152, 149–150f, 151t
  insulation value, 13
  in protection of vital organs, 13
  after spot reduction, 151–152
Adolescence
  fat cell development in, 146, 146–147f
  Recommended Dietary Allowance for protein, 17, 17t
ADP, as product of ATP energy release, 54, 55f
Aerobic conditioning
  age influence on decline, 243
  circuit weight training effect on, 205
  developing program for, 230–236
    continuous exercise training, 234–235
    determination of training intensity, 231–234, 232t, 233f
    guidelines for beginning, 231
    interval training, 235–236
  duration of training related to, 228–229
  evaluating cardiovascular capacity, 221–222
    classification of responses, 225–226, 225t
    prediction of maximal oxygen uptake, 224–226, 224f, 225t
    pulse rate measurements, 224
    Queens College step test, 222–223, 223t
    step up test, 221–222, 222f
    Techumseh step test, 226, 227t
  factors influencing, 226–230
  frequency of training related to, 228
  genetic influences, 228
  goals, 226, 227f
  initial level of cardiovascular capacity and, 227–228
  intensity of training related to, 229
  maintenance, 236
  specificity of training related to, 229–230
Aerobic energy metabolism, 55
  conditioning of, 220–236. *See also* Aerobic conditioning
  energy formation from, 59–61
  in interval training, 235
  lactic acid removal during, 72
  relative contribution during exercise, 72–74, 73f
  sports dependent upon, 217–219, 218f
Aging, 239–258
  and bodily functions, 240–243, 240f
  and cardiovascular function, 242
  coronary heart disease related to, 250–251, 257t
  exercise influence on decline of physiologic function, 240–241, 243
  exercise influence on extending lifetime, 243–246, 244f, 245f
  fatness changes with, 134t, 135
  and flexibility, 241
  and muscular strength, 241
  and nervous system function, 241–242
Alcohol, calories in beverages containing, 316
Aldosterone, 29
Amenorrhea
  exercise related to, 28–29
  fatness related to, 119–120
Amino acids
  absorption from intestinal tract, 40
  energy metabolism from, 58
  essential, 15
  optimal diet for exercise and sport, 40
  as protein building blocks, 14–15
  structure, 14, 14f
Anabolism, minerals role in, 23–24
Anaerobic energy metabolism, 55
  conditioning of, 219–220
  energy formation from, 57–59
  in interval training, 235
  relative contribution during exercise, 72–74, 73f
  sports dependent upon, 217–219, 218f
Anemia, iron deficiency, 25
Angina pectoris, 248. *See also* Coronary heart disease
Animals, fat cell development in, 145–146
Anorexia nervosa, behavior modification, 179–180
Aorta, 82–83, 83f

Appetite
exercise effect on, 170–173
training effect on, 172–173, 172t
Archery, energy expenditure in, 268–269t
Archimedes principle, application to body volume determination, 122–124, 123f
Arms, strengthening exercises, 329
Arterial system, 82–83, 82f, 83f
Arterioles, 83
Ascorbic acid. *See* Vitamin C
Asthma, exercise-induced, 80–81
Atherosclerosis. *See also* Coronary heart disease
exercise favorable effect on, 256
lipoproteins related to, 251
pathophysiology, 247–249, 249f
Athletes. *See also* Sports
amenorrhea in, 119–120
ATP
aerobic metabolism producing, 59–61, 60f, 61f
anaerobic metabolism producing, 58–59
as energy fuel, 53–55, 54f, 219
food metabolism to, 57–61, 58f
glycolysis producing, 58–59, 89–90
in muscle contraction, 55
resynthesis from creatine phosphate, 55–56
structure, 54, 54f
training to enhance energy system, 219–220

Back
extension, as warm-up exercise, 209f
strengthening exercises, 208, 330
Ballet
energy expenditure of, 106–107
in training for fitness, 106–107
Balloon, meteorologic, in oxygen consumption determination, 100, 100f
Barbells, in weight training, 210
Basal metabolic rate, 101–104
changes during caloric restriction, 167–168, 167f
Basketball
caloric intake associated with, 171t
energy expenditure in, 268–269t
maximal oxygen consumption in, 64f
Behavior, type A personality related to heart disease, 255
Behavior modification, 179
in anorexia nervosa, 179–180
of eating, 179–183. *See also* Eating behavior, modification
of exercise behavior, 183–186, 187t, 188–190
description of behavior to be modified, 185–186, 187t
providing positive reinforcement, 189–190
substituting alternate behaviors, 186, 188
techniques to maximize success, 188–189
steps in applying, 179–180
Bicycling. *See* Cycling
Bioelectrical impedance, in body composition measurement, 130
Biotin, 20t
Blood pressure, 85–86
body inversion effect on, 86
during exercise, 86
hypertension, 253. *See also* Hypertension
Body builders, female, 120, 121f
Body composition, 30
amenorrhea related to low body fat, 119–120
average values, 133, 134t, 135–136
body volume measurement in evaluation, 122–128
calculation of percent fat, 279–281, 282–289t
changes after diet plus exercise, 175–176, 175f
chemical analysis, 120–122
circumference measurements for body fat, 128–129, 278–281, 279f, 282–289t
computed tomography in evaluation, 132, 133f
evaluation, 115–136, 278–289
exercise effects on, 173, 175
fatfold technique for subcutaneous fat, 129
fatness versus overweight, 113, 115. *See also* Fatness of football players, 115
indirect measurement, 129–132, 133f
laboratory methods for, 120–129
minimal leanness standard, 117–118
minimal weight, 117–118
nutritional practices in pregnancy influencing, 147
optimal, 135–136
reference man and woman gross composition, 116, 117f
after spot reduction, 151–152
ultrasound determination, 130, 130f
underweight and thin, 118–119
x-ray measurement, 130, 131f, 132
Body inversion, blood pressure with, 86
Bomb calorimeter, 93–94, 94f
Bone
exercise influence on loss of mass with age, 243
exercise related to metabolism, 28–29
osteoporosis, 27–28
Boxing
caloric intake associated with, 171t
energy expenditure in, 268–269t
Breathing
during exercise, 76–77
mechanics, 75–77, 76f
Valsalva maneuver, 77
water loss in, 33
during weight lifting, 77
Bronchi, 74, 75f
Buttocks, strengthening exercises, 331

Calcium, 27–29
functions, 24
osteoporosis related to deficiency, 28
recommended daily allowance, 28
Caliper, in subcutaneous fat measurement, 129
Calisthenics, as warm-up exercises, 207–208, 209f
Calories, 93–97
counting, 162–165, 164t
daily requirement, 104
definition, 93
in foods, 94–97, 292–327
calculation, 95–96, 96t
determining intake, 162–165, 164t
digestive processes influencing, 95
measurement, 93–94, 94f
optimal contributions of major food components for active people, 40f
restriction diets causing weight loss, 165–170, 167f. *See also* Diet
Calorimetry, 93–94, 94f
body heat production measured by, 97–98, 97f
direct, 97–98, 97f
indirect, 98–101
Canoeing, energy expenditure in, 268–269t
Capillaries, 83
Carbohydrates, 4–9. *See also* Glucose
caloric value, 94–95
disaccharides, 5
as energy source, 12–13
before exercise, 47, 49–50
during exercise, 46–47
in food, 8–9, 8f, 292–327
functions, 7–8
in intense training, 45–46, 45f
loading to increase glycogen reserves, 47–49, 48t, 49t

monosaccharides, 4
optimal diet for exercise and sport, 41–42
polysaccharides, 5
in precompetition meal, 49–50
protein-sparing effects, 7–8
recommended daily allowance, 41–42
source, 6–7, 7f
storage as glycogen, 7
structure, 4, 4f
water absorption influenced by, 33–34
water production during metabolism, 31–32
Carbon
chemical bonds, 3
hydrogen and oxygen combined with, 3
nutrients containing, 3
Carbon dioxide
arterial pressure, 77, 78f
exchange in lung, 77–79, 78f
Cardiac output, 86–87, 88f, 89
training effect on, 86–87, 88f, 89
Cardiovascular system, 82–84, 83f, 84f. *See also* Heart
evaluating capacity, 221–226
in exercise in pregnancy, 236
Carotenes, 21
Carotid artery, pulse rate taken at, 85, 85f
Catabolism, minerals role in, 23
Cellulose, 5
Central nervous system, aging influence on, 241–242
Chemical bonding, 3
Chest, strengthening exercises, 330
Chest pain, angina pectoris, 248
Chlorophyll, 7
Cholesterol, 10
coronary heart disease related to, 251–252, 252f, 257t
dietary levels related to atherosclerosis, 248
in food, 11t
functions, 10
lipoprotein fractions containing, 11, 251, 252f
reduction in diet, 10–11
Cigarettes. *See* Smoking
Circuit training, energy expenditure in, 268–269t
Circulatory system, 81–89, 82f. *See also* Heart
blood pressure, 85–86
cardiovascular system, 82–84, 83f, 84f
functions during exercise, 81
in trained and untrained individual, 86–87, 88f, 89
Circumference measurements, 278–281, 279f, 282–289t
Clothing, for exercise, 231
Coenzyme, 19
Computed tomography, in body composition measurement, 132, 133f
Computer
in nutrient analysis of foods, 96
in oxygen consumption determination, 100–101, 101f
Computerized exercise plan, 170, 264–266
Computerized meal plan, 44, 169–170, 261–263, 265–266
Concentric contraction, 198–199, 198f
Conditioning, 193–196. *See also* Fitness; Training
aerobic, 220–236. *See also* Aerobic conditioning
anaerobic, 219–220
general principles, 194–196
individual differences principle, 195
medical checkup prior to, 196
for muscular strength, 197–214
overload principle, 194–195
physiologic, 194–196
reversibility principle, 195–196
specificity principle, 195
Conversions, 291
Cool-down period, 231
Coronary circulation, 246, 248f
atherosclerosis, 247–249, 249f
Coronary heart disease, 246–258. *See also* Heart disease
age, gender and heredity related to, 250–251
conditioning program in, 196
dietary saturated fat related to, 10
exercise influence in protection, 255–256
lipids related to, 11–12, 251–252, 252f
obesity related to, 254–255
pathophysiology, 247–249, 249f
personality related to, 255
risk factors, 249–250, 254f
assessment, 256, 257t, 258
smoking related to, 253–254
Creatine phosphate
energy derived from, 219
in energy storage, 55–57, 55f
training to enhance energy system, 219–220
Cycling
caloric intake associated with, 171t
energy expenditure in, 107t, 108, 270–271t
maximal oxygen consumption in, 65f
Cytochromes, 25

Dancing, energy expenditure in, 270–271t
Dehydration
water replacement in, 33–34
weight loss diets causing, 156–157, 176
Density
of human body, 124
percent body fat computed from, 124–125, 126f, 127–128
Diaphragm, in breathing, 75–76, 76f
Diastole, 85
Diet. *See also* Food; Nutrients
atherosclerosis related to, 248
body composition changes after food restriction, 175–176, 175f
carbohydrate in, 8–9, 156, 158t
loading, 47–49, 48t, 49t
computerized meal plan, 44, 169–170, 261–263, 265–266
endurance related to, 44–47
erroneous claims of weight loss, 155–156, 168–169
exercise combined with, 174–177
advantages over diet or exercise alone, 174–175
optimal duration, 175–177, 175f, 176f
fiber in, 5, 6t
glycogen storage modified by, 8
high-carbohydrate, low-fat, 158t
high-protein, 156–157, 158t
iron in, 25
low-carbohydrate, high-fat, 156, 158t
in obesity, 155–157, 158t. *See also* Weight control
metabolism changes during, 167–168, 167f
one-food-centered, 158t
optimal for exercise and sport, 39–51
carbohydrate loading, 47–49
computerized meal plans, 44
endurance performance, 44–47
four-food-group plan, 42, 42–43t, 44
nutrient recommendations, 39–42
precompetition meal, 49–50
protein-sparing modified fast, 158t
saturated fat in, 10
selection in weight control, 168–169
seven-day record, 162–164
starvation, 156
therapeutic fast, 156
thermogenesis induced by, 104
to unbalance energy balance equation, 165–170, 167f
vegetarian approach to sound nutrition, 18
Diffusion, in lung, 77
Disinhibition, strength improvement after, 201
Diving, caloric intake associated with, 171t

Eating behavior
factors influencing, 161–162
modification, 179–183
in anorexia nervosa, 179–180
describing behavior to be modified, 180–181
providing positive reinforcement, 182–183
substituting alternative behaviors, 182
techniques to control act of eating, 182
in weight control, 180–183, 181f
taste influencing, 161–162
Eccentric contraction, 197, 198f
Echocardiography, heart muscle thickness determined by, 89
Elderly. *See* Aging
Electrocardiogram, stress, 196
Electrolytes
functions, 24
replacement after exercise, 29–30
Endurance
carbohydrate needs in, 45–46, 45f
diet related to performance, 44–47
slow twitch fibers related to, 69
Endurance fitness, 221
Energy. *See also* Energy expenditure; Energy metabolism
aerobic reactions producing, 59–61
anaerobic reactions producing, 57–59
ATP as fuel for, 53–55, 54f
balancing input with output in weight control, 159–161, 160f. *See also* Weight control
biologic work requiring, 53
creatine phosphate in storage, 55–57, 55f
definition, 53
for exercise, 53–91
in food, 57–61, 93–97. *See also* Calories
digestive processes influencing, 95, 104
optimal contributions of major food components, 40f, 41
predominant sources for different kinds of exercise, 57
for short-duration high-intensity activities, 59
spectrum during exercise, 72–74
storage, creatine phosphate in, 55–57, 55f
transfer, in transition from rest to vigorous physical activity, 1
Energy balance equation, 159–161, 160f
unbalancing in weight control, 165–177
by diet, 165–170, 167f
by exercise, 170–177
Energy expenditure. *See also* Energy; Energy metabolism
of ballet, 106–107
body weight related to, 108, 268–277t
calculation during various physical activities, 105–106
carbohydrate requirements in training, 45–46, 45f
in circuit weight training, 204–205, 204t
daily rates, 108–110, 109–110t
during dieting, 166
exercise effects on, 173
in household and recreational activities, 268–277t
in hydraulic resistance exercise, 205–206
intensity of exercise related to, 174–175
METS, 111, 111t
of occupations, 106t
of physical activity, 105–106
basal metabolic rate, 101–104
heat production measurement, 97–98, 97f
oxygen consumption measurement, 98, 99–101f, 100–101
of rowing, 105
in sports, 107–108, 107t, 268–277t
in weight training, 203–205
Energy metabolism. *See also* Energy; Energy expenditure
aerobic, 59–61, 60f, 61f, 62f, 66
conditioning for, 220–236
in slow twitch muscle fibers, 68–69
anaerobic, 57–59, 66–68, 67f
conditioning for, 219–220
in fast twitch muscle fibers, 68
carbohydrates as fuel source, 7
conditioning anaerobic and aerobic utilization, 217–237. *See also* Aerobic conditioning
continuous exercise requirements, 221
fat as fuel source, 12–13
lactic acid as source, 72
phosphorus role in, 24
during physical activity, 105–106
training directed toward predominant system, 74
vitamins role in, 21–22
water production during, 31–32
Enzymes, 15
in energy release reactions from food, 57
Estrogen, osteoporosis related to deficiency, 28
Exercise
and aging of skeleton, 28–29
amenorrhea related to, 28–29, 119
and appetite, 170–173
in asthmatic, 80–81
behavior modification, 183–186, 187t, 188–190
description of behavior to be modified, 185–186, 187t
providing positive reinforcement, 189–190
substituting alternate behaviors, 186, 188
techniques to maximize success, 188–189
blood pressure during, 86
blood pressure lowered by, 253
body composition changes related to, 173, 175
bone mass loss with age influenced by, 243
breathing mechanics during, 76
carbohydrate drinks before, 47
carbohydrate drinks during, 46–47
cardiac output after, 86–87, 88f, 89
cardiovascular response in pregnancy, 236
changing personal habits in weight control, 162
circuit training, energy expenditure in, 268–269t
circulatory system functions during, 81
computerized plan in weight control, 264–266
concentric contraction, 198–199, 198f
conditioning, 193–196. *See also* Conditioning; Training
continuous training, 234–235
cool-down period, 231
and decline of function with age, 240–241
diet combined with, 174–177
advantages over diet or exercise alone, 174–175
optimal duration, 175–177, 175f, 176f
diet optimal for, 39–51
carbohydrate loading, 47–49
computerized meal plans, 44
endurance performance, 44–47
four-food-group plan, 42, 42–43t, 44
nutrient recommendations, 39–42
precompetition meal, 49–50
energy for, 12, 53–91
in continuous activity, 221
different sources for different sports, 57
expenditure in sports and recreational activities, 173, 268–277t
short-duration high-intensity activities, 59
spectrum, 72–74
and extension of lifetime, 243–246, 244f, 245f, 255–256
fat cell changes related to, 148–152, 149–150f, 151t
fluid and electrolyte replacement after sweating, 29–30
guidelines for beginning aerobic conditioning program, 231
heart disease risk reduced by, 239, 255–256
high-energy phosphates role in, 56–57
intensity related to energy expenditure, 174–175
interval training, 235–236
iron influence on capacity, 25–26, 27t
iron supplementation in, 26–27
lactic acid blood levels related to tolerance, 68
lipoproteins related to, 251–252
lung ventilation during, 79–80

minerals influence on performance, 29–30
motivating person to increase activity, 188–189
overload accomplished by, 194
oxygen consumption during, 61–66
lactic acid formation related to, 66, 67f, 68
maximal, 63–65, 63–65f
steady state, 61–63, 62f
during pregnancy, 236–237
recovery oxygen consumption after, 69–72, 70f
relative contributions of anaerobic and aerobic metabolism during, 72–74, 73f
resistance. *See* Strength, conditioning for
smoking effect on tolerance to, 81
in spot reduction, 150–152, 151t
straining-type. *See* Weight lifting
for strength training, 197, 329–331. *See also* Strength
to unbalance energy balance equation, 170–177
vitamins related to performance, 21–22
warm-up, 207–208, 209f, 231
water intake before, 33
water replacement during, 33–34
Exercise prescription, computerized, 170
Eye, body inversion effect on, 86

Farming, energy expenditure in, 270–271t
Fast
therapeutic, 156
in weight control, 158t
Fat, 9–14. *See also* Fatness
caloric value, 94–95
energy metabolism from, 12–13, 58
essential, 116
in food, 14, 292–327
functions, 12–13
hunger related to dietary levels, 13
hydrogenation, 12
optimal diet for exercise and sport, 41
recommended daily allowance, 41
saturated
coronary heart disease related to, 10
in food, 11t
sources, 12
versus unsaturated, 9–10, 9f
source, 12
storage, 116–120
structure, 9, 9f
types, 9–10
unsaturated, 12
vitamin utilization related to, 13
Fat cells. *See also* Adipose tissue; Fatness
changes, 147–152
exercise effects, 148–152, 149–150f, 151t
nutritional influences, 147–148
development, 146–147f
animal studies, 145–146
human studies, 146–147, 146–147f
early childhood nutrition effects on, 147–148
size and number
determination, 139–140, 141f
in obesity, 139, 140–142, 142f, 143f
after weight gain, 144, 145f
after weight reduction, 142–144, 143f
Fatfold technique, 129
Fatness. *See also* Body composition; Obesity
acceptable limits for normal body composition, 157, 159
age related to, 134t, 135, 242–243
amenorrhea related to low level, 119–120
average values, 133, 134t, 135
chemical methods of measurement, 120–122
circumference measurements for, 128–129, 278–281, 279f, 282–289t
determination of, 278–289
subcutaneous, 129
distribution related to obesity health risk, 139
health risks, 113
minimal standard in health, 117–118
in obesity, 138. *See also* Obesity
optimal, 135–136
percent computed, 124–125, 126f, 127–128, 279–281, 282–289t
prediction from circumference measurements, 128–129
of reference man and woman, 116, 117f
x-ray determination, 130, 131f, 132
Fatty acid, 9
saturated versus unsaturated, 9–10, 9f
Feces, water loss in, 33
Female. *See also* Gender
amenorrhea related to fatness, 119–120
average fatness, 133, 134t, 135
body builders, 120, 121f
conversion constants to predict percent body fat in, 282–285t
minimal weight, 118
reference, 116, 117f
strength training in, 202–203
Fencing, maximal oxygen consumption in, 64f
Fetus
exercise effect on, 236–237
fat cell development in, 146, 146–147f
Fiber
in foods, 5, 6t
gastrointestinal disease related to dietary content, 5
Fitness. *See also* Conditioning; Training
aerobic conditioning related to initial level, 227–228
ballet as exercise for, 106–107
cardiovascular, 221
circuit weight training effect on, 205
conditioning for, 193–196
definition, 193
developing aerobic conditioning program, 230–236
continuous exercise training, 234–235
determination of training intensity, 231–234, 232t, 233f
guidelines for beginning, 231
interval training, 235–236
evaluating cardiovascular capacity, 221–226
heredity of, 66
maintenance, 236
Flexibility
aging influence on, 241
exercises, as warm-up, 208, 209f
Folic acid, 20t
Food(s). *See also* Diet
calories in, 94–97, calories in, 292–327
calculation, 95–96, 96t
digestive processes influencing, 95
carbohydrate in, 8–9, 8f
cholesterol in, 11t
determining caloric intake from, 162–165, 164t
energy value, 57–61, 93–97. *See also* Calories
fast, 316–327
fat in, 14
fiber content, 5, 6t
four-group plan, 42, 42–43t, 44
intake related to exercise, 170–173, 171t, 172t
measuring portions for calorie counting, 162–163
minerals in, 24–29
nutrients in, 3–35
nutritive value, 290–327
protein in, 16–17, 16f
saturated fat in, 11t
water content, 31
Football
body composition of players, 115
energy costs, 107t
Four-Food-Group Plan, 42, 42–43t, 44
Fractures, in osteoporosis, 27–28

Fructose, 4
Fruit, measuring portions, 162–163

Galactose, 4
Gardening, energy expenditure in, 272–273t
Gas exchange, in lung, 77–79
Gastrointestinal tract
 dietary fiber related to disorders, 5
 protein absorption in, 40
Gender
 coronary heart disease related to, 250–251
 and fat storage, 116–117
 fatness related to, 134t, 135
 minimal weight related to, 117–118
 strength differences between men and women, 202–203
Genetics. *See* Heredity
Glucolipids, 10
Gluconeogenesis, 6
Glucose. *See also* Carbohydrates
 glycogen conversion to, 6
 metabolism
  aerobic, 59–61, 60f, 61f
  ATP formation from, 57–61
  glycolysis, 57–59, 89–90
 structure, 4, 4f
Glycerol, 9
Glycogen, 6
 carbohydrate loading to increase reserves, 47–49, 48t, 49t
 depletion during intense training, 45–46, 45f
 diet influence on storage, 8, 45–48, 45f, 48t, 49t
Glycogenesis, 6
Glycogenolysis, 6
Glycolysis, energy production from, 58–59, 89–90
Gymnastics
 caloric intake associated with, 171t
 energy expenditure in, 272–273t

Heart, 81–89
 aging influence on, 242
 athlete's, 89
 cardiac output, 86–87, 88f, 89
 coronary circulation, 246, 248f
 functions, 82–83, 83f
 in trained and untrained individual, 86–87, 88f, 89
Heart disease, 246–258. *See also* Coronary heart disease
 cholesterol reduction and, 10–11
 exercise reducing risk, 239–240
 obesity as risk factor, 139
 saturated fat related to, 10
 statistics on, 246, 247f
Heart failure, 85
Heart rate
 age influence on maximal response to exercise, 232t, 242
 in circuit-type training program, 205
 measurement after exercise, 224
 in omnikinetic exercise, 205–206
 response to exercise as measure of cardiovascular fitness, 221–222, 222t, 224–225, 224f
 target of exercise intensity for aerobic conditioning, 229, 232–234, 232t, 233f
Heat production, 97–101
 calorimetric measurement, 97–98
 dietary-induced, 104
 oxygen consumption measurement, 98, 99–101f, 100–101
 regulation, fat as insulator in, 13
Hemoglobin, 16, 25
 oxygen transport in blood, 79
Heredity
 and aerobic conditioning, 228
 and coronary heart disease, 250–251, 257t
 fitness capacity related to, 66
Hockey, caloric intake associated with, 171t
Honey, nutritional value, 5
Hormones, 16
 minerals role in action of, 24
Humidity, relative, 32
Hydraulic resistance exercises
 circuit for, 212, 213f
 energy cost of, 205–206
Hydrogen, carbon and oxygen combined with, 3
Hydrogenation, 12
Hydrostatic weighing, 125, 126f
Hyperlipoproteinemia, 251–252, 252f
Hypertension, 85, 253
 exercise effect on, 253
 sodium intake related to, 29
Hypoglycemia, 8
Hypothalamus, in setpoint theory, 166–168

Inactivity, obesity associated with, 183–185, 184t
Interval training, 235–236
Intraocular pressure, body inversion effect on, 86
Inversion, blood pressure with, 86
Iodine, dietary deficiency, 24–25
Iron, 25–27
 absorption, vitamin C influence on, 25
 deficiency, 25
 and exercise capacity, 25–26, 27t
 in foods, 292–327
 plant versus animal sources, 25–26
 recommended dietary allowance, 25, 26t
 supplementation for exercise training, 26–27
Isokinetic training, 200
Isometric contraction, 198f, 199
Isometric training, 199–200
Isotonic contraction, 199

Jogging, as warm-up exercise, 207, 209f

Keratin, 16
Krebs cycle, 59–61, 60f, 61f

Laboratory, body composition studies, 120–129
Lactic acid
 blood level related to exercise tolerance, 68
 conversion to pyruvic acid, 71–72
 as energy source, 72
 formation during anaerobic metabolism, 66–68
 oxygen consumption related to formation, 66, 67f, 68
 during recovery from exercise, 71–72
 removal during aerobic submaximal exercise, 72
 sports dependent upon energy from production, 218–219, 218f
 training for increasing production in energy metabolism, 220
Lactose, 5
Lean body weight, calculation, 124–125, 127–128, 279–281
Leanness, minimal standards for, 117–118
Lean tissue mass, protection in exercise plus diet weight loss program, 175
Leg, strengthening exercises, 331
Leg-raising, as warm-up exercise, 209f
Lifestyle
 exercise influence on extending lifetime, 243–246, 244f, 245f
 risk factors for coronary heart disease, 249–250
Linoleic acid, 41
Lipids. *See also* Fat
 coronary heart disease related to, 251–252, 252f, 257t
 dietary levels related to atherosclerosis, 248
Lipoproteins, 10, 251–252, 252f
 cholesterol combined with, 11, 251–252, 252f

and coronary heart disease, 11–12
exercise effects on, 251–252
high-density versus low-density, 11, 251–252, 252f
Lung, 74–81
anatomy, 74–75, 75f
during exercise, 79–80
gas exchange in, 77–79
mechanics of breathing, 75–77, 76f

Magnesium, 24
Male. *See also* Gender
average fatness, 133, 134t, 135
conversion constants to predict percent body fat in, 285–289t
minimal weight, 117–118
reference, 116, 117f
Maltose, 5
Meal plan, computerized, 169–170, 261–263, 265–266
Megavitamins, 22
Men. *See* Gender; Male
Menstrual cycle, fatness related to, 119–120
Menu
carbohydrate loading, 49t
computerized meal plans, 44
four-food-group plan, 43t, 44
precompetition meal, 49–50
MET, 111, 111t
Metabolism, 3. *See also* Energy metabolism
basal rate, 101–104
changes during caloric restriction, 167–168, 167f
surface area related to, 102
Minerals, 23–30
calcium, 27–29
exercise performance related to, 29–30
in food, 24–29
functions, 23–24
importance, 23
iron, 25–27
sources, 23
Mitochondria, energy reactions in, 59, 60f
Monosaccharides, 4
Movement, aging influence on, 241–242
Muscle(s)
aging influence on, 241
anatomic factors influencing strength, 201–202
contraction
ATP role, 55
concentric, 198–199, 198f
eccentric, 197, 198f
isometric, 198f, 199
isotonic, 199
energy metabolism related to type of muscle fiber, 68–69
fast versus slow twitch fibers, 68–69
glycogen stores influenced by diet, 45–48, 45f, 48t, 49t
hypertrophy after overload training, 202
protein content after training, 15
strength. *See* Strength
Myocardial infarction
pathophysiology, 248
physical activity reducing risk, 239
Myoglobin, 25

Nautilus, energy costs, 107t
Neck, strengthening exercises, 329
Nerve conduction velocity, aging influence on, 241
Niacin, 20t, 21
Nitrogen, carbon, hydrogen and oxygen combined with, 3
Nutrients. *See also* Diet; Food
body processes dependent on, 3
carbohydrates, 4–9. *See also* Carbohydrates
categories, 3
chemical differences between, 3–4
energy required in digesting, absorbing and assimilating, 104
fats, 9–14. *See also* Fat
in food, 3–35
minerals, 23–30. *See also* Minerals
organic building blocks, 3
protein, 14–17. *See also* Protein
vitamins, 18–23. *See also* Vitamin
water, 30–34. *See also* Water
Nutrition. *See also* Diet; Nutrients
fat cell changes related to, 147–148
four-food-group plan, 42, 42–43t, 44
Recommended Dietary Allowance for protein, 17, 17t
in vegetarian, 18

Obesity, 137–152
acceptable limits of fatness above which weight reduction indicated, 157, 159
behavior modification in, 180–183, 181f
describing behavior to be modified, 180–181
providing positive reinforcement, 182–183
results, 180, 181f
substituting alternative behaviors, 182
techniques to control act of eating, 182
definition, 138–139
diets in, 155–157, 158t. *See also* Diet; Weight control
difficulty in achieving weight loss, 180
difficulty in maintaining weight loss, 157
early prevention versus treatment, 150
etiology, 137–138
exercise behavior modification in, 183–190. *See also* Exercise, behavior modification
fasting in, 158t
fat cell size and number in, 140–142, 142f, 143f
as criterion, 139
after weight reduction, 142–144, 143f
grading of, 138
health risks of, 113, 139, 254–255, 257t
high-carbohydrate, low-fat diet in, 158t
high-protein diet in, 156–157, 158t
magnitude of problem, 137, 254
one-food-centered diet in, 158t
percent body fat as criterion, 138
physical activity associated with, 183–185, 184t
protein-sparing modified fast in, 158t
starvation diet in, 156
surgical treatment, 158t
weight control, 155–177. *See also* Weight control
Occupations, energy expenditure associated with, 106t, 109–110,110t, 268–277t
Omnikinetic exercise, heart rate and metabolic response to, 205–206
Organic acid, 14
Osteoporosis, 27–28
Overload, 194–195
in strength training, 212, 214
in weight training, 210
Oxygen
arterial pressure, 77, 78f
carbon and hydrogen combined with, 3
delivery, 63
ventilation, 74–81
energy-release reactions dependent on, 55. *See also* Exercise, aerobic
exchange in lung, 77–79, 78f
hemoglobin binding, 79
transport in blood, 79
utilization, 63

Oxygen consumption
in basal metabolic rate determination, 101–102, 104
cardiac output related to, 87, 88f
computerized instrumentation in measurement, 100–101, 101f
during exercise, 61–66
maximal, 63–65, 63–65f
steady state, 61–63, 62f
in hydraulic resistance exercise, 205–206
lactic acid formation related to, 66, 67f, 68
maximal, 63–65, 63–65f
as basis for determining training intensity in aerobic conditioning program, 231–232
predicted values from Queens College step test, 223–226, 223t, 224f, 225t
measurement, 98, 99–101f, 100–101
MET measure, 111, 111t
meteorologic balloon in measurement, 100, 100f
recovery, 69–72, 70f
spirometry in measurement, 98, 99f, 100, 100f
training influence on relationship between pulmonary ventilation and, 79–80, 80f
Oxygen debt, 69–72, 70f

Pantothenic acid, 20t
Personality, heart disease related to, 255
Phosphate, 24
in anaerobic energy, 219–220
high energy bonds, 54. *See also* ATP
Phospholipids, 10
Phosphorus. *See* Phosphate
Photosynthesis, 6–7, 7f
Physical activity. *See also* Exercise
daily energy expenditure rates, 108–110, 109–110t
determining profile, 185–186, 187t
energy metabolism during, 105–106
sports, 107–108, 107t
in obese individuals, 183–185, 184t
work, 110–111, 111t
Physical fitness. *See* Fitness
Polysaccharides, 5
Potassium, replacement after exercise, 30
Pregnancy
exercise during, 236–237
cardiovascular response, 236
fetal effects, 236–237
nutritional practices influencing fetus body composition, 147
Protein, 14–17
caloric value, 94–95
calorie-burning effect of ingestion, 104
carbohydrate role in limiting use as energy source, 7–8
complete versus incomplete, 16
energy metabolism from, 58
in enzymes, 15
in foods, 16–17, 16f, 292–327
functions, 15–16
optimal diet for exercise and sport, 39–40
recommended daily allowance, 17, 17t, 39–40
source, 15
in strengthened muscle, 15
structure, 14–15, 14f
in vegetarian diet, 18
Protein-sparing, in exercise plus diet weight loss program, 175
Protein-sparing modified fast, 158t
Provitamins, 21
Psychologic factors
in eating behavior, 162. *See also* Eating behavior, modification
personality related to heart disease, 255
strength influenced by, 201
Pulse, 85, 85f
Pulse rate. *See* Heart rate

Pyridoxine, 20t
Pyruvic acid, lactic acid formation from, 66, 67f

Queens College step test, 222–223, 223t
predicting maximal oxygen uptake from, 224–226, 224f, 225t

Radial artery, pulse rate taken at, 85, 85f
Radiography, in body composition measurement, 130, 131f, 132
Recommended daily allowance
for calcium, 28
for carbohydrates, 41–42
for fat, 41
for iron, 25, 26t
for protein, 17, 17t, 39–40
for sodium, 29
Resistance training. *See* Strength, conditioning for
Respiration. *See* Breathing
Respiratory system, 74–75, 75f
Reversibility principle, 195–196
Riboflavin
in foods, 292–327
function, 20t
Risk factors for heart disease, 249–250, 254f
assessment, 256, 257t, 258
RISKO, 256, 257t, 258
Rowers, maximal oxygen consumption in, 64f, 65f
Rowing exercise, energy cost, 206
Running
caloric intake associated with, 171t
cardiovascular response compared with swimming, 233–234
continuous exercise training for, 234–235
energy expenditure in, 274–275t
interval training, 235
maximal oxygen consumption in, 64f, 65f

Salt. *See* Sodium
Scurvy, 19
Setpoint theory, 166–168, 167f
Sex. *See* Gender
Shoulders, strengthening exercises, 329
Side bender, as warm-up exercise, 209f
Sit-ups, spot reduction after, 151, 151t
Skating, maximal oxygen consumption in, 64f, 65f
Skiing
cross country
caloric intake associated with, 171t
maximal oxygen consumption in, 64f, 65f
energy expenditure in, 107t, 274–275t
Skin, water loss through, 32
Smoking
exercise and, 81
heart disease related to, 253–254, 257t
Soccer, caloric intake associated with, 171t
Sodium
recommended daily allowance, 29
replacement after exercise, 29–30
Specific gravity, 123
Specificity, 195
of strength, 206–207
of training, aerobic conditioning related to, 229–230
Spirometry
in oxygen consumption determination, 98, 99f, 100, 100f
portable, 98, 99f, 100
Sports
caloric intake in athletes, 171–173, 171t, 172t
diet optimal for, 39–51
energy costs of, 107–108, 107t, 173, 268–277t
energy sources for, 57

energy systems predominantly required in various activities, 217–219, 218f
extension of lifetime related to participation in, 244, 244f
fast versus slow twitch muscle fibers in various athletes, 69
maximal oxygen consumption in athletes, 64–65, 64f, 65f
meal prior to competition, 49–50
relative contributions of anaerobic and aerobic metabolism during, 72–74, 73f
Spot reduction, 150–152, 151t
Starch, 5
Starvation diet, 156
Step up test, 221–222, 222f
Queens College step test, 222–223, 223t
Techumseh test, 226, 227t
Strength
aging influence on, 241
back exercises, 208
CNS inhibitions influencing, 201
comparison between men and women, 202–203
conditioning for, 197–214
goals, 210
household items used for, 210, 211f, 212
isokinetic training, 200
isometric training, 197–200, 198f
metabolic stress of, 203–205
muscular adaptations with, 200–202
organizing, 207–214
overload in, 212, 214
selecting exercises, 212
selecting proper weight, 208, 210
specificity principle applied to, 207
steps in planning workout, 210, 211f, 212, 213f, 214
types, 197–200, 198f
weight training, 197–199, 198f
in women, 202–203
exercises for, 329–331
muscular anatomic factors influencing, 201–202
psychologic factors influencing, 201
specificity, 206–207
Stress electrocardiogram, 196
Stretching, as warm-up exercises, 208, 209f
Stroke, 85
Stroke volume, 86–87, 88f, 89
Sucrose, 5
Sugar, 4–5. *See also* Carbohydrates
Surface area
basal metabolism related to, 102
nomogram for, 103, 103f
Surgery, in weight control, 158t
Sweating
cooling effect, 32
fluid and electrolyte replacement after, 29–30
water loss in, 32
Swimming
cardiovascular response compared with running, 233–234
energy costs, 107t, 108, 274–277t
interval training, 235
maximal oxygen consumption in, 64f, 65f
target heart rate for use in aerobic conditioning program, 233–234
Systole, 85

Taste, and eating behavior, 161–162
Techumseh step test, 226, 227t
Temperature
fat as insulator in control, 13
during recovery from exercise, 71–72
Temporal artery, pulse rate taken at, 85, 85f
Tennis, energy costs, 107t, 108
Thiamine
in foods, 292–327
function, 20t
Thinness, 118–119
Thyroid gland goiter, 25
Tobacco. *See* Smoking
Toe touch, as warm-up exercise, 209f
Tomography, computed, in body composition measurement, 132, 133f
Training. *See also* Conditioning
aerobic, 220–236. *See also* Aerobic conditioning
amenorrhea related to, 119
appetite related to, 172–173, 172t
for ATP-CP energy capacity, 219–220
ballet in, 106–107
carbohydrate needs in, 45–46, 45f
cardiac output after, 86–87, 88f, 89
continuous exercise, 234–235
developing aerobic conditioning program, 230–236
continuous exercise training, 234–235
determination of training intensity, 231–234, 232t, 233f
guidelines for beginning, 231
interval training, 235–236
duration related to aerobic conditioning, 228–229
frequency related to aerobic conditioning, 228
individual differences principle, 195
intensity related to aerobic conditioning, 229, 231–234, 232t, 233f
interval, 235–236
isokinetic, 200
isometric, 199–200
for lactic acid production, 220
for muscular strength, 197–214
back exercises, 208
goals, 210
household items used for, 210, 211f, 212
isokinetic, 200
isometric, 199–200
muscular adaptations with, 200–202
organizing, 207–208, 209f, 210, 211f, 212, 213f, 214
overload in, 212, 214
selecting exercises, 212
selecting proper weight, 208, 210
steps in planning workout, 210, 211f, 212, 213f, 214
types, 197–200, 198f
weight, 197–199, 198f
overload principle, 194–195
principles of physiologic conditioning, 194–196
protein content of muscle after, 15
reversibility principle, 195–196
specificity principle, 195
related to aerobic conditioning, 229–230
stroke volume after, 86–87, 88f, 89
ventilation influence on oxygen consumption after, 79–80, 80f
weight, 197–199, 198f
Treadmill exercise, energy cost, 206
Triglyceride, 9
Type A personality, 255

Ultrasound, in body composition measurement, 130, 130f
Underweight, 118–119
Urine, water output in, 32

Valsalva maneuver, 77
Vegetables, measuring portions, 162–163
Vegetarian, protein nutrition in, 18
Veins, 83, 84f
Ventilation, 74–81
during exercise, 79–80
oxygen consumption related to, 79–80, 80f

Vitamin(s), 18–23
B complex
in exercise, 21
function, 20t
classification, 19
discovery, 18–19
exercise performance related to, 21–22
fat role in utilization, 13
fat soluble, 19
functions, 20–21t, 21
source, 19, 21
supplementation, 22–23
synthesis, 19, 21
toxicity, 19
water soluble, 19
Vitamin A, 19
carotenes conversion to, 21
in foods, 292–327
function, 20t
toxicity, 19
Vitamin B12, 20t
Vitamin C
excessive doses, 22
in foods, 292–327
function, 21t
iron absorption related to, 25
in training, 22
Vitamin D, 19, 20t
Vitamin E
excessive doses, 22
function, 20t, 22
Vitamin K, 19, 20t
Volleyball, energy costs, 107t, 108, 276–277t
Volume
determination in evaluating body composition, 122–128
equivalents for measuring, 290

Walking, energy expenditure in, 276–277t
Warm-up, 231
before strength exercises, 207–208, 209f
Water, 30–34
balance, 30–33, 31f
body composition, 30
carbohydrate influence on absorption, 33–34
distribution in body, 30
energy metabolism producing, 31–32
extra intake before exercise, 33
in feces, 33
in food, 31
intake, 30–32
loss during weight reduction program, 156–157, 175–176, 175f
output, 32–33
replacement, 33–34
after exercise, 29–30
in respiration, 33
skin losses, 32
urinary output, 32
Weight
aging influence on, 242–243
body composition versus, 113, 115
desirable, 135–136
equivalents for measuring, 290
hydrostatic, 125, 126f
minimal, 117–118
stability, 155
underweight and thin, 118–119
Weight control, 155–177
balancing energy input with energy output, 159–161, 160f
ballet in, 106–107
calculation of fat weight to lose, 280–281
caloric equivalent of each kilogram lost, 176–177, 176f
changing physical activity lifestyle, 162
combination of diet and exercise, 174–177
dieting, 155–157, 158t, 165–170, 167f
computerized meal plan, 169–170, 261–263, 265–266
with erroneous claims, 155–157
exercise with, 174–177
high-carbohydrate, low-fat diet, 158t
high-protein diet in, 156–157, 158t
one-food-centered diet, 158t
protein-sparing modified fast, 158t
selecting diet plan, 168–169
starvation diet, 156
difficulty in maintaining weight loss, 157
eating behavior modification, 162, 180–183, 181f
exercise, 170–173
computerized plan, 264–266
frequency, 228
with diet, 174–177
fasting, 158t
fatness limit above which weight reduction indicated, 157, 159
lean tissue mass preservation in exercise plus diet program, 175
setpoint theory acting against, 166–168, 167f
surgery, 158t
target loss of fat desirable, 174
unbalancing energy balance equation, 165–177
Weight gain, fat cell size and number after, 144, 145f
Weight lifting. *See also* Weight training
blood pressure in, 86
fainting due to inadequate venous return in, 84
protein preparations in diet for, 40
Valsalva maneuver in, 77
Weight loss
calories equivalent to kilograms lost during weight reduction program, 176–177, 176f
difficulty in maintaining, 157
fat cell size and number after, 142–144, 143f
low-carbohydrate diet in, 156, 158t
percentage composition after food restriction plus exercise, 175–176, 175f
spot reduction, 150–152, 151t
by unbalancing energy balance equation, 160–161, 160f
Weight training, 197–199, 198f. *See also* Weight lifting
circuit, 204–205, 204t, 212, 213f, 214
concentric contraction, 198–199, 198f
eccentric contraction, 197, 198f
energy cost, 203–205
isometric contraction, 198f, 199
selecting proper weight, 208, 210
Women. *See* Female; Gender
Work
classification, 110–111, 111t
intensity, 111, 111t

X-rays, in body composition measurement, 130, 131f, 132